Clinical Manual of Implant Dentistry

Clinical Manual of Implant Dentistry

Mithridade Davarpanah
Henry Martínez

Myriam Kebir
Jean-François Tecucianu

in cooperation with
Richard J. Lazzara
Renato Celletti
Daniel Etienne
Curtis Jansen
Karl Donath

Translation by
Marie Pascale Hippolyte

quintessence books

Quintessence Publishing Co, Ltd

London, Chicago, Berlin, Tokyo, Copenhagen, Paris, Milan, Barcelona, Istanbul, São Paulo, New Delhi, Moscow, Prague, and Warsaw

British Library Cataloging-in-Publication Data

Clinical manual of implant dentistry
1. dental implants
I. Davarpanah, Mithridade
617.6'92

ISBN 1850970491

Quintessence Publishing Co, Ltd
Grafton Road
New Malden
Surrey KT3 3AB
United Kingdom
www.quintpub.co.uk

ISBN 1-85097-049-1

Printed in Germany

Contents

Foreword

Since the early 1980s, oral implants have provided a new dimension to all fields of dentistry. Reliable procedures have developed rapidly and gained an important place in treatment planning. In periodontics, the usual, despairingly conservative treatment is moderated by a rational implant option. In prosthodontics, esthetic and functional restorations have certainly benefited from implant therapy. In orthodontics, an implant abutment may be used to facilitate tooth movement in some situations.

Successful implant treatment relies on a knowledge of anatomy, an understanding of tissue physiology, and a skillful surgical technique. This textbook is intended for the use of students, practitioners, and clinicians who are new to implant dentistry, as well as for those who want to improve their technique.

Each chapter offers a detailed approach to implant treatment using diagrams and clinical illustrations to provide the reader with comprehensive information on each given situation. From preimplant diagnosis, which guides treatment decision making, to the different types of edentulism, clinical situations are addressed from both surgical and prosthetic perspectives. Submerged and nonsubmerged implants, implant diameters, and specific surgical procedures, such as bone grafts, osteotomies, sinus lift and grafting, soft tissue management, and guided bone regeneration, are described in separate chapters.

New prospects are the future of implant dentistry. However, advances are rapid; therefore the basic principles of this discipline must be well understood. This textbook is intended to be practical and contemporary, from diagnosis to technique, from knowledge to application, and is recommended for all dentists.

Henri S. Koskas

Editors

Mithridade Davarpanah
Lecturer in Periodontics
Division of Research in Stomatology and Maxillofacial Surgery
Pitié-Salpêtrière Hospital
Paris, France

Henry Martínez
Associate Professor
University of Paris 7;
Lecturer
Department of Surgery
Hôtel-Dieu Hospital
Paris, France

Myriam Kebir
Former Lecturer
Department of Dentistry
Max Forestier Hospital
Nanterre, France

Jean-François Tecucianu
Professor
Department of Education and Research in Stomatology and Maxillofacial Surgery;
Chairman
Department of Periodontology
Division of Research in Stomatology and Maxillofacial Surgery
Pitié-Salpêtrière Hospital;
Chairman
Division of Dentistry and Stomatology
American Hospital of Paris
Paris, France

Contributors

Gil Alcoforado
Professor
Department of Periodontology
University of Lisbon
Lisbon, Portugal

Grégoire Audi
Paris, France

Keith D. Beaty
Chief Executive Officer
Implant Innovations
Palm Beach Gardens, Florida

Philippe Bouchard
Assistant Professor
University of Paris 7;
Division of Periodontology
Department of Dentistry
Hôtel-Dieu
Paris, France

Jean-Pierre Bressand
Paris, France

Renato Celletti
Professor
Department of Prosthodontics
University G. d'Annunzio
Chieti, Italy

Edouard Cohen
Division of Dentistry and Stomatology
American Hospital of Paris
Paris, France

Karl Donath
Professor and Chairman
Department of Oral Pathology
University of Hamburg
Hamburg, Germany

Daniel Etienne
Assistant Professor
University of Paris 7;
Division of Periodontology
Department of Dentistry
Hôtel-Dieu
Paris, France

Olivier Fromentin
Former Assistant Professor
Division of Prosthodontics
University of Paris 7
Paris, France

Eric Hazan
Paris, France

Curtis Jansen
Monterey, California

Francis Lamond
Paris, France

Richard J. Lazzara
Chairman of the Board
Implant Innovations
Palm Beach Gardens, Florida

Patrick Missika
Assistant Professor
University of Paris 7;
Division of Surgery
Department of Dentistry
Hôtel-Dieu Hospital
Paris, France

Stephan S. Porter
West Palm Beach, Florida

Christophe Raygot
Paris, France

Pierre Raygot
Paris, France

Jean-Luc Sauvan
Former Assistant Professor
University of Paris 5
Paris, France

CHAPTER 1

Considerations for Implant Treatment Planning

M. Davarpanah/H. Martínez/K. Donath/M. Kebir

I. Tooth conservation versus implants: Treatment decision criteria

The dental surgeon must frequently face the dilemma of extracting or conserving a tooth. Previously, teeth showing an unfavorable prognosis were often preserved in order to delay the wearing of a removable denture. Today, implant therapy is often too rapidly preferred.[1,2] Before deciding on a treatment choice, the practitioner must establish the etiologic diagnosis, determine the prognosis of the remaining teeth, and visualize the final esthetic and functional results. Prognosis for the different treatment options must be carefully assessed.[3,4]

A conservative treatment choice must always be prevalent in the clinician's mind. However, a poor prognosis must lead to consideration of tooth extraction. Preserving compromised teeth may lead to extensive tissue loss. Alveolar bone collapse limits treatment options, greatly increases treatment time, and may jeopardize the final outcome.

A. Diagnosis

Longevity of teeth directly depends on the periodontal tissue state.[3,5] Different etiologic factors such as trauma, endodontic problems, caries, developmental anomalies, and bone defects may lead to tooth loss. Tooth loss is frequently associated with bone resorption.[6]

The radiographic diagnosis is mainly based upon the long-cone status analysis. Computed tomography scans allow evaluation of the implant option before deciding if extraction of compromised teeth is necessary. The different periodontal, prosthetic, and endodontic criteria allow assessment of the value of a tooth or a dental abutment for possible prosthetic treatment. These criteria determine the choice of preserving a tooth or not.

1. Bone loss extent

The periodontal diagnosis allows evaluation of bone loss around the affected teeth and establishment of a prognosis. It is essential to assess furcation involvement and anatomy in order to decide the treatment option (preservation, regeneration, tunnel procedure, root amputation, hemisection, or extraction) (Figs 1-1 to 1-3).[3,7–13]

2. Root length (clinical crown:root ratio)

The clinical crown:root ratio is assessed on periapical radiographs. Tooth lengthening may compromise the adjacent teeth, and an unfavorable clinical crown:root ratio may thus occur.[3] Tooth extraction and implant options must be considered if this ratio is unfavorable.

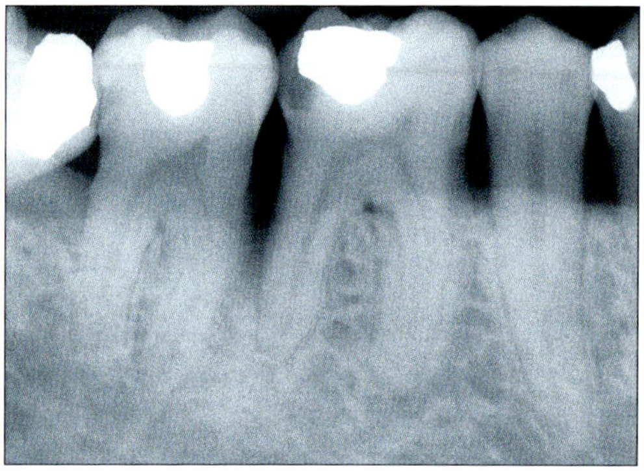

Fig 1-1 Radiograph showing intrabony defects on the distal aspect of the mandibular right first and second molars.

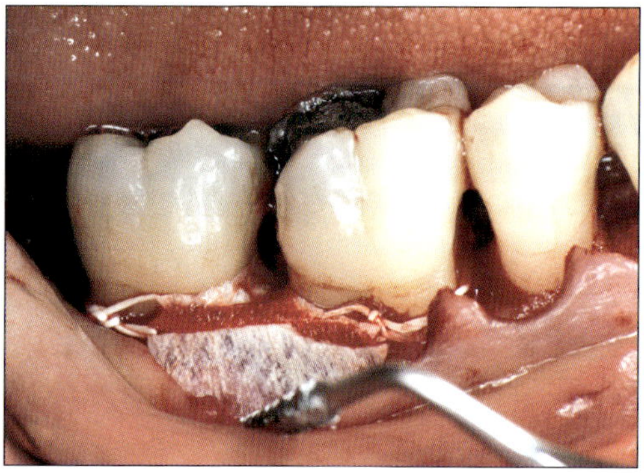

Fig 1-2 Clinical view following strategic extraction of mandibular right third molar and guided tissue regeneration using a Gore-Tex membrane placed between the first and second molars.

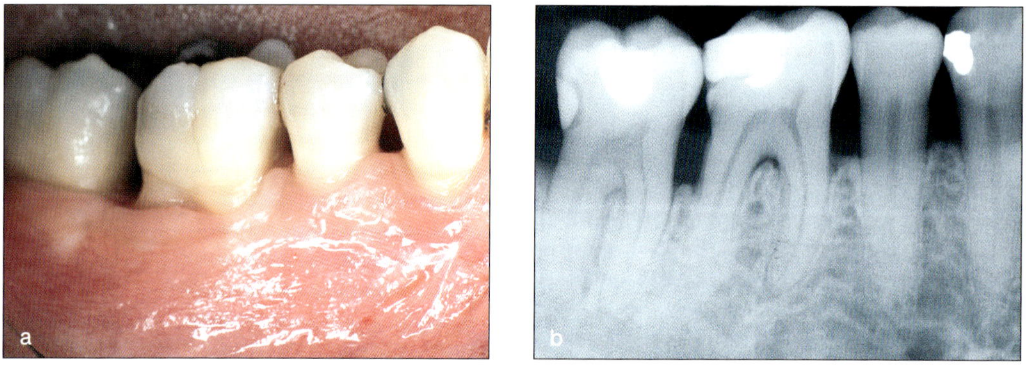

Figs 1-3a and 1-3b Clinical and radiographic views at 2 years. Note the good regeneration on the distal aspect of the first and second molars.

Preprosthetic orthodontics (forced eruption) must also be considered (Figs 1-4 to 1-6).

3. Clinical crown height

A tooth showing insufficient clinical crown height is too often restored with subgingival preparations that violate the biologic width and/or with large root posts that weaken the tooth.[14] Violation of the biologic width leads to chronic inflammation, attachment loss, or gingival recession at teeth with thin periodontal tissue. In the case of a short clinical crown, the indications for preprosthetic surgery must be considered (Figs 1-7 and 1-8).

4. Endodontic assessment

In the presence of a periapical defect, the endodontic-periodontal differential diagnosis must be established.[15] If the etiology is endodontic, root canal treatment must be per-

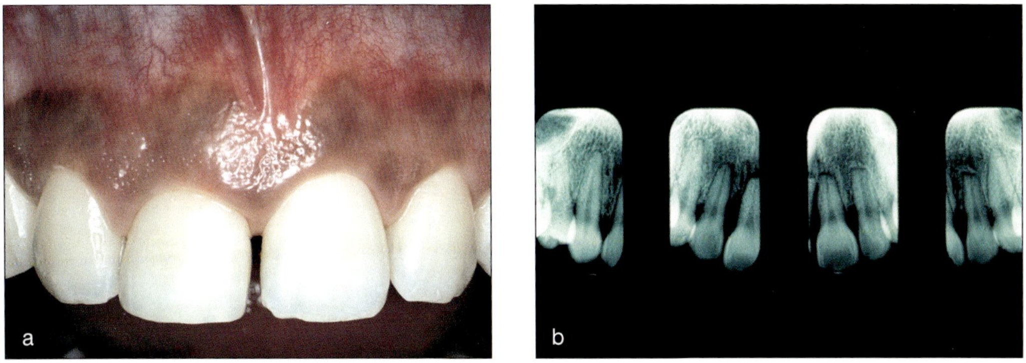

Figs 1-4a and 1-4b Clinical and radiographic views of an 18-year-old female patient showing a severe advanced periodontal defect on the maxillary right central incisor.

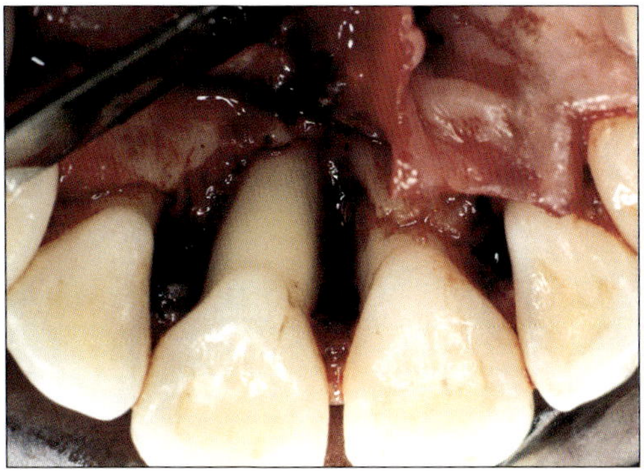

Fig 1-5 Exploration flap confirming the need for strategic extraction of the central incisor.

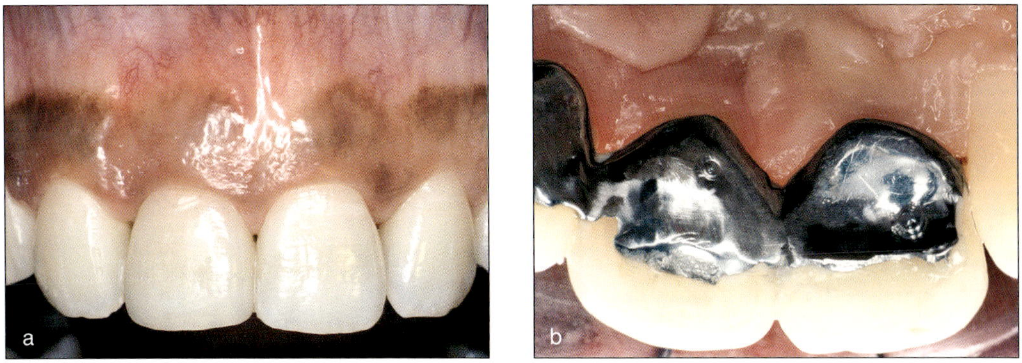

Figs 1-6a and 1-6b Buccal and palatal views at 2 years of the bonded denture replacing the right central incisor.

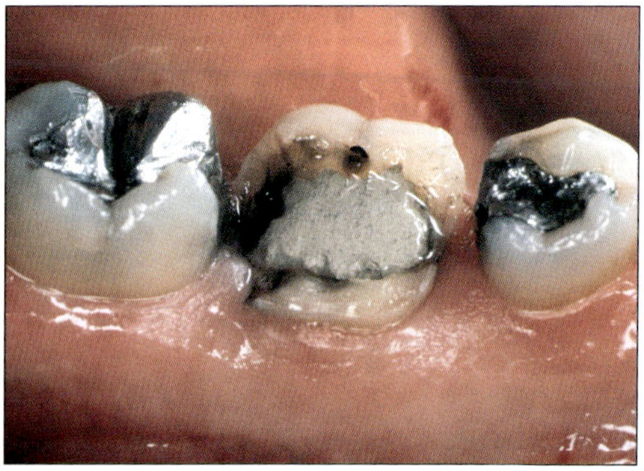

Fig 1-7 Insufficient residual clinical crown height following the lingual wall fracture of the mandibular left first molar.

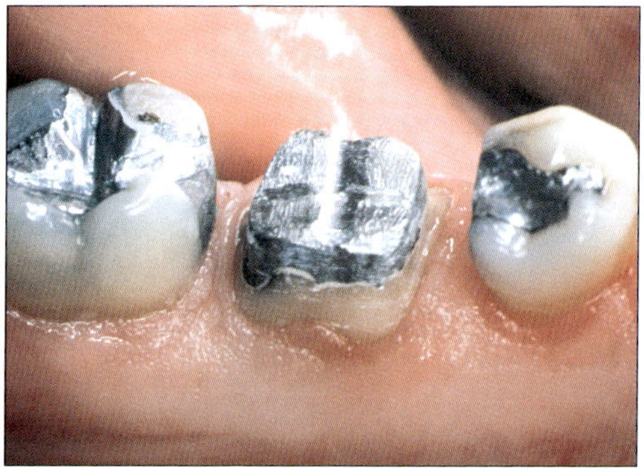

Fig 1-8 Clinical view of the preparation 2 months after crown lengthening.

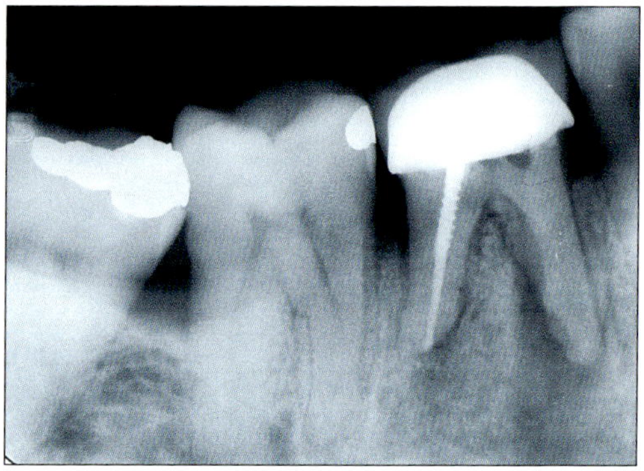

Fig 1-9 Radiograph of a terminal endodontic defect on the mandibular right first molar. Extraction is indicated.

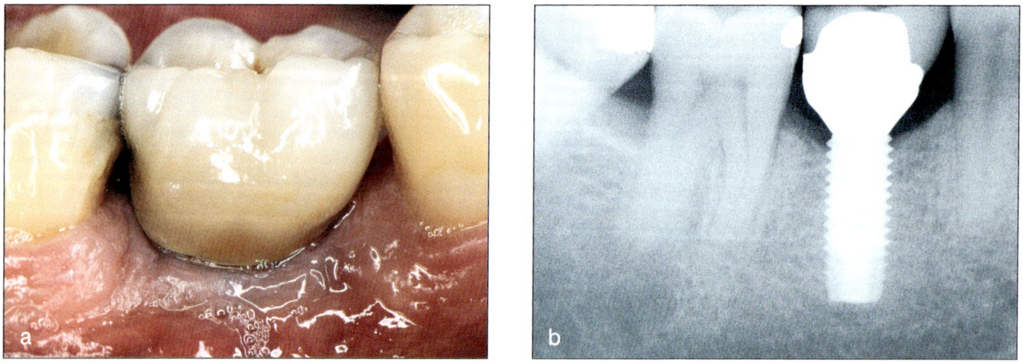

Figs 1-10a and 1-10b Clinical and radiographic views of implant treatment after 1 year.

formed. A healing period of several months is often necessary before starting the periodontal surgical treatment (Figs 1-9 and 1-10).

5. *Esthetic demands*

The patient's esthetic demands, the location of the site to be restored (anterior region), and the type of smile are determining factors for treatment choice and planning.[4,14,16]

B. Prognosis

The aim of the practitioner must be to preserve teeth within the parameters of a good local and general state of health. Prognosis is the prediction of the treatment outcome over time following a pathology. Anticipating the progression of periodontally affected teeth is sometimes uncertain. In order to select the best treatment option for tooth preservation, the prognosis must be established.[14] This also allows selection of the restorative choice (fixed, removable, or implant-supported prosthesis).[17]

The longevity of a tooth directly depends on the periodontal tissue status. The overall prognosis is based on assessment of different factors (general, local, and psychologic; Tables 1-1 to 1-3). A recently developed genetic test has allowed assessment of the individual's susceptibility to periodontal disease. Kornman et al[18] have demonstrated that specific genetic markers combined with increased interleukin-1 production indicate a strong susceptibility to severe adult periodontitis. This information allows detection of subjects at risk for rapidly progressive periodontitis and adaptation of the periodontal treatment. The genetic test completes the information provided until now by microbiologic and immunologic tests. It is important to stress that this genetic test does not allow diagnosis. It is simply a means to confirm the periodontal prognosis. It allows the clinician to educate the patient on the "controllable" risk factors concerning periodontal disease (oral hygiene, tobacco smoking, stress). In the presence of some systemic disorders (diabetes, Down syndrome, Papillon-Lefèvre syndrome), tissue and immunity changes occur. Several exogenous factors must also be carefully assessed (nutritional deficiencies, medications, tobacco smoking). These parameters may dramatically modify the patient's dental prognosis (Table 1-1). The different local factors (bacterial plaque, occlusal trauma, endodontic problems, caries, bone loss, etc) are assessed during the clinical and radiographic diagnosis (Table 1-2).

Psychologic factors are essential for establishing the prognosis and consequently for the treatment strategy (Table 1-3). Several epidemiologic studies have shown the relationship between stress and periodontal disease. The patient's psychologic state may influence his or her treatment demand (adapted or unrealistic) and oral hygiene. Indeed, patient cooperation and motivation are determining factors in prognosis. In 1996, Wilson[19] studied patient motivation for plaque control and professional maintenance. He stated that the maintenance protocol is rarely followed by patients affected with chronic types of disorders. Most studies concerning daily bacterial plaque control and maintenance report less than 50% patient follow-up. Studies on control and maintenance performed in hospital-university institutions and in specialized dental offices report even higher failure rates.

Table 1-1 General factors and prognosis[3]

Factors to consider	Unfavorable prognosis	Favorable prognosis
Patient's general state of health	At-risk patient	Good health
Medical history	Significant	None
Immune system	Immunosuppressed	Stable
Genetic test (periodontitis)	Positive	Negative
Tobacco smoking	Yes	No
Medication intake	Cyclosporine, phenantoin	None
Nutrition	Protein deficiency	Adequate
Drug addiction	Yes	No

Table 1-2 Local factors and prognosis[3]

Factors to consider	Unfavorable prognosis	Favorable prognosis
Bacterial flora	Pathologic	Physiologic
Attachment loss	Significant	Absent
Pocket activity	Bleeding, pus	Physiologic
Bone loss	> 50%	< 50%
Disease development	Acute	Chronic
Furcation involvement	Affected	Absent
Mobility	Increased	Physiologic
Plaque control	Insufficient	Adequate
Residual teeth	Few and isolated	Majority
Crown:root ratio	Inadequate	Favorable
Occlusal trauma	Present	Absent
Parafunction	Present (bruxism)	Absent
Tooth position	Malposition	Adequate
Root anatomy	Inadequate	Favorable
Caries	Present	Absent
Restorations	Poorly adapted	Well adapted
Endodontic criteria	Complicated	Favorable

Table 1-3 Psychologic factors and prognosis[3]

Factors to consider	Unfavorable prognosis	Favorable prognosis
Patient motivation	Low	Excellent
Treatment demand	Unrealistic	Adapted
Stress	Significant	Absent

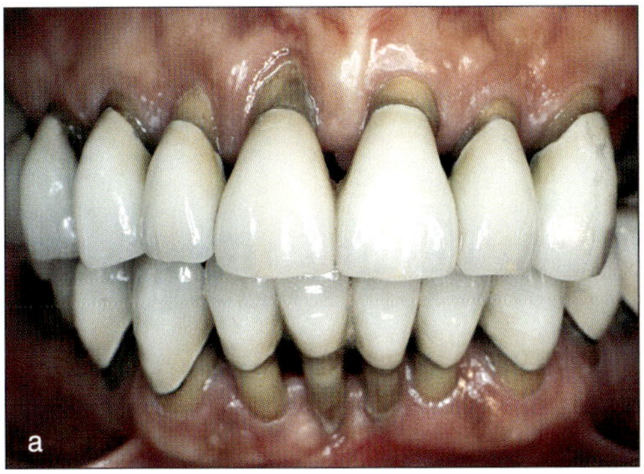

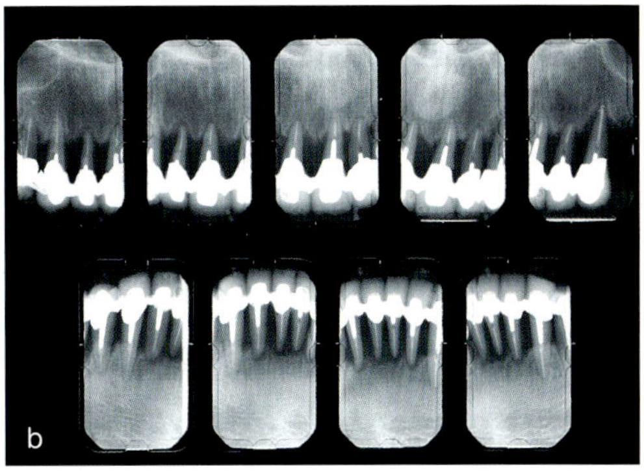

Figs 1-11a and 1-11b Clinical and radiographic views of advanced periodontitis.

C. Advanced periodontal diseases

Advanced periodontal diseases are often characterized by tooth mobility, associated with partially edentulous situations (Fig 1-11). The use of combined tooth and implant components in a patient affected with advanced periodontitis is much debated.[20] Indeed, the differences in tooth mobility between the implant and the tooth imply specific biomechanical considerations. For some specific cases, some authors[21,22] advocate the use of complete-arch combined dentures. The aim of this prosthesis is to control tooth mobility and to oppose chewing forces. This type of restoration requires perfect occlusal adjustment, excellent patient cooperation, and regular professional controls.

According to Langer and Sullivan,[23] this type of prosthesis built on natural abutments is limited in its effectiveness, and survival rates do not exceed 5 to 10 years. The main reasons for failure are caries and vertical abutment fracture. Failures are most often of a biomechanical nature; sometimes they may be due to periodontal disease aggravation. According to the same authors, the decision for tooth conservation must be mainly based on biomechanical factors. A tooth is preserved if no mobility is observed and if it does not require endodontic treatment or crown restoration. According to Langer and Sullivan,[23] four implants appropriately distributed on the arch and splinted to the residual teeth are sufficient to fabricate a complete denture. The anterior teeth are preferably preserved in order to maintain esthetics and avoid functional problems.

D. Strategic extraction

An extraction is considered strategic if it significantly improves the prognosis of the adjacent teeth.[3] The recent classifications concerning periodontitis and the notion of disease activity make the concept of strategic extraction more delicate to apply. This notion is based on a strict analysis of "tooth-by-tooth" prognosis. From a prosthetic point of view, it is preferable to extract teeth that may to lead to complications. Teeth with a compromised prognosis that are located in a bone site that is likely to receive implants must be extracted. These strategic extractions thus allow placement of a greater number of longer implants with better prosthetic positioning. It may be necessary to temporarily preserve some residual teeth for psychologic reasons or to support provisional restorations.

Table 1-4 Long-term results of multidisciplinary studies: Posterior teeth[24]

Author, year	Observation period (y)	No. of teeth observed	Success rate (%)
Hirschfeld and Wasserman, 1978[9]	15	1,464	98
Ross, 1978[24]	5–24	387	97
McFall, 1982[12]	15–29	163	65
Goldman, 1980[25]	15–34	636	93
Wood, 1989[26]	10–34	164	86
Wang et al, 1994[27]	8	87	66

E. Remarks

Periodontal disease type, patient age, bone loss extent, number of residual teeth, available bone volume, patient demand, and treatment reliability are factors that determine tooth conservation or extraction.[3] Conventional treatments for periodontal disease have shown their efficacy (Table 1-4). However, extraction of a tooth with a limited or unfavorable prognosis must be considered (Figs 1-12 to 1-14).[28]

Prior to the use of endosseous implants, teeth showing advanced periodontal defects were treated with sometimes heroic therapies. Today, these teeth are frequently extracted and replaced by dental implants. The reasons for this treatment choice are variable and include a limited periodontal treatment prognosis or an implant option offering a better long-term prognosis than the natural abutments. This attitude may verge on overtreatment, however, if an accurate diagnosis and a carefully considered treatment plan have not been established.

The rapidly progressive periodontitis group represents a specific situation (Figs 1-15 to 1-17).[29] Periodontal reevaluation is essential, because the treatment choice is very difficult for these patients. Great caution is recommended before extracting a tooth.

Several reasons may lead to compromises in the treatment decision making for either a conservative approach or implant placement:

—state of patient's oral and general health
—treatment time
—patient's motivation and prosthetic demand
—prognosis for different treatment options

II. Indications for dental implants

These indications are (Fig 1-18):

—lack of retention of a removable denture
—instability of a removable denture
—functional discomfort wearing removable dentures
—psychologic refusal to wear a removable denture
—parafunctional habits that compromise the stability of a removable denture
—inadequate location and number of residual abutments
—absence of dental abutments to fabricate a fixed restoration
—single-tooth replacement with healthy adjacent teeth
—tooth agenesis
—demand for a conservative treatment (patient's refusal to mutilate sound teeth)

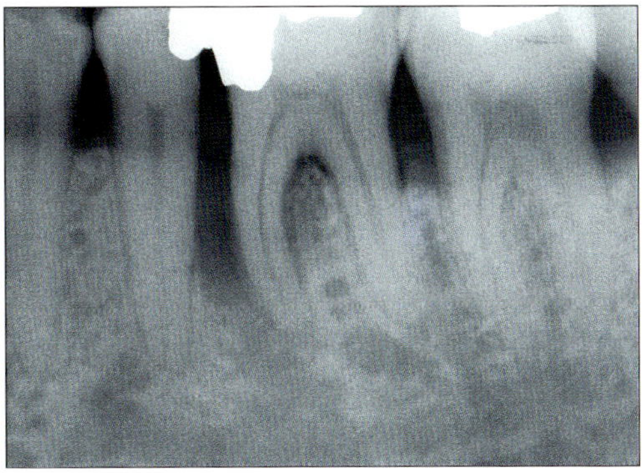

Fig 1-12 Circumferential intrabony defect in the interproximal aspect of the mandibular left first molar and second premolar.

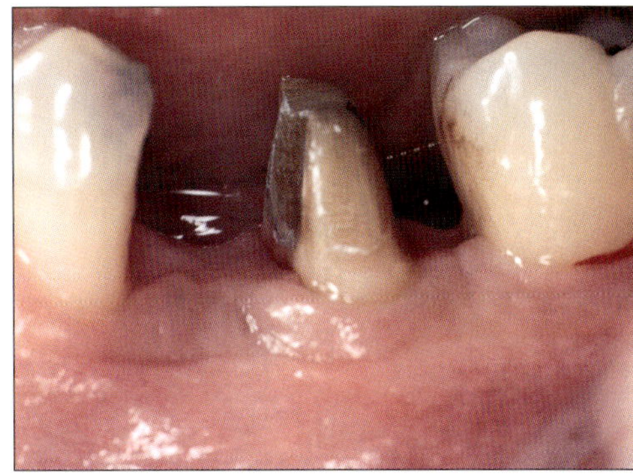

Fig 1-13 Clinical view 2 months following the mesial root amputation of the first molar.

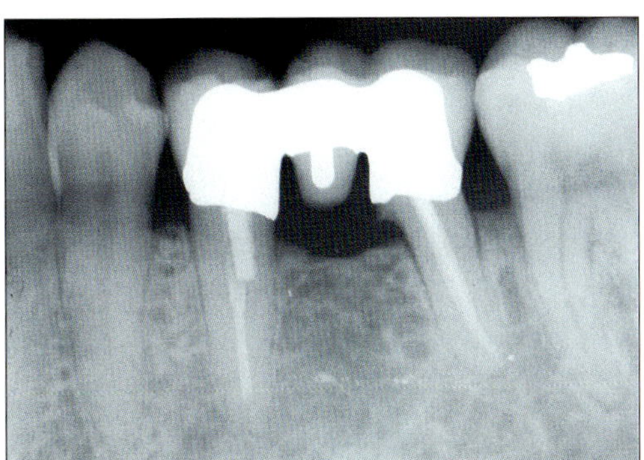

Fig 1-14 Radiograph of the left mandibular fixed partial denture.

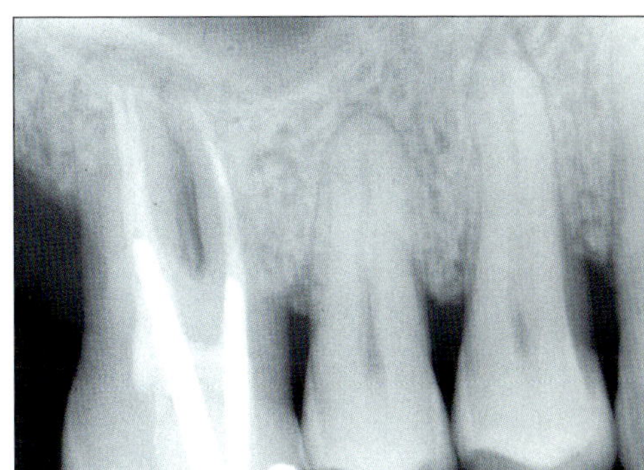

Fig 1-15 Radiograph of a patient diagnosed with adult periodontitis. Scaling and root planing as well as open-flap debridement were performed.

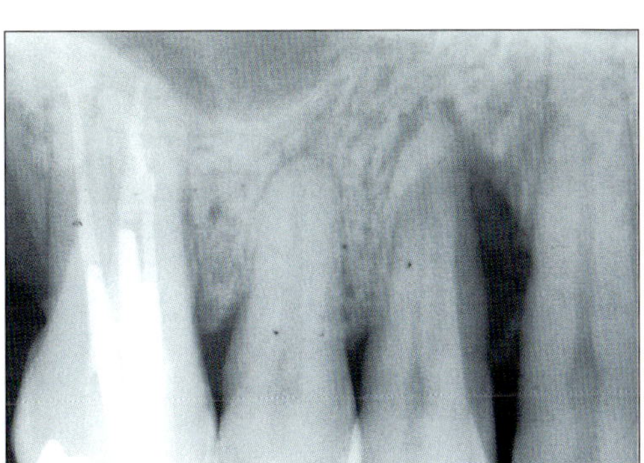

Fig 1-16 Radiographic control at 1 year. Note the bone loss aggravation on the maxillary right first premolar despite the performed treatment.

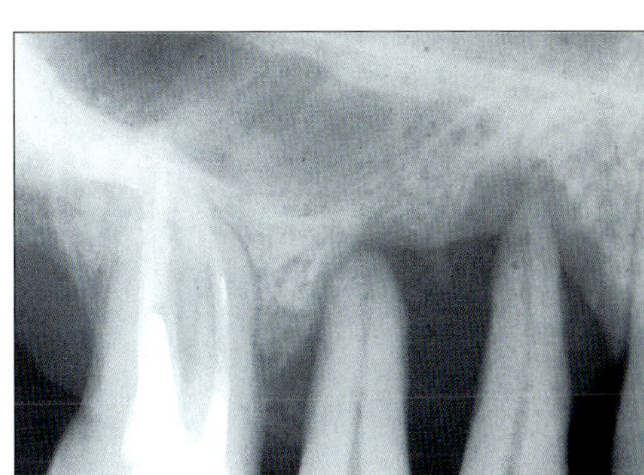

Fig 1-17 Radiographic control at 2 years showing the terminal bone loss on the first and second premolars.

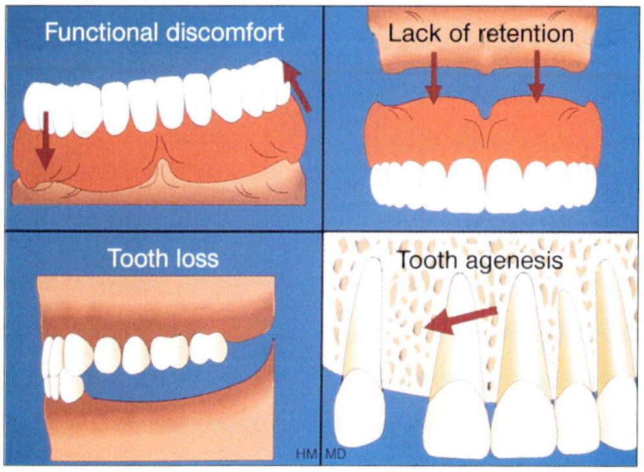

Fig 1-18 Indications for dental implants.

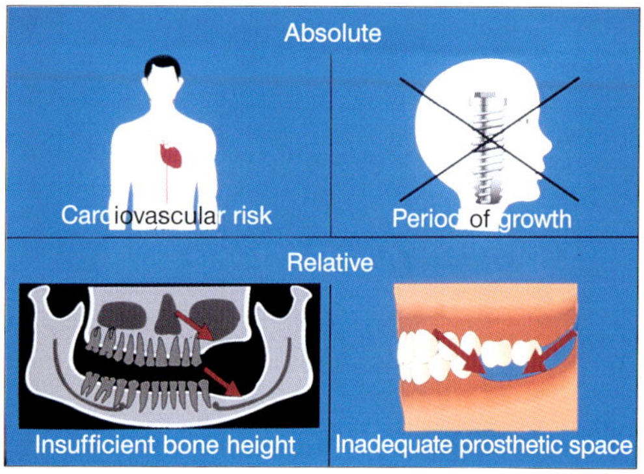

Fig 1-19 Contraindications for dental implants.

III. Contraindications for dental implants

Contraindications for dental implants can be absolute or relative (Fig 1-19).

A. Absolute contraindications

—major psychologic disorders
—risk of heart pathologies
—uncontrolled systemic disorders
—alcohol or medication dependence
—patient age (young patient in growth period)

B. Relative contraindications

—insufficient bone volume and/or poor bone quality
—insufficient interocclusal space
—at-risk patient (irradiated patient, bruxism, uncontrolled periodontitis, tobacco smoking)

IV. Minimum bone volume for implant placement

Placement of endosseous implants 3.75 mm in diameter and 10 mm in length requires a minimum volume in the three dimensions of space.

A. Buccolingual aspect

Crestal ridge width required equals the implant diameter plus 2 mm (in order to have 1 mm of bone on either side of the implant; Fig 1-20).

B. Apicocoronal aspect

In the mandible (Fig 1-21), the ridge height required is at least 12 mm (implant length plus 2 mm). A 2-mm security zone is recommended above the infraalveolar nerve. In the maxilla, the ridge height required is at least 10 mm (implant length) (Fig 1-21). No security zone is needed below the maxillary sinus.

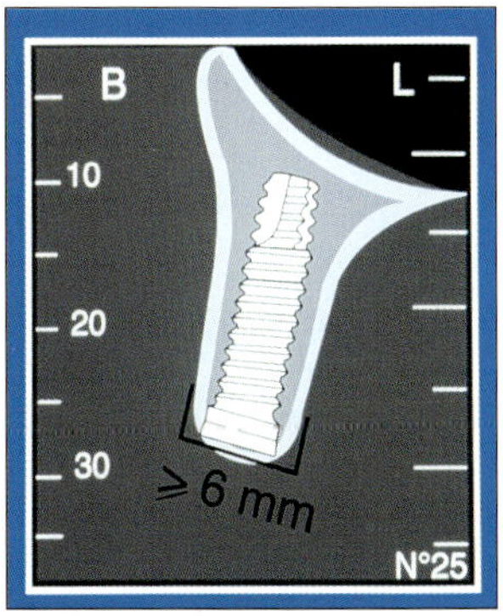

Fig 1-20 Oblique CT scan reconstruction showing the minimal bone volume needed for placement of a standard (3.75 mm) implant.

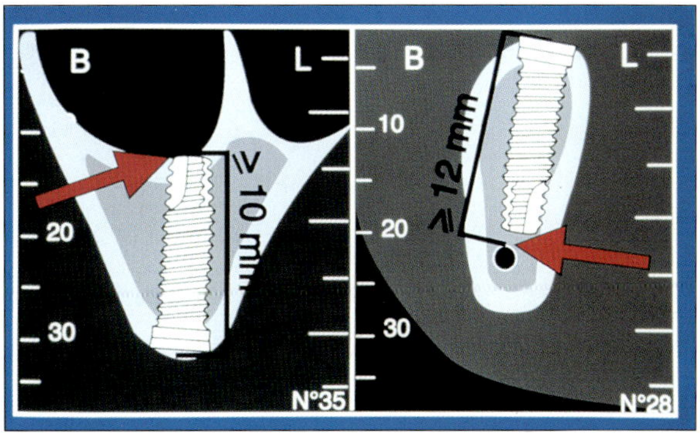

Fig 1-21 Oblique CT scan reconstructions showing the minimal amount of bone height needed for placement of a 10-mm implant.

C. Mesiodistal aspect

For a single implant, the bone available mesiodistally must be greater than 7 mm. In a partially edentulous situation, the following formula should be used (Fig 1-22):

$$\text{No. of implants} = \frac{\text{mesiodistal distance} - 1\text{ mm}}{\text{implant diameter} + 3\text{ mm}}$$

Three millimeters should be allowed between two implants for the prosthetic components; 2 mm should be allowed between implant and tooth in order to preserve bone and ligament. For complete edentulism, the residual bone volume and the prosthetic design determine implant size and type.

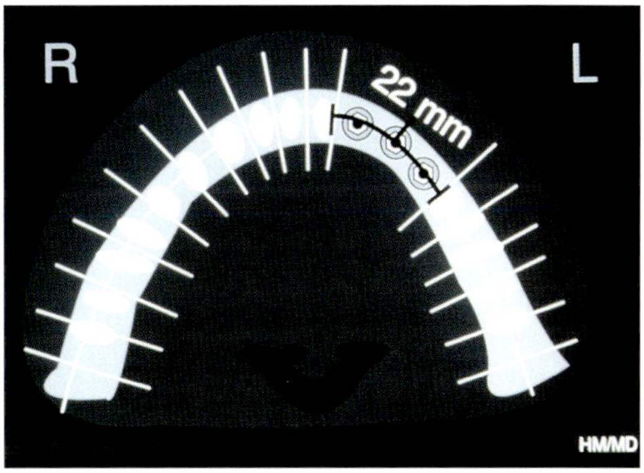

Fig 1-22 Axial cut showing the minimal mesiodistal space necessary for placement of three standard implants.

V. Longitudinal studies

A. Success factors in implant dentistry

To be considered a success, an implant must meet several criteria:

—functional (chewing and speaking)
—psychologic (absence of pain and discomfort, esthetic result)
—physiologic (achievement and maintenance of osseointegration, no tissue inflammation)

An inability to meet one of these criteria is considered a failure, even if the other conditions are fulfilled.

The most commonly used success criteria are those of Albrektsson et al[30]:

—no clinical mobility on a free-standing, non-connected implant
—no peri-implant radiolucency
—vertical bone loss less than 0.2 mm per year after 1 year of implant loading (marginal bone loss must be less than 1.5 mm during the first year of loading)
—no irreversible signs or symptoms of pain, infection, neuropathy, paresthesia, or mandibular nerve canal perforation

The authors suggest that, in order to be considered reliable, an implant system must fulfill the conditions stated above in 85% of the cases over 5 years and 80% of the cases after 10 years.[30]

B. Implant success rate

Implant success rates vary according to the location, bone quality, and edentulous site. Four anatomic regions have been classified according to decreasing success rate:

—The anterior region of the mandible (limited by the mental foramina) has an average success rate of 90% or more over 5 years; this is based on the edentulous patient restored with a fixed prosthesis. Overdenture treatment and treatment of the partially edentulous patient are lacking long-term data.
—The anterior region of the maxilla (limited to the region anterior to the medial aspect of the maxillary sinuses) has an average success rate of 85% or more over 5 years for the edentulous patient restored with a fixed prosthesis. Overdenture treatment and treatment of the partially edentulous patient are lacking long-term data.
—In the posterior mandible (distal to the mental foramina), long-term data are lacking, although short-term data are promising.
—In the posterior maxilla (restricted to the region under the sinus cavity and in the tuberosity), short-term data are limited. Further assessments are needed.

C. Statistical results in implantology

Analysis of the various statistical data allows assessment of surgical and prosthetic success rates. The reliability of the different implant systems must be confirmed by longitudinal multicenter studies. For some studies, results are difficult to analyze. Success criteria (surgical and prosthetic) must be clearly established before interpreting the obtained data.

1. Implant success criteria (new suggestion)

Implant success criteria have been well defined by Zarb and coworkers.[30,31] However, in 1993 the same group suggested a new assessment.[32] Implants are precisely classified in four categories.

Implant success: An implant is considered successful when it presents:

—no mobility after prosthesis removal
—no peri-implant radiolucency
—no peri-implant bone instability
—no pain

Functional implant: An implant is considered "functional" when the overall success criteria cannot be objectively assessed.

Nonassessed implant: The third category concerns "nonassessed" implants in patients who have died or who fail to come to the maintenance recall appointments.

Implant failure: A removed implant is considered a failure.

Although more precise, this new classification remains limited. For example, how should we classify implants showing a bone loss that is greater than the critical threshold (1.5 mm after the first year of loading) despite a perfect clinical stability? Moreover, we must mention implants left submerged because of angulation or implant proximity problems. These implants should obviously be considered failures.

2. *Prosthetic success criteria*

Most of the long-term studies report excellent success rates for implant-supported prostheses.[33–38] However, prosthetic success or failure criteria have not been standardized.[39]

According to most longitudinal studies, only the cases in which the patient had to abandon his or her implant-supported prosthesis and have it replaced by a conventional removable denture are considered failures.[32,33,39–41] This concept of prosthetic failure seems totally subjective. It would be more logical to consider the following as prosthetic failures:

- —changes in the prosthetic treatment plan because of inadequately positioned implants
- —inability to achieve the prosthetic option offered to the patient
- —prosthetic restorations refabricated several times because of mechanical complications (screw loosening or fracture of the different components)
- —patient dissatisfaction with the esthetic result
- —persisting speech problems
- —hygiene and maintenance problems because of inadequate prosthetic design

The implant success criteria defined by Albrektsson et al in 1986[30] require removal of the prosthetic components once a year in order to check for the absence of implant mobility. Nevertheless, this assessment renders maintenance difficult, possibly even unrealistic, while the radiographic control is satisfactory. Cemented prosthetic restorations limit the effectiveness of this particular success criterion.

The reliability of a study depends on respect and selection of the success criteria, number of patients assessed, selected indications, techniques performed, and clinical and radiographic follow-up. Albrektsson and Zarb[32] reported a minimum sampling of 50 patients regularly followed during 5 years by two different centers.

Roos et al[42] review the literature concerning the different endosseous implant systems. According to these authors:

- —Most implant systems lack sufficient follow-up.
- —Results are often presented in two groups: implant failures and "functional" implants grouped together with successful implants.
- —In some studies, the period of implant assessment is quite variable.
- —The statistical analyses specify little or no information concerning implant sites, failures, and patients lost during the implant follow-up (nonassessed implants).
- —Very few studies report the radiographic bone level assessment.
- —Success criteria are not always reported.
- —Very few systems present a reliable clinical and radiographic assessment over 5 years.

Evolution of surgical and prosthetic components in an implant system renders data analysis more difficult. Implant success rates are detailed in Tables 1-5 to 1-14 and Figs 1-23 to 1-32.

Table 1-5 Surgical success rates in completely edentulous patients (fixed restorations)*

Author, year	Type of study	Total No. of implants	Observation period (y)	Mandible I	Mandible L	Mandible S (%)	Maxilla I	Maxilla L	Maxilla S (%)
Adell et al, 1981[40]	Retrospective	2,768	3	423	38	91	472	89	82
Lindquist et al, 1987[43]	Longitudinal	314	3–6	272	2	99	42	2	95
Albrektsson, 1988[44]	Multicenter	3,643	3	1,029	41	96	164	18	89
			5	195	14	93	11	0	100
Adell et al, 1990[33]	Multicenter	4,636	5	480	43	91	524	84	84
			10		53	89		99	81
			15		67	86		115	78
Wyatt and Zarb, 1998[45]	Longitudinal	274	5–9	234	30	87	28	0	100
Jemt, 1991[46]	Retrospective	2,199	1	1,613	11	99	586	25	96
Quirynen et al, 1992[37]	Longitudinal	589	0–6	320	12	96	269	22	92
Hemmings et al, 1994[47]	Longitudinal comparative	132	5	132	14	89	–	–	–
Henry et al, 1995[34]	Prospective	83	10	83	0	100	–	–	–
Brånemark et al, 1995[48]	Retrospective	882	10	406	30	93	476	102	79

*Implant success rates reported in relation to fixed restorations (between 1 and 10 years) range from 87% to 100% in the mandible and from 79% to 100% in the maxilla (in studies reporting on more than 83 implants). Success rates are lower between 10 and 15 years observation (see Fig 1-23).
I = number of implants; L = number of lost implants; S = success rate.

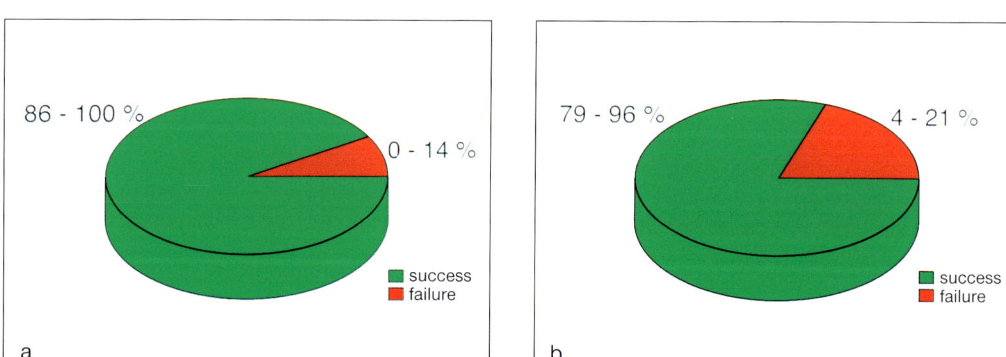

Fig 1-23 Surgical success rates in edentulous patients: a = implant-supported denture in the mandible; b = implant-supported denture in the maxilla. Data taken from studies reporting on more than 50 implants.

Table 1-6 Surgical success rates in completely edentulous patients (overdenture)*

Author, year	Type of study	Total No. of implants	Observation period (y)	Mandible I	Mandible L	Mandible S (%)	Maxilla I	Maxilla L	Maxilla S (%)
Engquist et al, 1988[49]	Retrospective multicenter	339	0–3	148	9	94	191	58	70
Johns et al, 1992[50]	Prospective multicenter	510	0–1	198	11	94	100	21	79
Jemt et al, 1992[51]	Retrospective	430	1	–	–	–	430	69	84
Hemmings et al, 1994[47]	Longitudinal comparative	68	5	68	4	94	–	–	–
Spiekermann et al, 1995[52]	Longitudinal	300	1–10	300	19	93	–	–	–
Hutton et al, 1995[53]	Prospective multicenter	510	0–3	393	11	97	117	29	75
Jemt et al, 1996[54]	Prospective multicenter	510	0–5	393	14	96	117	30	74
Ekfeldt et al, 1997[55]	Retrospective	221	0–8	43	13	70	178	69	61
Bergendahl and Engquist, 1998[56]	Prospective	122	3–10	68	1	98	54	16	70

*Implant success rates reported in relation to overdentures (between 1 and 10 years) range from 70% to 100% in the mandible and from 61% to 84% in the maxilla (in studies reporting on more than 68 implants). Success rates are clearly greater in the maxilla (see Fig 1-24).

I = number of implants; L = number of lost implants; S = success rate.

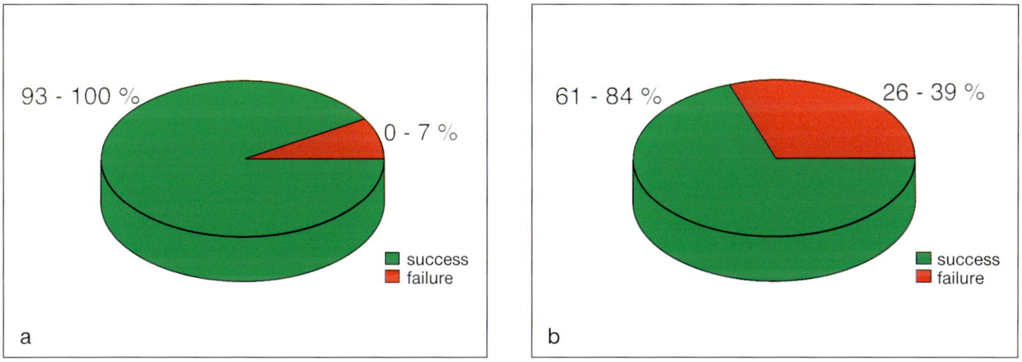

Fig 1-24 Surgical success rates in edentulous patients: a = overdenture in the mandible; b = overdenture in the maxilla. Data taken from studies reporting on more than 50 implants.

Table 1-7 Surgical success rates in partially edentulous patients (fixed restorations)*

Author, year	Type of study	Total No. of implants	Observation period (y)	Mandible I	Mandible L	Mandible S (%)	Maxilla I	Maxilla L	Maxilla S (%)
Jemt et al, 1989[35]	Retrospective	876	1-5	210	1	99	238	13	95
			6–15	19	5	74	24	3	88
van Steenberghe et al, 1990[57]	Prospective multicenter	558	1	338	12	96	220	11	95
Jemt et al, 1992[58]	Prospective	354	1	217	2	99	137	3	98
Pylant et al, 1992[59]	Retrospective	102	0–4	74	9	88	28	3	89
Zarb and Schmitt, 1993[60]	Prospective	105	2–7	64	5	92	41	1	98
Zarb and Schmitt, 1993[61]	Prospective	94	2–8	44	5	88	50	3	94
Lekholm et al, 1994[36]	Prospective multicenter	558	1–5	338	19	94	220	17	92
Wyatt and Zarb, 1998[45]	Longitudinal	230	1–12	129	8	94	101	6	94

*Implant success rates reported in relation to fixed restorations (between 1 and 8 years) range from 88% to 99% in the mandible and from 89% to 98% in the maxilla (in studies reporting on more than 98 implants). Success rates are equivalent in the mandible and the maxilla (see Fig 1-25).
I = number of implants; L = number of lost implants; S = success rate.

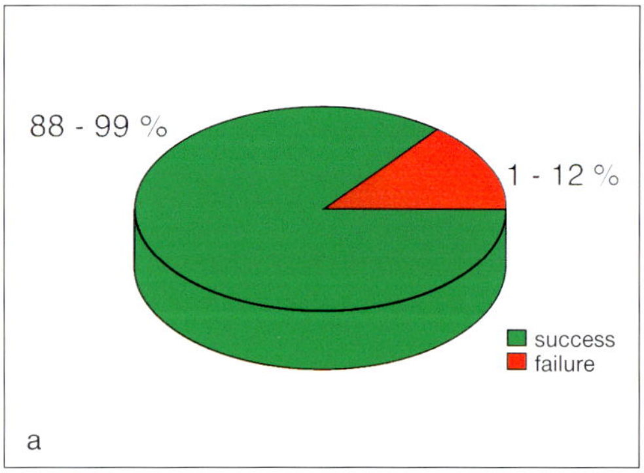

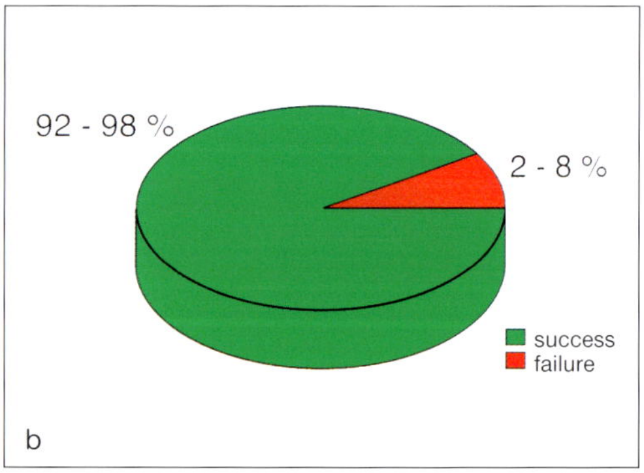

Fig 1-25 Surgical success rates in partially edentulous patients: a = implant-supported fixed partial denture in the mandible; b = implant-supported fixed partial denture in the maxilla. Data taken from studies reporting on more than 50 implants.

Table 1-8 Surgical success rates in patients with a single missing tooth (fixed restorations)*

Author, year	Type of study	Total No. of implants	Observation period (y)	Mandible I	Mandible L	Mandible S (%)	Maxilla I	Maxilla L	Maxilla S (%)
Jemt et al, 1990[62]	Longitudinal	23	3	2	0	100	21	2	90
Jemt et al, 1991[63]	Prospective	107	1	19	0	100	88	3	97
Haas et al, 1995[64]	Retrospective	76	1–6	17	0	100	59	1	98
Engquist et al, 1995[65]	Retrospective	82	1–5	8	1	88	74	1	99
Henry et al, 1996[66]	Prospective multicenter	107	1–5	19	0	100	88	3	97
Avivi-Arber and Zarb, 1996[67]	Prospective	49	1–8	14	0	100	35	1	97
Levine et al, 1997[68]	Retrospective multicenter	174	> 0.5	110	0	100	64	1	98
Scheller et al, 1998[69]	Multicenter	99	1–5	12	2	83	87	2	98

*Implant success rates reported in relation to fixed restorations (between 1 and 8 years) range from 88% to 100% in the mandible and from 90% to 99% in the maxilla (in studies reporting on more than 23 implants). Success rates of 83% in the mandible result from the small number of implants (12). Great success rates characterize the treatment of single missing teeth (see Fig 1-26).
I = number of implants; L = number of lost implants; S = success rate.

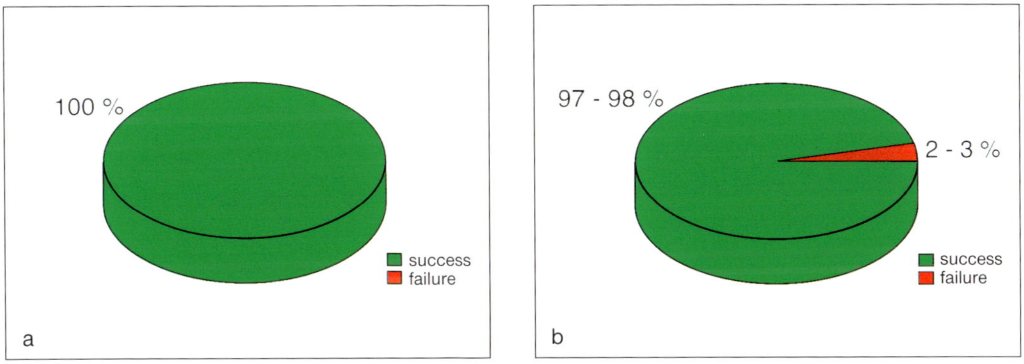

Fig 1-26 Surgical success rate in the patient with a single missing tooth: a = implant-supported crown in the mandible; b = implant-supported crown in the maxilla. Data taken from studies reporting on more than 50 implants.

Table 1-9 Implant success rates and bone quality*

Author, year	Bone types I to III I	Bone types I to III S (%)	Type IV bone I	Type IV bone S (%)
Engquist et al, 1988[49]	141	89	198	74
van Steenberghe et al, 1990[57]	491	96	67	94
Jaffin and Berman, 1991[70]	952	97	102	65
Johns et al, 1992[50]	453	96	57	72
Bahat, 1992[71]	44	93	28	93
Hutton et al, 1995[53]	254	91	40	50
Jemt et al, 1996[54]	118	97	15	80

*Implant success rates reported in relation to bone quality range from 89% to 97% in types I, II, and III bone and from 50% to 94% in type IV bone. Failure rates are greater in poor-density bone (see Fig 1-27).
I = number of implants; S = success rate.

Table 1-10 Implant success rates and implant length*

Implant length (mm)	van Steenberghe et al (1990)[53] I = 514 (1y follow-up) Maxilla I	Maxilla S (%)	Mandible I	Mandible S (%)	Lekholm et al (1994)[32] I = 558 (5y follow-up) 3.75 mm I	3.75 mm S (%)	4 mm I	4 mm S (%)	Wyatt and Zarb (1998)[41] I = 229 (5y follow-up) completely edentulous I	S (%)
7	28	89	81	100	109	94	11	94	12	75
10	85	95	140	94	224	90	21	100	93	92
13	50	96	35	91	86	94	4	100	58	95
15	40	100	26	100	74	100	0	100	53	98
18	4	100	16	100	20	100	0	100	12	100
20	2	100	7	100	9	100	0	100	1	100
Total	209	96	305	96	522	93	36	97	229	94

*Implant success rates range from 91% to 100% for implants more than 10 mm long (see Fig 1-28).
I = number of implants; S = success rate.

Table 1-11 Prosthetic success rates in completely edentulous patients (implant-supported dentures)*

Author, year	Prosthesis type	Total No. of prostheses	Observation period (y)	Mandible P	Mandible F	Mandible S (%)	Maxilla P	Maxilla F	Maxilla S (%)
Adell et al, 1990[29]	Fixed	163	5	83	1	99	80	3	96
			10		1	99		4	95
			15		1	99		6	93
Zarb and Schmitt, 1989[31]	44 fixed, 5 overdenture	49	4–9	43	0	100	6	0	100
Jemt, 1991[46]	Fixed	391	1	292	0	100	99	2	98
Arvidson et al, 1992[72]	Fixed	54	3	54	0	100			
Quirynen et al, 1992[37]	Fixed	99	0–6	57	1	96	42	3	90
Henry et al, 1995[34]	Fixed	15	10	15	0	100			
Brånemark et al, 1995[48]	Fixed	156	10	79	0	100	84	7	92

*For implant-supported complete dentures, success rates (0 to 10 years) in the mandible range from 96% to 100% and in the maxilla from 90% to 100%. These prosthetic success rates are stable at 10 and 15 years (see Fig 1-29).
P = number of prostheses; F = number of prosthetic failures; S = success rate.

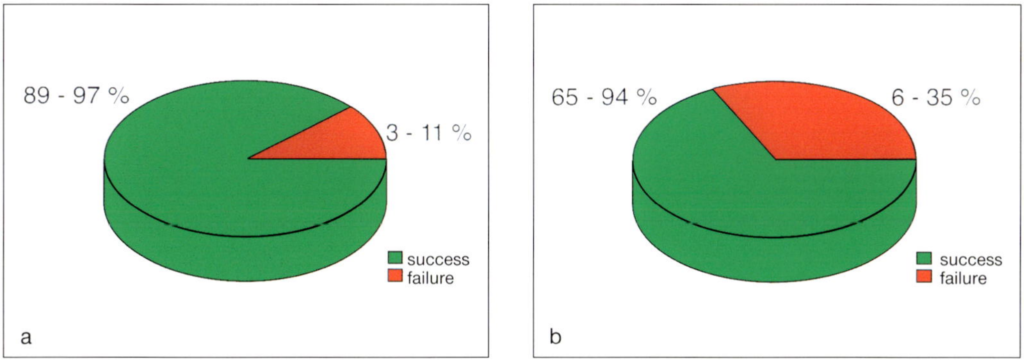

Fig 1-27 Surgical success rate and bone quality: a = types I, II, and III bone; b = type IV bone. Data taken from studies reporting on more than 50 implants.

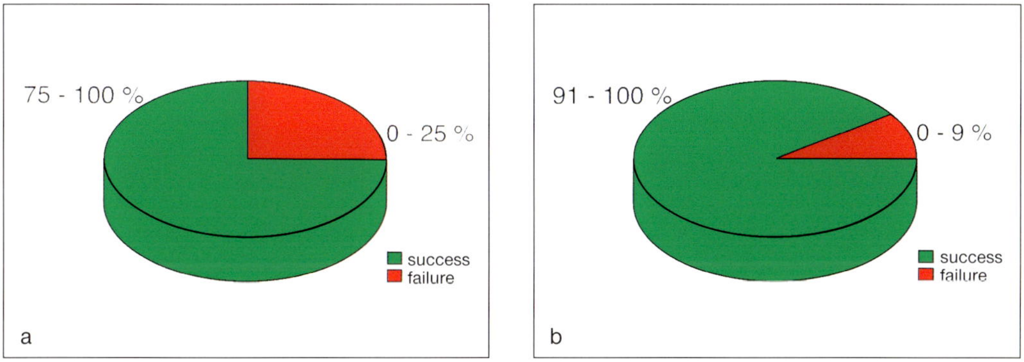

Fig 1-28 Surgical success rate and implant length: a = 7-mm implant length; b = 10- to 20-mm implant length. Data taken from studies reporting on more than 50 implants.

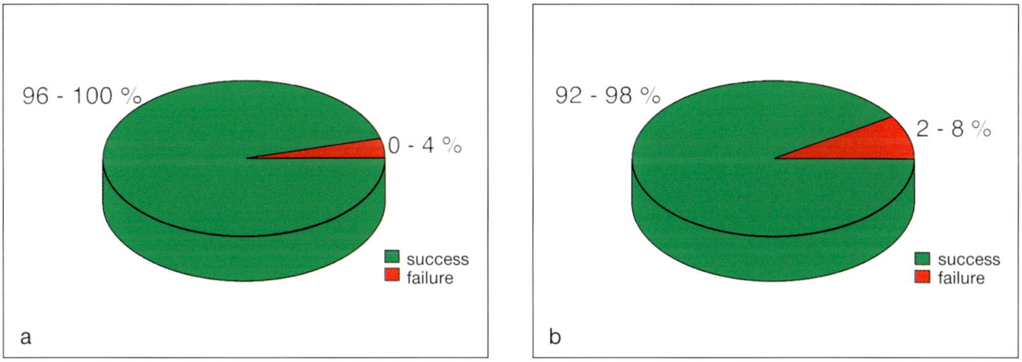

Fig 1-29 Prosthetic success rate in the completely edentulous patient: a = implant-supported denture in the mandible; b = implant-supported denture in the maxilla. Data taken from studies reporting on more than 30 prostheses.

Table 1-12 Prosthetic success rates in completely edentulous patients (overdenture)*

Author, year	Type of study	Total No. of prostheses	Observation period (y)	Mandible P	Mandible F	Mandible S (%)	Maxilla P	Maxilla F	Maxilla S (%)
Johns et al, 1992[50]	Prospective multicenter	127	0–1	98	0	100	29	4	86
Jemt et al, 1992[51]	Retrospective	92	1	–	–	–	92	7	92
Naert et al, 1994[73]	Prospective	36	0–2	36	0	100			
Hutton et al, 1995[53]	Prospective multicenter	120	0–3	91	3	97	29	8	72
Jemt et al, 1996[54]	Prospective multicenter	133	0–5	103	0	100	30	6	80
Ekfeldt et al, 1997[55]	Retrospective	43	0–8	9	1	89	34	9	74
Bergendal and Engquist, 1998[56]	Prospective	50	3–10	32	0	100	18	5	72

*For overdentures, success rates (1 to 8 years) in the mandible range from 89% to 100% and in the maxilla from 72% to 92% (in studies reporting on more than 43 prostheses). The prosthetic failure rates are greater in the maxilla (see Fig 1-30).
P = number of prostheses; F = number of prosthetic failures; S = success rate.

Table 1-13 Prosthetic success rates in partially edentulous patients (implant-supported fixed partial dentures)*

Author, year	Type of prosthesis	Total No. of prostheses	Observation period (y)	Mandible P	Mandible F	Mandible S (%)	Maxilla P	Maxilla F	Maxilla S (%)
Jemt et al, 1989[35]	Fixed	293	1–5	76	0	100	91	3	97
Jemt et al, 1992[58]	Fixed	127	1	53	0	100	43	0	100
Zarb and Schmitt, 1993[60]	Fixed posterior	46	2–7	29	0	100	17	0	100
Zarb and Schmitt, 1993[61]	Fixed anterior	31	2–8	15	0	100	16	0	100
Lekholm et al, 1994[36]	Fixed	197	1–5	121	7	94	76	4	94

*For fixed partial prostheses, success rates (1 to 8 years) in the mandible range from 94% to 100% and in the maxilla from 94% to 100% (in studies reporting on more than 31 prostheses). The prosthetic success rates are equivalent in the mandible and the maxilla for the partially edentulous patient (see Fig 1-31).
P = number of prostheses; F = number of prosthetic failures; S = success rate.

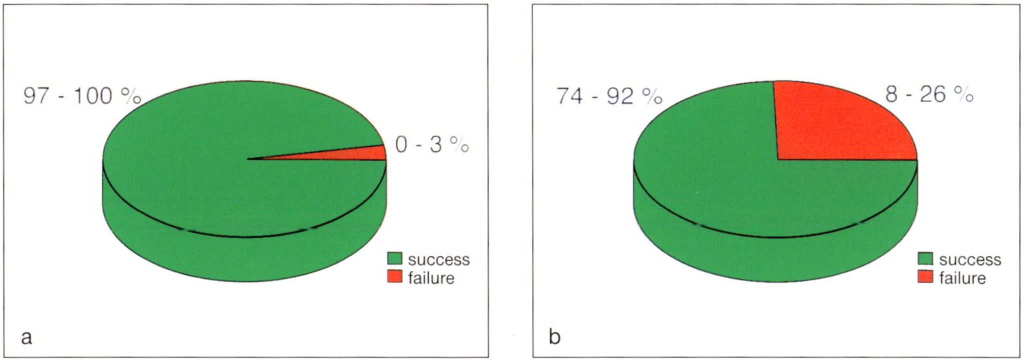

Fig 1-30 Prosthetic success rate in the completely edentulous patient: a = overdenture in the mandible; b = overdenture in the maxilla. Data taken from studies reporting on more than 30 prostheses.

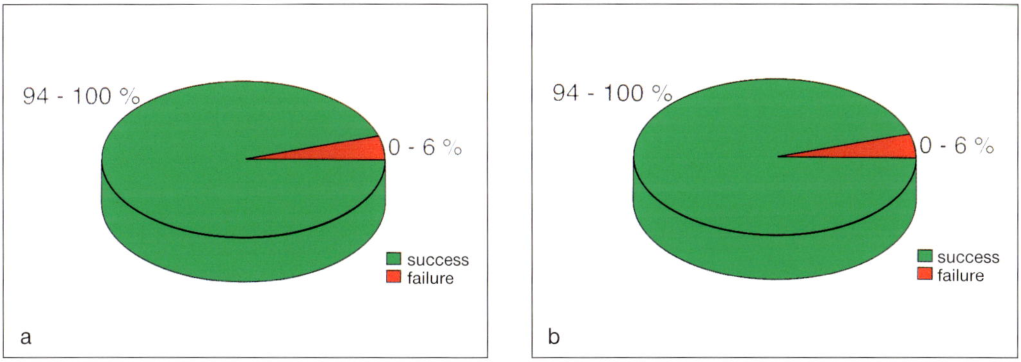

Fig 1-31 Prosthetic success rate in the partially edentulous patient: a = implant-supported fixed partial denture in the mandible; b = implant-supported fixed partial denture in the maxilla. Data taken from studies reporting on more than 30 prostheses.

Table 1-14 Surgical success rates for different implant systems*

Author, year	Type of implant	Total No. of implants	Observation period (y)	Mandible I	Mandible S (%)	Maxilla I	Maxilla S (%)
Quirynen et al, 1992[37]	Brånemark (CE, FR)	589	0–6	320	96	269	92
De Bruyn et al, 1992[74]	Screw-Vent (CE, PE)	85	> 0.5	23	100	62	90
Fugazzotto et al, 1993[75]	IMZ (CE, PE, ST)	2,023	0–5	1,032	98	991	96
Wedgwood et al, 1992[76]	ITI (CE, PE, ST)	352	0–3	286	92	66	78
Lekholm et al, 1994[36]	Brånemark (PE)	558	1–5	338	94	220	92
Leimola-Virtanen et al, 1995[77]	ITI (CE mandible)	153	3–10	153	92		
Khayat and Nader, 1995[78]	Screw-Vent (CE, PE, ST)	200	4	100	98	60	97
Buchs et al, 1995[79]	Steri-Oss (CE, PE, ST)	2,372	0–6	1,444	96	856	93
Haas et al, 1996[80]	IMZ (CE, PE, ST)	1,920	1–9	1,436	97	484	91
Jemt et al, 1996[54]	Brånemark (CE, OD)	510	0–5	393	96	117	74
Saadoun and Le Gall, 1996[81]	Steri-Oss (PE, CE)	1,499	0–8	783	96	716	95
Lazzara et al, 1996[82]	3i (CE, PE, ST)	1,969	0–5	936	96	935	97
Gomez-Roman et al, 1997[83]	Frialit-2 (ST)	696	0–5	331	97	365	97
Buser et al, 1997[84]	ITI (CE, PE, ST)	2,359	1–8	1,808	94	551	87
Makkonen et al, 1997[85]	Astra (CE mandible)	155	0–5	155	98		

*Several of these studies do not specify the success rate according to the different indications. The results obtained are similar for the different implant systems. However, the success criteria are not always identical, the observation period is quite variable, and very few studies report reliable clinical and radiographic assessment over 5 years (see Fig 1-32).
CE = completely edentulous; FR = fixed restoration; PE = partially edentulous; ST = single-tooth implant; OD = overdenture; I = control implants; S = success rate.

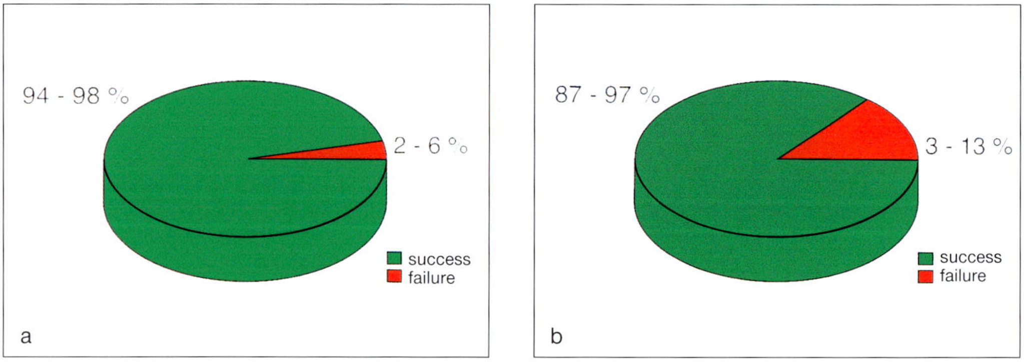

Fig 1-32 Surgical success rate for different implant systems: a = in the mandible; b = in the maxilla. Data taken from studies reporting on more than 300 implants.

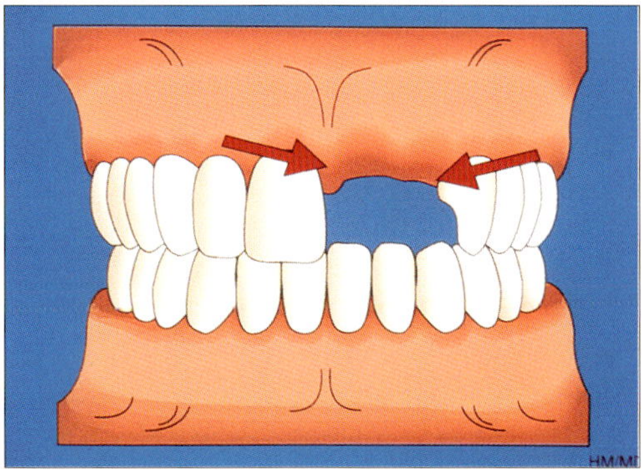

Fig 1-33 Different treatment options for partial edentulism.

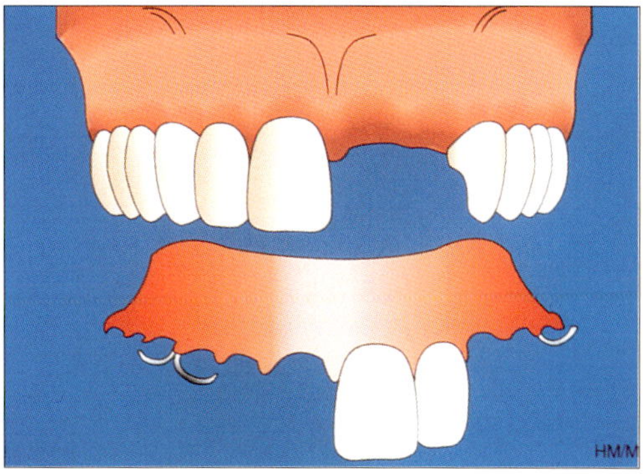

Fig 1-34 Removable partial denture.

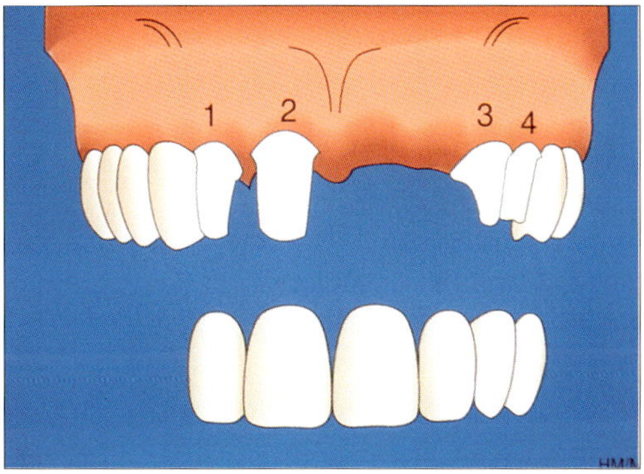

Fig 1-35 Fixed prosthesis (bridge).

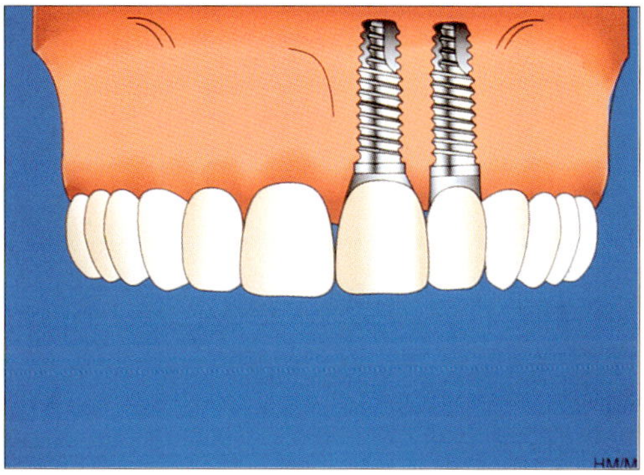

Fig 1-36 Implant-supported prosthesis.

VI. Implant treatment decision making and planning overview

The different prosthetic options must be explained to the patient (Figs 1-33 to 1-36). The benefit:risk ratio as well as the treatment advantages must be assessed.[86]

The practitioner must advise the patient on the most appropriate option according to his or her demands, age, and general and oral health status. The implant assessment confirms or contraindicates implant treatment.[87,88] A treatment plan is proposed to the patient. Treatment time, treatment alternatives, visualization of the future functional and esthetic outcome, as well as the prognosis must be specified. The different surgical and prosthetic treatment stages must be explained to the patient, as should the stresses that may occur during the treatment.

References

1. Lewis S. Treatment planning: Teeth versus implants. Int J Periodontics Restorative Dent 1996;16:367–377.
2. Wilson TG, Kornman KS, Newman MG. Advances in Periodontics. Chicago: Quintessence, 1992.
3. Davarpanah M, Mattout C, Kebir M, Martínez H. Conserver ou extraire: Un défi en parodontologie. J Parodontol Implantol Orale 1998;17:43–55.
4. Davarpanah M, Martínez H, Tecucianu JF, Fromentin O, Celletti R. To conserve or implant: Which choice of therapy? Int J Periodontics Restorative Dent 2000; 20:413–422.
5. Rateitschak HEM, Wolf HF, Hassell TM. Color Atlas of Periodontology. New York: Thieme Medical, 1989.
6. Atwood DA. Bone loss of edentulous alveolar ridges. J Periodontol 1979;50:11–21.
7. Basten C, Ammons WF, Persson R. Long-term evaluation of root-resected molars: A retrospective study. Int J Periodontics Restorative Dent 1996;16:207–219.
8. Carnevale G, Gianfranco DF, Tonelli MP, Marin C, Fuzzi MA. A retrospective analysis of the periodontal-prosthetic treatment of molars with interradicular lesions. Int J Periodontics Restorative Dent 1991; 11:188–205.
9. Hirschfeld L, Wasserman B. A long-term survey of tooth loss in 600 treated periodontal patients. J Periodontol 1978;5:225–237.
10. Lindhe J. Pathogenesis of plaque-associated periodontal disease. In: Textbook of Clinical Periodontology. Copenhagen: Munksgaard, 1989:153–190.
11. Lindhe J. Treatment of furcation-involved teeth. In: Textbook of Clinical Periodontology. Copenhagen: Munksgaard, 1989:515–532.
12. McFall WT. Tooth loss in 100 treated patients with periodontal disease. A long-term study. J Periodontol 1982;53:539–549.
13. Ramfjord SP, Knowles JW, Nissle RR, Burgett FG, Schick RA. Results following three modalities of periodontal therapy. J Periodontol 1975;46:522–526.
14. Fugazzotto PA, Parma-Benfenati S. Preprosthetic periodontal considerations. Crown length and biologic width. Quintessence Int 1984;15:1247–1256.
15. Cohen A, Machtou P. Endo-periodontal lesions: Biologic and mechanical considerations. J Parodontol 1996;15:235–250.
16. Missika P, Khayat P. Etude esthétique pré-implantaire. Cah Prothet 1990;71:106–121.
17. Nyman S, Lindhe J. A longitudinal study of combined periodontal and prosthetic treatment of patients with advanced periodontal disease. J Clin Periodontol 1979;4:163–169.
18. Kornman KS, Crane A, Wang HY, et al. The interleukin-1 genotype as a severity factor in adult periodontal disease. J Clin Periodontol 1997;24:72–77.
19. Wilson TS. Compliance and its role in periodontal therapy. Periodontol 2000 1996;12:16–23.
20. Nyman SR, Lang NP. Tooth mobility and the biological rationale for splinting teeth. Periodontol 2000 1994;4:15–22.
21. Lindhe J. Clinical Periodontology and Implant Dentistry. Copenhagen, Munksgaard, 1998.
22. Genon P, Genon-Romagna C. Apport des implants dans le traitement des parodontites avancées. J Parodontol Implantol Orale 1997;16:177–189.
23. Langer B, Sullivan DY. Osseointegration: Its impact on the interrelationship of periodontics and restorative dentistry. Part III. Periodontal prosthesis redefined. Int J Periodontics Restorative Dent 1989;9:241–261.
24. Ross IF, Thompson RH Jr. A long-term study of root retention in the treatment of maxillary molars with furcation involvement. J Periodontol 1978;49:238–244.
25. Goldman HM, Cohen DW. Periodontal Therapy, ed 6. St Louis: Mosby, 1980:1133–1135.
26. Wood WR, Greco GW, McFall WT Jr. Tooth loss in patients with moderate periodontitis after treatment and long-term maintenance care. J Periodontol 1989; 60:516–520.
27. Wang HL, Burgett FG, Shyr Y, Ramfjord S. The influence of molar furcation involvement and mobility on future clinical periodontal attachment loss. J Periodontol 1994;65:25–29.
28. Carnevale G. Effets à long terme des résections et/ou amputations radiculaires. Presented at Communication Europerio 1, Paris, May 1994.
29. Wilson TG. Les parodontites réfractaires existent-elles? J Parodontol 1994;13:133–138.
30. Albrektsson T, Zarb GA, Worthington P, Eriksson AR. The long-term efficacy of currently used dental implants: A review and proposed criteria of success. Int J Oral Maxillofac Implants 1986;1:11–25.
31. Zarb GA, Schmitt A. The longitudinal clinical effectiveness of osseointegrated dental implants: The Toronto study. Part II: The prosthetic results. J Prosthet Dent 1989;64:53–61.
32. Albrektsson T, Zarb GA. Current interpretation of the osseointegrated response: Clinical significance. Int J Prosthodont 1993;6:95–105.
33. Adell R, Eriksson B, Lekholm U, Brånemark P-I, Jemt T. A long-term follow-up study of osseointegrated implants in the treatment of totally edentulous jaws. Int J Oral Maxillofac Implants 1990;5:347–359.
34. Henry JP, Bower C, Wall D. Rehabilitation of the edentulous mandible with osseointegrated dental implants. Aust Dent J 1995;40:1–9.
35. Jemt T, Lekholm U, Adell R. Osseointegrated implants in the treatments of partially edentulous patients: A preliminary study on 875 consecutively placed fixtures. Int J Oral Maxillofac Implants 1989;4:211–217.

36. Lekholm U, van Steenberghe D, Herrmann I, et al. Osseointegrated implants in the treatment of partially edentulous jaws: A prospective 5-year multicenter study. Int J Oral Maxillofac Implants 1994;9:627–635.
37. Quirynen M, Naert I, van Steenberghe D. A study of 589 consecutive implants supporting complete fixed prostheses. Part I: Periodontal aspects. J Prosthet Dent 1992;68:655–663.
38. Zarb GA, Schmitt A. The longitudinal clinical effectiveness of osseointegrated dental implants: The Toronto study. Part III: Problems and complications encountered. J Prosthet Dent 1990;64:185–194.
39. Naert I, Quirynen M, van Steenberghe D, Darius P. A study of 589 consecutive implants supporting complete fixed prostheses. Part II: Prosthetic aspects. J Prosthet Dent 1992;68:949–956.
40. Adell R, Lekholm U, Rockler B, Brånemark P-I. A 15-year study of osseointegrated implants in the treatment of edentulous jaws. Int J Oral Surg 1981;10: 387–416.
41. Naert I, Quirynen M, van Steenberghe D, Darius P. Six-year prosthodontic study of 509 consecutively-inserted implants for the treatment of facial edentulism. J Prosthet Dent 1992;67:236–245.
42. Roos J, Sennerby L, Albrektsson T. An update on the clinical documentation on currently used bone anchored endosseous oral implants. Dent Update 1997;24:194–200.
43. Lindquist L, Carlsson G, Glantz P. Rehabilitation of the edentulous mandible with a tissue-integrated fixed prosthesis: A six-year longitudinal study. Quintessence Int 1987;18:89–96.
44. Albrektsson T. A multicenter study of osseointegrated oral implants. J Prosthet Dent 1988;60:75–84.
45. Wyatt CC, Zarb GA. Treatment outcomes of patients with implant-supported fixed partial prostheses. Int J Oral Maxillofac Implants 1998;13:204–211.
46. Jemt T. Failures and complications in 391 consecutively inserted fixed prostheses supported by Brånemark implants in edentulous jaws: A study of treatment from the time of prosthesis placement to the first annual checkup. Int J Oral Maxillofac Implants 1991;6:270–275.
47. Hemmings KW, Schmitt A, Zarb GA. Complications and maintenance requirements for fixed prostheses and overdentures in the edentulous mandible: A 5-year report. Int J Oral Maxillofac Implants 1994;9: 191–196.
48. Brånemark P-I, Svensson B, van Steenberghe D. Ten-year survival rates of fixed prosthesis on four or six implants ad modum Brånemark in full edentulism. Clin Oral Implants Res 1995;6:227–231.
49. Engquist B, Bergendal T, Kallus T, Linden U. A retrospective multicenter evaluation of osseointegrated implants supporting overdentures. Int J Oral Maxillofac Implants 1988;3:129–134.
50. Johns RB, Jemt T, Heath MR. A multicenter study of overdentures supported by Brånemark implants. Int J Oral Maxillofac Implants 1992;7:513–522.
51. Jemt T, Book K, Linden B, Urde G. Failures and complications in 92 consecutively inserted overdentures supported by Brånemark implants in severely resorbed edentulous maxillae: A study from prosthetic treatment to first annual checkup. Int J Oral Maxillofac Implants 1992;7:162–167.
52. Spiekermann H, Jansen UK, Richter EJ. A 10-year follow-up of IMZ and TPS implants in the edentulous mandible using bar-retained overdentures. Int J Oral Maxillofac Implants 1995;10:231–243.
53. Hutton JE, Heath R, Chai JY, et al. Factors related to success and failure rates at 3-year follow-up in a multicenter study of overdentures supported by Brånemark implants. Int J Oral Maxillofac Implants 1995;10:33–42.
54. Jemt T, Chai J, Harnett J, et al. A five-year prospective multicenter follow-up report on overdentures supported by osseointegrated implants. Int J Oral Maxillofac Implants 1996;11:291–298.
55. Ekfeldt A, Johansson LA, Isaksson S. Implant-supported overdenture therapy: A retrospective study. Int J Prosthodont 1997;10:366–374.
56. Bergendal T, Engquist B. Implant-supported overdentures: A longitudinal prospective study. Int J Oral Maxillofac Implants 1998;13:253–262.
57. van Steenberghe D, Lekholm U, Bolender C. The applicability of osseointegrated oral implants in the rehabilitation of partial edentulism: A prospective multicenter study on 588 fixtures. Int J Oral Maxillofac Implants 1990;5:272–281.
58. Jemt T, Linden B, Lekholm U. Failures and complications in 127 consecutively placed fixed partial prostheses supported by Brånemark implants: From prosthetic treatment to first annual checkup. Int J Oral Maxillofac Implants 1992;7:40–44.
59. Pylant T, Triplett RG, Key MC, Brusvold MA. A retrospective evaluation of endosseous titanium implants in the partially edentulous patient. Int J Oral Maxillofac Implants 1992;7:195–202.
60. Zarb GA, Schmitt A. The longitudinal effectiveness of osseointegrated implants in posterior partially edentulous patients. Int J Prosthodont 1993;6:189–196.
61. Zarb GA, Schmitt A. The longitudinal effectiveness of osseointegrated implants in anterior partially edentulous patients. Int J Prosthodont 1993;6:180–188.
62. Jemt T, Lekholm U, Grondahl K. Single implant restorations ad modum Brånemark. A 3-year follow-up study of the development group. Int J Periodontics Restorative Dent 1990;5:341–349.

63. Jemt T, Laney WR, Harris D, et al. Osseointegrated implants for single tooth replacement: A 1-year report from a multicenter prospective study. Int J Oral Maxillofac Implants 1991;6:29–36.
64. Haas R, Mensdorff-Pouilly N, Mailath G, Watzek G. Brånemark single tooth implants: A preliminary report of 76 implants. J Prosthet Dent 1995;73:274–279.
65. Engquist B, Nilson H, Astrand P. Single-tooth replacement by osseointegrated Brånemark implants. Clin Oral Implants Res 1995;6:238–245.
66. Henry JP, Laney WR, Jemt T, et al. Osseointegrated implants for single-tooth replacement: A prospective 5-year multicenter study. Int J Oral Maxillofac Implants 1996;11:450–455.
67. Avivi-Arber L, Zarb GA. Clinical effectiveness of implant-supported single-tooth replacement: The Toronto study. Int J Oral Maxillofac Implants 1996;11: 311–321.
68. Levine RA, Clem DS, Wilson T Jr, Higginbottom F, Saunders SL. A multicenter retrospective analysis of the ITI implant system used for single-tooth replacements: Preliminary results at 6 or more months of loading. Int J Oral Maxillofac Implants 1997;12: 237–242.
69. Scheller H, Urgell JP, Kultje C, et al. A 5-year multicenter study on implant-supported single crown restorations. Int J Oral Maxillofac Implants 1998; 13:212–218.
70. Jaffin R, Berman C. The excessive loss of Brånemark fixtures in type IV bone: A 5-year analysis. J Periodontol 1991;62:2–4.
71. Bahat O. Osseointegrated implants in the maxillary tuberosity: Report on 45 consecutive patients. Int J Oral Maxillofac Implants 1992;7:459–467.
72. Arvidson K, Bystedt H, Frykholm A, Konow L, Lothigius E. A 3-year clinical study of Astra dental implants in the treatment of edentulous mandibles. Int J Oral Maxillofac Implants 1992;7:321–329.
73. Naert I, Quirynen M, Hooghe M, van Steenberghe D. A comparative prospective study of splinted and unsplinted Brånemark implants in mandibular overdenture therapy: A preliminary report. J Prosthet Dent 1994;71:486–492.
74. De Bruyn H, Callaert B, Linden U, Flygare L. A comparative study of the clinical efficacy of Screw-Vent implants versus Brånemark fixtures installed in a periodontal clinic. Clin Oral Implants Res 1992;3:32–41.
75. Fugazzotto PA, Gulbransen HJ, Wheeler SL, Lindsay JA. The use of IMZ osseointegrated implants in partially and completely edentulous patients: Success and failures of 2,032 implant cylinders up to 60+ months in function. Int J Oral Maxillofac Implants 1993;8:617–621.
76. Wedgwood D, Jennings KJ, Critchlow HA, et al. Experience with ITI osseointegrated implants at five centers in the UK. Br J Oral Maxillofac Surg 1992;30:377–381.
77. Leimola-Virtanen R, Peltola J, Oksala E, Helenius H, Happonen RP. ITI titanium plasma-sprayed implants in the treatment of edentulous mandibles: A follow-up study of 39 patients. Int J Oral Maxillofac Implants 1995;10:373–378.
78. Khayat PG, Nader NA. Intérêt et indications d'un implant vissé à hexagone interne: Le Screw Vent (deuxième partie). J Parodontol 1995;14:31–41.
79. Buchs AU, Hanh J, Vassos DM. The prospective clinical study of 2,372 Steri-Oss HA-coated threaded implants—Six year post-restoration update results. Presented at the 1995 Steri-Oss International Conference, July 1995.
80. Haas R, Mensdorff-Pouilly N, Mailath G, Watzek G. Survival of 1,920 IMZ implants followed for up to 100 months. Int J Oral Maxillofac Implants 1996;11: 581–588.
81. Saadoun A, Le Gall MG. An 8-year compilation of clinical results obtained with Steri-Oss endosseous implants. Compendium 1996;17:669–688.
82. Lazzara RJ, Siddiqui AA, Binon P, et al. Retrospective multicenter analysis of 3 endosseous dental implants placed over a five-year period. Clin Oral Implants Res 1996;7:73–83.
83. Gomez-Roman G, Schulte W, d'Hoedt B, Axman-Krcmar D. The Frialit-2 Implant system: Five-year clinical experience in single-tooth and immediately postextraction applications. Int J Oral Maxillofac Implants 1997;12:299–309.
84. Buser D, Mericske-Stern R, Bernard JP, Behneke A, Behneke N, Hirt HP, et al. Long-term evaluation of non-submerged ITI implants. Clin Oral Implants Res 1997;8:161–172.
85. Makkonen TA, Holmberg S, Niemi L, Olson C, Tammisald T, Peltola J. A 5-year prospective clinical study of Astra Tech dental implants supporting fixed bridges or overdentures in the edentulous mandible. Clin Oral Implants Res 1997;8:469–475.
86. Assémat-Tessandier X, Amzalag G. La Décision en Implantologie. Paris: CdP, 1993.
87. McKiney RV. Endosteal Dental Implants. St Louis: Mosby Year Book, 1991.
88. Worthington P, Lang BR, Lavelle WE. Osseointegration in Dentistry. An Introduction. Chicago: Quintessence, 1994.

CHAPTER 2

Implant Diameters

H. Martínez/M. Davarpanah/R. Lazzara/K. Beaty/D. Etienne

During the last 10 years, the development of new surgical and prosthetic components has allowed optimization of functional and esthetic outcomes. Different implant diameters have been suggested since the end of the 1980s (Fig 2-1). The residual bone quantity and quality, type of prosthesis, esthetics, and biomechanical factors determine the choice of implant diameter. Indications and limits of the different implant diameters are presented in this chapter.

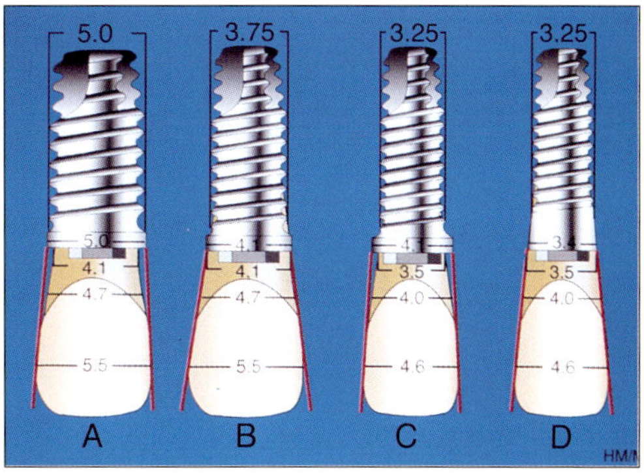

Fig 2-1 Implant diameter influences the functional and esthetic result: a = large-diameter (5 and 6 mm) 3i implant with a neck corresponding to the implant diameter; b = standard 3i implant (3.75 and 4 mm) with a 4.1-mm neck; c = small-diameter (3.25 mm) 3i implant with a 4.1-mm reduced collar; d = small-diameter (3.25 mm) 3i implant with a 3.4-mm reduced collar.

I. Small-diameter implants

Positioning of a standard implant in borderline anatomic conditions increases the risks for implant complications and failures. The small-diameter implant (from 3 to 3.4 mm) is indicated in the presence of a thin alveolar ridge or a mesiodistal space of less than 7 mm. In some cases, small-diameter implants prevent the need for more extensive surgical procedures (bone grafting, guided bone regeneration [GBR], ridge augmentation) or widening of the prosthetic mesiodistal space and/or bony space (orthodontics) (Figs 2-2 and 2-3). However, all the biomechanical risk factors must be strictly assessed before using a small-diameter implant.

A. Review of literature

Several types of small-diameter implants have been marketed since the late 1980s (Calcitek, IMZ, Nobel Biocare, Implant Innovations, ITI). To date, more papers have been published on this type of implant,[1–3] but no longitudinal multicenter studies have been reported on small-diameter implants. Most authors who have assessed the reliability of different implant systems mention their results with small-diameter implants (Table 2-1).[1–9]

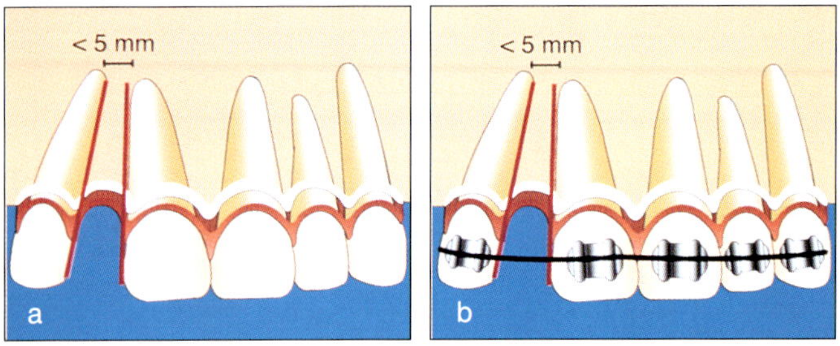

Figs 2-2a and 2-2b Reduced inter-root space: an indication for orthodontic treatment.

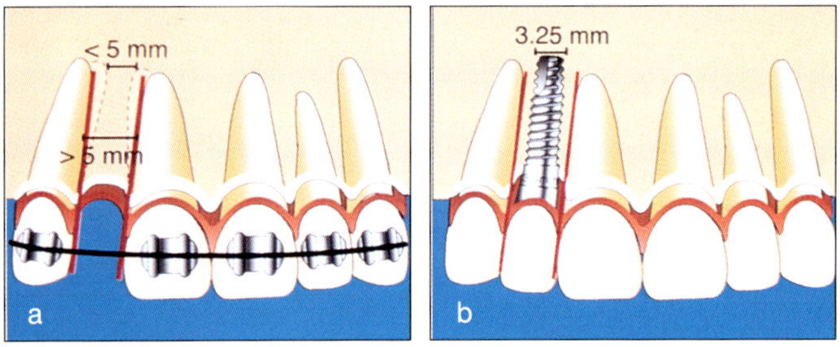

Figs 2-3a and 2-3b Restoring an inter-root space greater than 5 mm and placing a small-diameter implant.

In a clinical and radiographic report over 8 years on 1,374 impacted hydroxyapatite-coated implants (Integral), Block and Kent[4] have reported very good results for 238 3.25-mm-diameter implants. Complications and failures are not described.

Spiekermann et al[5] studied the clinical and radiographic results (1 to 10 years, mean 5.7 years) for 300 IMZ implants (3.3- to 4-mm diameter) stabilizing mandibular overdentures in 136 patients. One hundred twenty-seven small-diameter implants were placed in 61 patients. The small-diameter implants were placed in thin ridges. Over 5 years, the authors showed a 95% success rate for the 3.3-mm-diameter implants.

In 1996, Saadoun and Le Gall[6] published the clinical results over 8 years on 1,499 Steri-Oss implants placed in 605 patients to treat different types of edentulism. Four different types of implants were used. Three hundred six small-diameter implants of different lengths (8, 10, 12, 14, and 16 mm) were placed; 296 were loaded. The authors report 34 failures (success rate 89%). It is interesting to mention that of the 34 failures, 16 implants were 8 mm long (failure rate 43.2%). The authors did not advise the use of short, small-diameter implants.

Lazzara et al,[8] in a retrospective, multicenter study, showed the results at 5 years on 1,871 3i implants. Two hundred two impacted implants (titanium plasma sprayed) of 3.3-mm diameter were placed. Twenty implants were excluded from the study because of lack of follow-up. The success rates obtained in the mandible and in the maxilla were 96% and 95%, respectively. Of the eight reported failures, five were implants 7 mm long. Etiology of failure was the absence of osseointegration for six implants and excessive bone loss for two implants.

Buser et al[9] analyzed the results at 8 years for 2,359 ITI implants placed in 1,003 patients. Four different types of implants were used:

Table 2-1 Studies reporting results on small-diameter implants

Author, year	Implant type	Follow-up period (y)	Implant diameter (mm)	Small-diameter implants	Failures	Success rate (%)
Block and Kent, 1993[4]	Integral	8	3.25, 4.0	238	2	99
Spiekermann et al, 1995[5]	IMZ	1–10	3.3, 4.0	127	8	95
Saadoun and Le Gall, 1996[6]	Steri-Oss	8	3.25, 3.80, 4.50	306	34	89
Sethi et al, 1996[7]	Osteo Ti	3	2.75, 3.00, 3.75, 4.50	51 58	0 0	100 100
Lazzara et al, 1996[8]	3i	5	3.3, 4.0	202	8	96
Buser et al, 1997[9]	ITI	8	3.3, 4.1	213	Not specified	Not specified

—solid-screw implant, 4.1-mm diameter (n = 1,141)
—hollow-screw implant, 4.1-mm diameter (n = 639)
—cylindric hollow implant (n = 366)
—solid-screw implant, 3.3-mm diameter (n = 213)

The follow-up was less than 5 years, and the authors failed to report results for the small-diameter implants.

In the beginning of the 1990s, Nobel Biocare marketed a 3-mm-diameter implant. The 20% decrease of the standard implant diameter (from 3.75 to 3 mm) leads to a reduced resistance to fracture of about 50%. A preliminary report on a multicenter study started in 1988 shows a 93% success rate for 201 implants placed in 106 patients. Unfortunately, no study has been published to date, and this implant has been removed from the market.

B. Indications

Indications for small-diameter implants are[1]:

—reduced inter-root bone space
—thin alveolar crest
—limited prosthetic cervical diameter

1. Reduced inter-root bone space

In the anterior segments, a less than 7-mm inter-root distance contraindicates the use of 3.75-mm-diameter single-tooth implants. The risk for adjacent root damage must be kept in mind. In the presence of a 5- to 7-mm mesiodistal bone space, several treatment options may be considered: space management using orthodontics, placing a small-diameter implant, or conventional prosthetic options. Treatment choice should be guided by edentulous segment location, bone crest width, time required for possible orthodontic treatment, and occlusal forces (Figs 2-4 to 2-7).

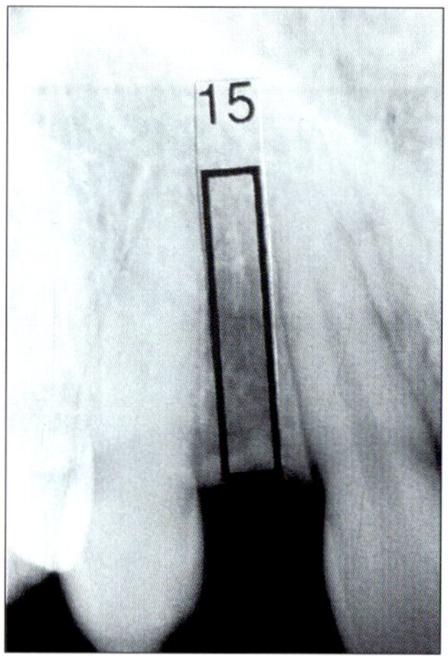

Fig 2-4 Periapical radiograph showing a reduced inter-root bone space.

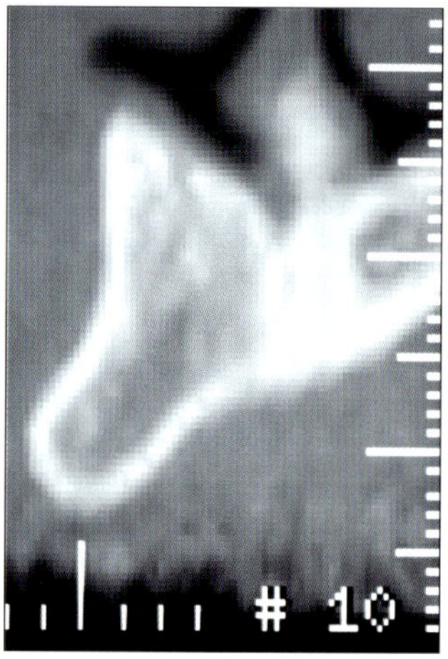

Fig 2-5 Oblique computed tomographic (CT) scan showing an adequate buccopalatal bone volume.

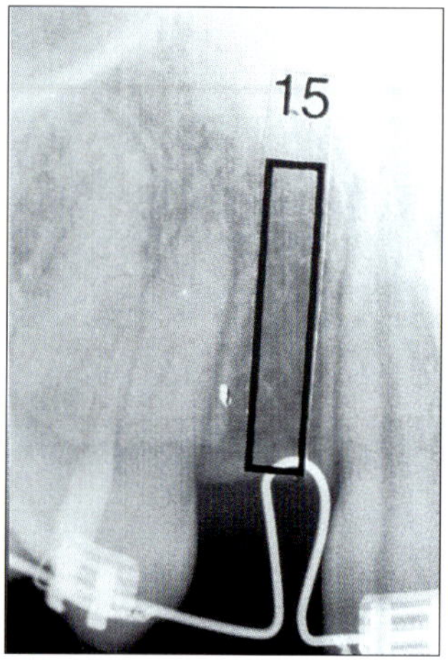

Fig 2-6 Adequate inter-root bone space following orthodontic treatment.

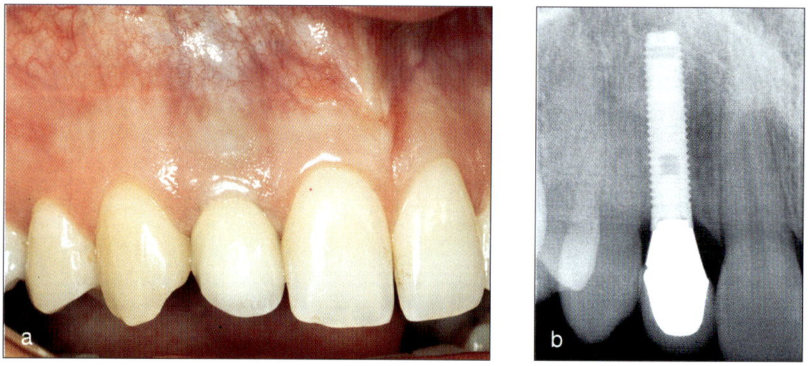

Figs 2-7a and 2-7b Clinical and radiographic views after 1 year of loading (prosthetic work, Dr Picard's department).

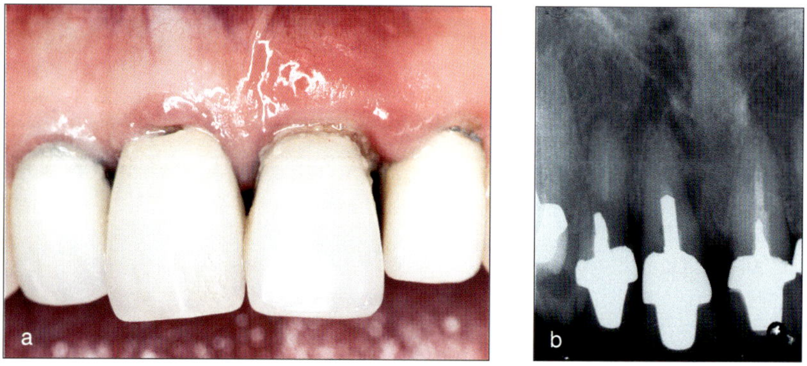

Figs 2-8a and 2-8b Clinical and radiographic views of four maxillary incisors. Note the advanced endodontic-periodontal defects.

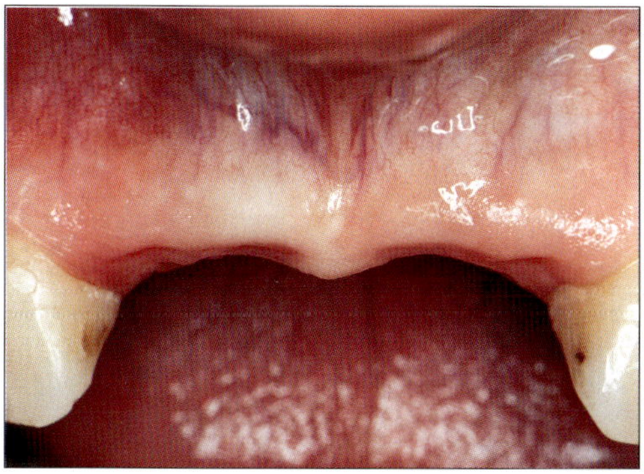

Fig 2-9 Clinical view following tooth extraction.

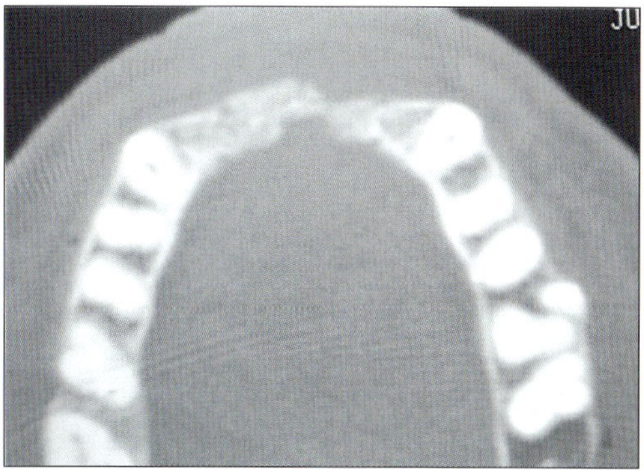

Fig 2-10a Axial CT scan showing the anterior edentulous segment.

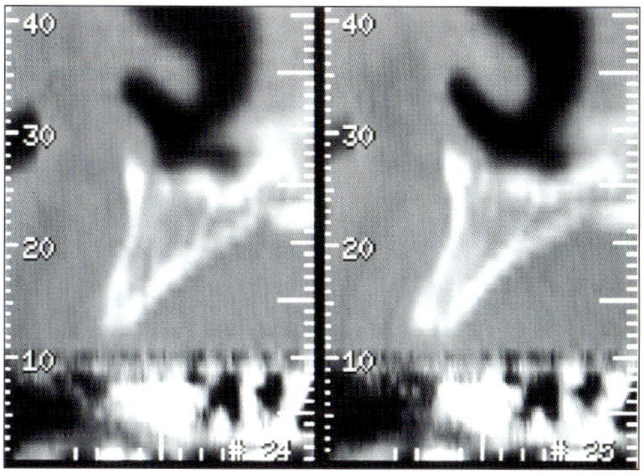

Fig 2-10b Oblique scan demonstrating a thin alveolar ridge.

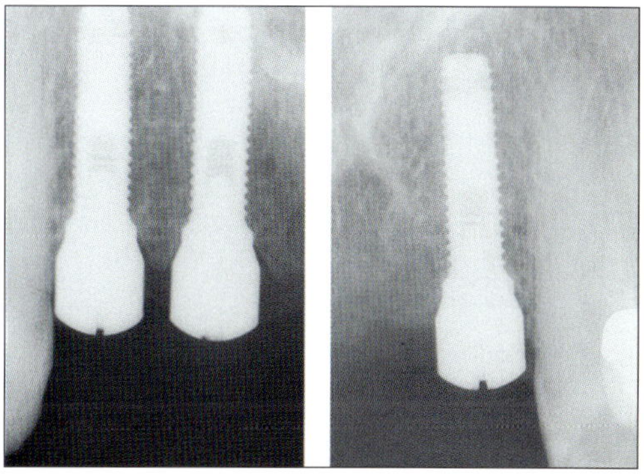

Fig 2-11 Periapical radiograph showing abutment placement. Note the perfect osseointegration of the implants.

2. Thin alveolar ridge

In the presence of a thin alveolar ridge less than 6 mm wide, the use of a small-diameter implant may be considered (Figs 2-8 to 2-12). The coronal emergence point has a decisive effect on the esthetic result. A buccal concavity or an extensive centripetal resorption may lead to an emergence point located too lingually. In some situations, maxillary bone loss must be treated using bone-reconstructive procedures.

3. Reduced mesiodistal prosthetic space

Implant selection for a reduced prosthetic space will depend on the crown's cervical and coronal diameter and on the implant's emergence profile. For the mandibular incisors, and sometimes for the maxillary lateral incisors, the mesiodistal prosthetic space is less than 4.5 mm. An appropriate esthetic result is often impossible to achieve using a standard implant (cervical diameter 4.1 mm). In the cervical aspect, the mesiodistal implant diameter must be slightly less than that of the future

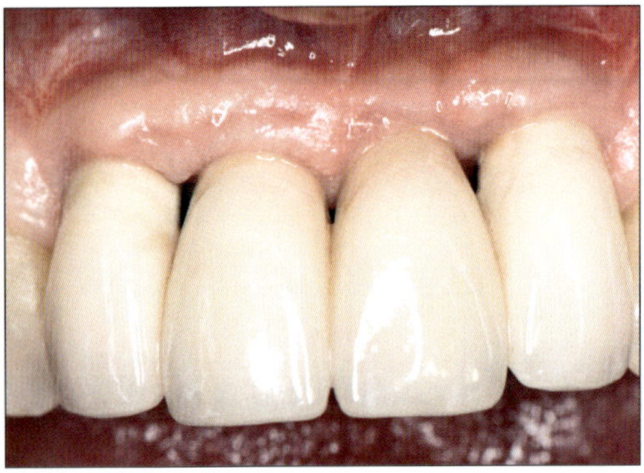

Fig 2-12a Clinical view of the final prosthetic result.

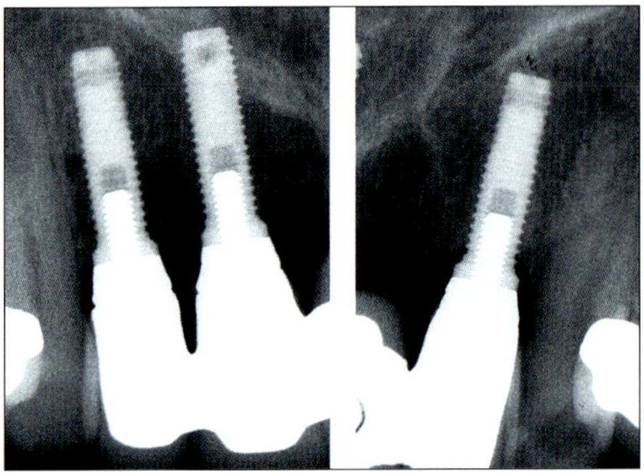

Fig 2-12b Radiographic view after 1 year of loading (prosthodontic work, Dr E. Cohen).

prosthetic tooth. A better esthetic result may thus be obtained. Moreover, in the apicocoronal aspect, the implant must be placed 2 to 4 mm under the cementoenamel junction of the adjacent teeth. At this level, the root diameter is less than the cementoenamel junction diameter. For a single-tooth replacement offering a mesiodistal cervical diameter equal to or less than 4 mm, an implant with a small-diameter neck (less than 4 mm) should be used. A more natural emergence profile will likely result.

C. Esthetics and tooth morphology

The choice of implant diameter has a major effect on the final esthetic result. Very often, in tooth agenesis (of the maxillary lateral incisor), the available bone and/or mesiodistal prosthetic space is limited. A possible root or crown convergence of the adjacent teeth may be managed using orthodontics before placing a small-diameter implant.

In the anterior region, the morphology of the future prosthetic tooth must match the contralateral tooth. A major anatomic difference may lead to an esthetic failure. Concerning the incisors, and sometimes the premolars, the mean cervical and coronal measurements may suggest the choice of a small-diameter implant (Table 2-2).[10]

D. Biomechanical considerations

Small-diameter implants offer reduced anchoring surface and resistance to fracture compared to standard implants. Before considering the use of this type of implant, occlusal forces must be appropriately assessed. The Nobel Biocare firm has taken the 3-mm-diameter implant off the market because of its insufficient biomechanical properties. A new small-diameter implant (3.3 mm) is now available. The biomechanical characteristics are optimized compared to those of the 3-mm-diameter implant. According to Forsmalm,[11] however, the fracture risk for the 3.3-mm-diameter implants is increased. Their resistance to fracture is 25% less than that of the standard implant.

In the beginning of the 1990s, several research teams studied the biomechanical stresses applied to bone using implants of different diameters. Matsushita et al[12] assessed the bone stresses applied by cylindric implants of 3-, 4-, 5-, 6-, 7-, and 8-mm diameters. Vertical and lateral forces of 100 N were applied to the implants. For both types of forces, the most important stresses are locat-

Table 2-2 Mean measurements (mm) of the anterior teeth (modified according to Wheeler[10])

Tooth	Coronal mesiodistal diameter	Coronal buccolingual diameter	Cervical mesiodistal diameter	Cervical buccolingual diameter
Maxillary central incisor	8.5	7.0	7.0	6.0
Maxillary lateral incisor	6.5	6.0	5.0	5.0
Maxillary first premolar	7.0	9.0	5.0	8.0
Maxillary second premolar	7.0	9.0	5.0	8.0
Mandibular central incisor	5.0	6.0	3.5	5.3
Mandibular lateral incisor	5.5	6.5	3.8	5.8
Mandibular first premolar	7.0	7.5	5.0	6.5
Mandibular second premolar	7.0	8.0	5.0	7.0

ed at the cortical bone level around the implant neck. According to these authors, force distribution is less favorable using small-diameter implants. Curiously, according to Rieger et al,[13] the small-diameter implant enhances the stresses transmitted to the bone.

Block et al[14] studied in the dog the tensile forces needed to remove impacted hydroxyapatite-coated implants (Calcitek) after 15 weeks of osseointegration. Different lengths (4, 8, and 15 mm) and diameters (3.0, 3.3, and 4.0 mm) were assessed. The removal torque increase is proportional to the implant length increase. However, the tensile strength forces reported do not vary, regardless of implant diameter. In 1992, Sendax[15] assessed the soft tissue environment around 50 implants; 3.25-mm-diameter (25 implants) and 4.0-mm-diameter hydroxyapatite-coated implants (25 implants) were used. Clinical assessment over 3 years shows a better tissue response around the small-diameter implants. According to Sendax, a critical implant diameter could exist, beyond which risk of bone loss may predispose peri-implant inflammation. Increase of stresses in the cervical level, combined with reduced bone vascularization, is suggested to justify this assumption.

Unfortunately, all the studies of different implant diameters fail to result in a consensus for biomechanical considerations. Research protocols were often very different and were mainly developed using bone-substitute laboratory models. Only long-term clinical results will be able to determine the reliability of small-diameter implants in terms of bone stability.

1. Occlusal force control

Small-diameter implants offer reduced anchoring surface and resistance to fracture compared to the standard implant. Occlusal forces must be well controlled.

2. Contraindications

The small-diameter implant is contraindicated for canine and molar replacement (Fig 2-13).

II. Large-diameter implants

In 1987, Langer developed the 5-mm-diameter implant starting from the basic concepts of osseointegration: the importance of the anchoring surface and primary stabilization of the implant. This large-diameter implant is appropriate for specific situations of insuffi-

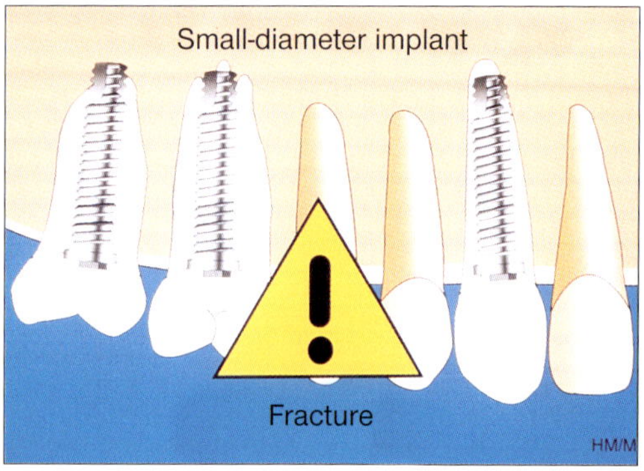

Fig 2-13 Contraindication for small-diameter implants.

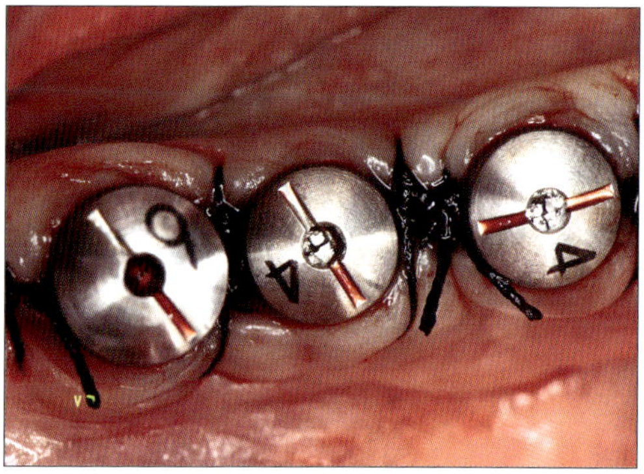

Fig 2-14 Stage-two surgery: placement of three healing abutments adapted to the diameters of the prosthetic teeth. A large-diameter implant has been used distally.

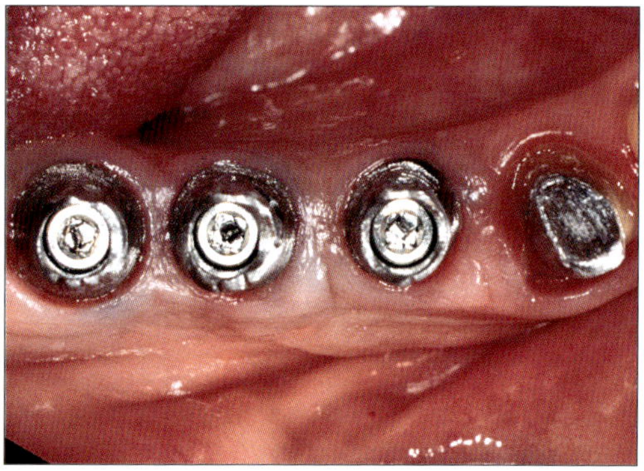

Fig 2-15a Occlusal view of the abutments adapted to the diameter of the prosthetic teeth. Note the larger diameter of the distal implant.

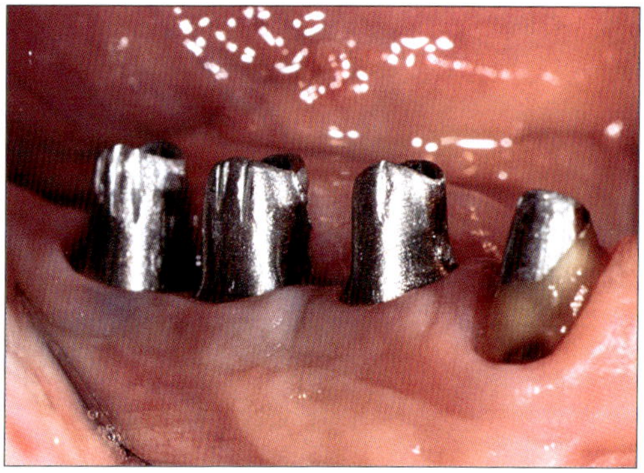

Fig 2-15b Buccal view of the UCLA abutments torqued to 32 N.

cient bone quality and/or height (Figs 2-14 to 2-17).[16–19]

A. Review of literature

A great number of manufacturers market large-diameter implants (Implant Innovations, ITI, Frialit, Nobel Biocare, Screw-Vent, Steri-Oss). However, few studies have been published to date (Table 2-3). Results fail to specify peri-implant bone loss and prosthetic complications. In a multicenter prospective study, Langer et al[19] were to report results concerning 140 implants of 5-mm diameter placed in patients aged from 40 to 75 years old. A provisional report of the Nobel Biocare multicenter study (13 countries, 35 clinics) using the 5-mm implant shows a 97.7% success rate for 977 implants placed in 614 patients (605 maxillary and 372 mandibular). Twenty-two failures were reported, with no cause-related details. No final statistical results have been published to date.

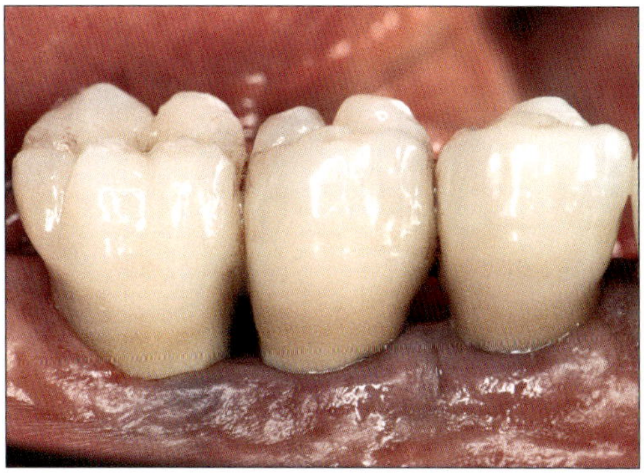

Fig 2-16a Buccal view of the three splinted crowns.

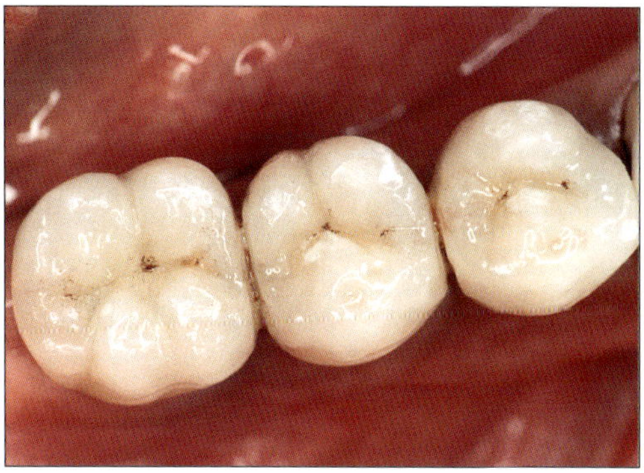

Fig 2-16b Occlusal view of the final prosthetic result.

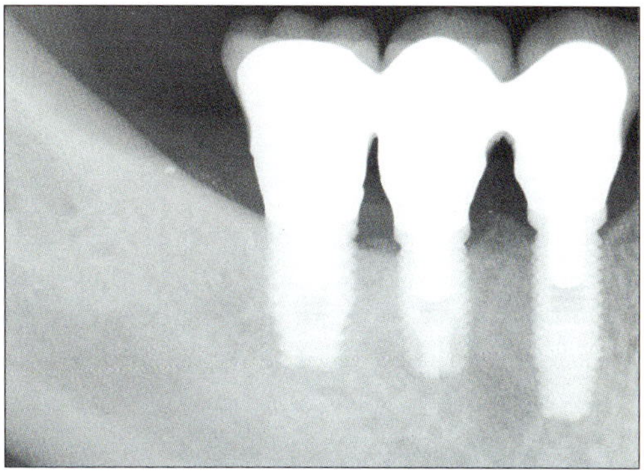

Fig 2-17 Periapical radiograph after 1 year of loading (prosthodontics, Dr P. Raygot).

Table 2-3 Mean measurements (mm) of the anterior teeth (modified according to Wheeler[10])

Author, year	Implant type	Study type	Follow-up period	No. of patients	Mx I	Mx F	Md I	Md F	Success rate (%)	Prosthetic complications	Tissue complications
Graves et al, 1994[20]	3i 5–6 mm	Prospective	1–2 y	196	110	2	158	9	95.9	Not specified	Not specified
Davarpanah et al, 1995[16]	Brånemark 5 mm	Prospective	2 y	30	29	1	27	1	96.3	Not specified	Specified
Barrachina et al, 1994[21]	Brånemark 5 mm	Prospective	1 y	51	48	5	36	1	88.2	Not specified	Not specified
Barrachina et al, 1996[22]	Brånemark 5 mm	Prospective	1–4 y	179	156	21	104	7	89.2	Not specified	Not specified
Bahat and Handelsman, 1996[23]	Brånemark 5 mm	Prospective	3–26 mo	90	46	0	95	4	97.1	Not specified	Not specified

Mx = maxilla; Md = mandible; I = number of implants; F = number of failures.

Graves et al[20] report a 95.9% success rate over 2 years in a prospective study started in 1992. Two hundred sixty-eight 3i implants of 5- and 6-mm diameter were placed in 196 patients. Eleven failures occurred during the second surgical stage and were attributed to poor bone quality. The authors published no statistical analysis.

Davarpanah et al[16] presented statistical results over 2 years on 56 Brånemark implants of 5-mm diameter placed in 30 partially edentulous patients. After healing, 53 of 55 functional implants were loaded. Forty-three were loaded for more than 18 months, and 48 for more than 12 months. A 96% success rate is observed over 12 and 18 months. The authors reported two-thread bone loss around five implants and a three-thread bone loss around one implant when put into function. This loss is stable in the clinical and radiographic controls over 6, 12, and 18 months.

Barrachina et al[21] reported the clinical follow-up of 84 large-diameter Brånemark implants placed in 51 patients. Over 1 year, six implants were cited as failures. According to these authors, most failures are due to poor bone quality. An 88.2% success rate was obtained over 1 year for 51 implants. In 1996, the same authors[22] reported clinical results from 1 to 4 years on 320 implants placed in 179 patients. They reported 28 failures for 260 implants put into function (89.2% success rate). The observation time for the 260 implants was very variable. Stability and peri-implant bone loss are not recorded in this study.

Bahat et al[23] studied 133 large-diameter Brånemark implants, some combined with standard implants to treat posterior edentulous regions. The authors described four failures in the mandible. A 97% overall success rate was obtained. The authors failed to specify possible prosthetic complications or peri-implant bone loss.

B. Indications

1. Insufficient bone quality

The use of large-diameter implants must be considered in the presence of poorly corticalized bone (Fig 2-18). The alveolar ridge width must, however, be greater than or equal to 8 mm.[17,24] Moreover, during the first surgical stage, primary stability of the implant must be sufficient. Indeed, in type IV bone, implants with diameters of 3.75 or 4 mm do not offer good primary stability. The use of a 5-mm-diameter implant must then be considered.

2. Insufficient ridge height

In the posterior regions, it is common to observe insufficient bone height associated with a ridge width equal to or greater than 8 mm (Fig 2-19). Short large-diameter implants offer an anchoring surface larger than that of standard implants. The length decrease is compensated for by the implant diameter increase. In some situations, this approach may prevent the need for extensive surgical procedures (bone grafts, sinus elevation and grafting, mandibular nerve repositioning).

3. Implant osseointegration failure

Implant osseointegration failure dramatically delays implant treatment time. If this occurs, an additional bone healing period of 4 to 8 months may be required before loading an implant within the same site. In the presence of sufficient alveolar ridge width, the large-diameter implant allows avoidance of this healing period, with immediate replacement of the standard implant. The implant is removed, and the peri-implant soft tissue is thoroughly debrided. In most situations, site widening is not necessary. The implant placement is often performed using self-tapping or threaded implants according to bone quality.

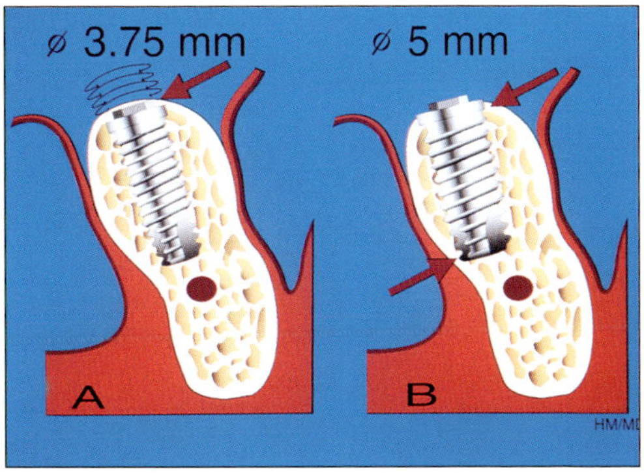

Fig 2-18 Large-diameter implant allowing better stability in poor bone-quality situations.

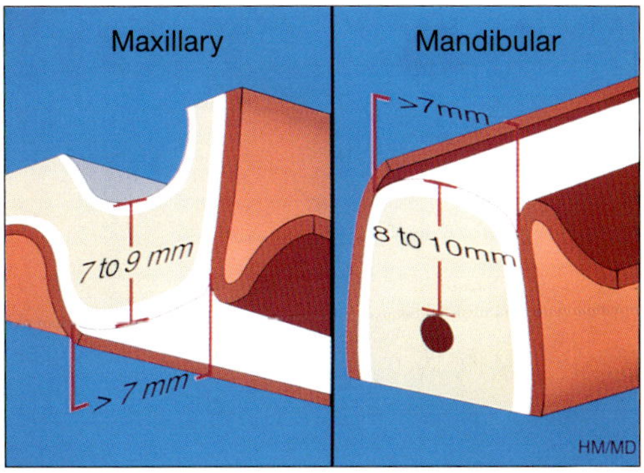

Fig 2-19 The large-diameter implant is indicated for insufficient ridge-height situations.

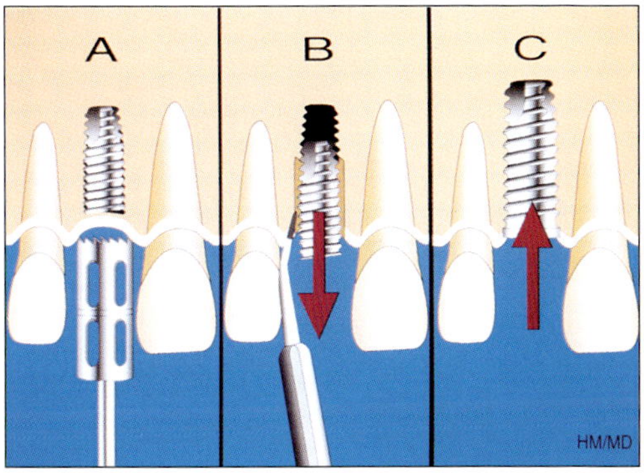

Fig 2-20 Removal of a fractured implant and immediate placement of a large-diameter implant.

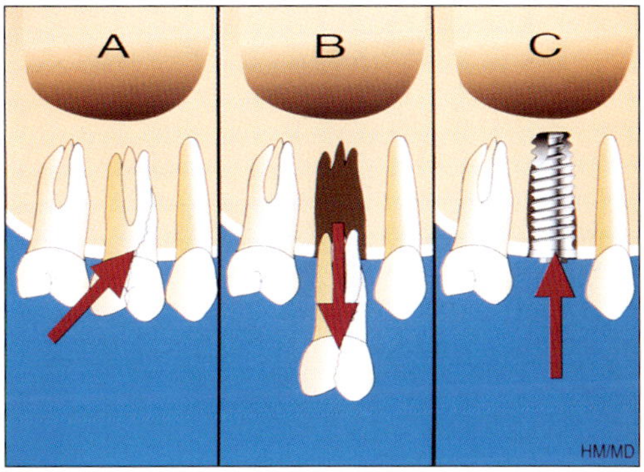

Fig 2-21 Tooth extraction and immediate placement of a large-diameter implant.

4. Implant fracture

Immediate replacement of a fractured standard implant by a large-diameter implant may be considered (Fig 2-20). Adapting intermediate abutments on a fractured implant is often delicate, and is associated with major risks of inflammation or chronic infection. An adapted trephine is used to remove the fractured implant. It is recommended not to drill down to the implant apex in order to preserve maximum available bone volume. A thin dissector completes the implant-bone separation. The fractured implant may then be easily removed. The implant site may be tapered, and a large-diameter implant placed.

5. Immediate implant placement after extraction

Immediate placement of a large-diameter implant (5 or 6 mm) after extraction was first suggested by Lazzara.[25] The socket is often larger than the standard implant and prevents primary stability. The alveolar space is filled owing to the implant diameter increase (Fig 2-21).

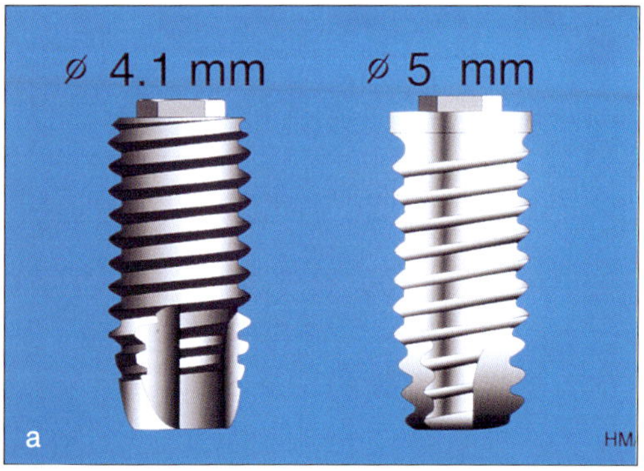

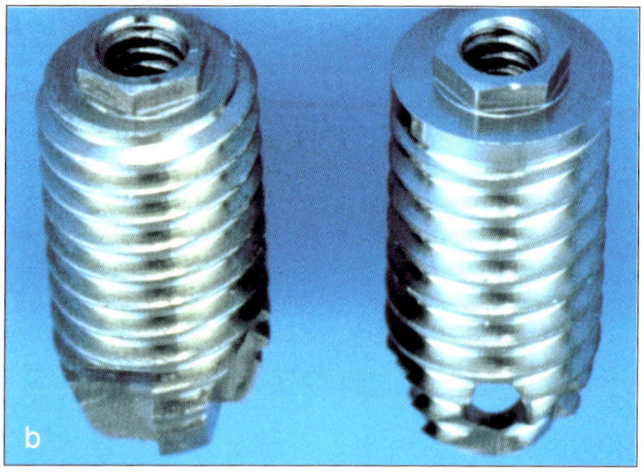

Figs 2-22a and 2-22b Left: diameter of a first-generation large-diameter Nobel Biocare implant (4.1 mm). Right: diameter of a 3i (5 mm) implant. Note the difference in the prosthetic base between the two implants.

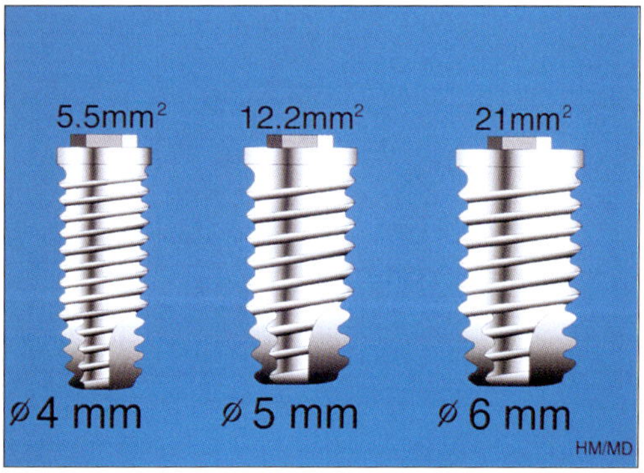

Fig 2-23 The prosthetic base surface area varies according to the diameter of the implant neck (3i implant).

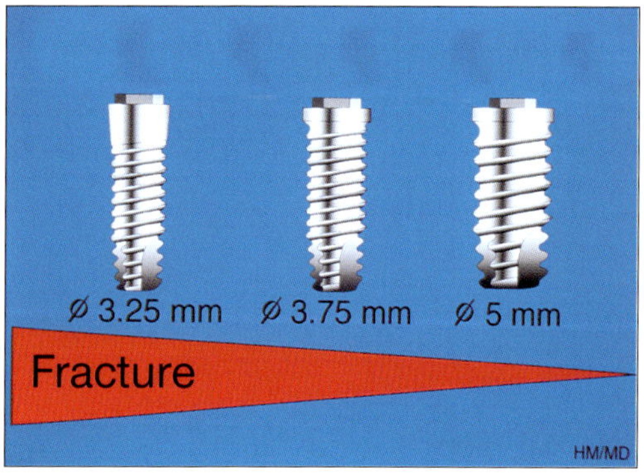

Fig 2-24 Resistance to fracture dramatically increases with the large-diameter 3i implants.

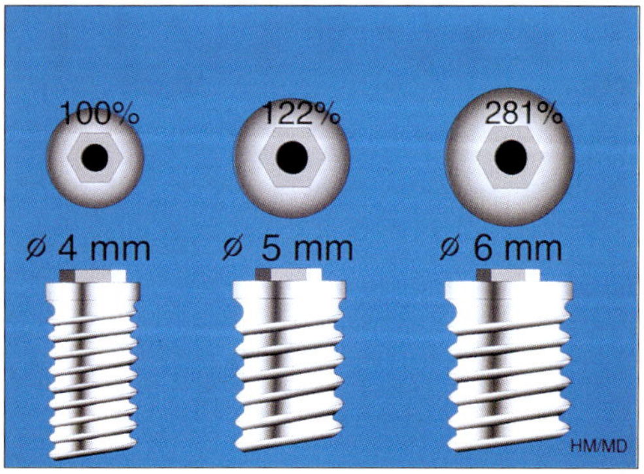

Fig 2-25 Percentage increase of the prosthetic base surface area of the large-diameter 3i implants compared to the standard implant.

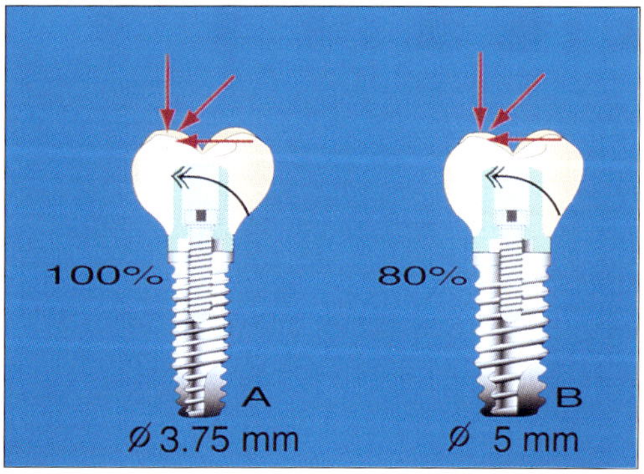

Fig 2-26 Increasing the prosthetic base surface area reduces the tensile forces on the abutment screw.

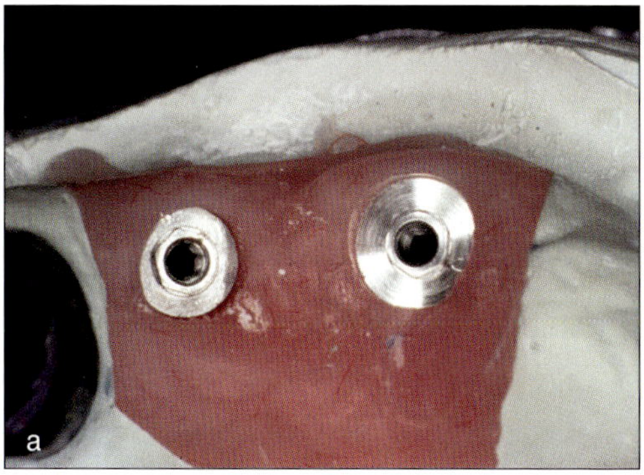

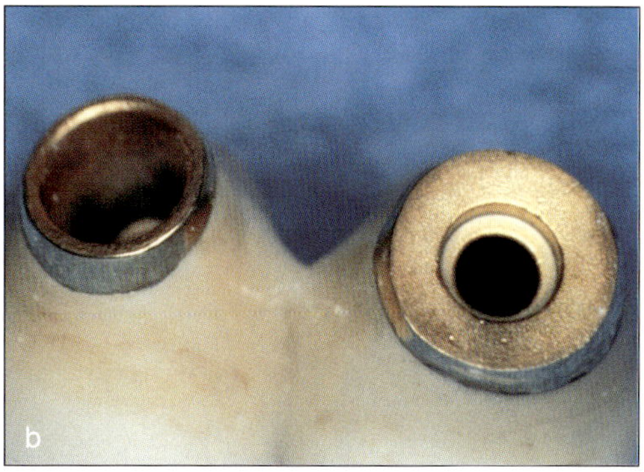

Figs 2-27a and 2-27b Study cast and prosthetic work demonstrating the difference in prosthetic base for a standard implant and a 6-mm-diameter 3i implant.

C. Concept development

The 5-mm (Nobel Biocare) implant developed by Langer et al[19] does not offer a smooth neck as does the standard implant (Fig 2-22). The threads of the implant body go down to the hexagonal base. This feature was intended to use as much of the residual bone volume as possible. The cortical anchorage of the implant at the alveolar ridge level is facilitated by the coronal threads. A greater marginal bone loss, compared to standard implants, was reported when using this implant. It has been recently replaced by a new large-diameter implant.

In the beginning of the 1990s, 3i developed large implants of 5- and 6-mm diameters. These implants have a neck diameter that is identical to that of the implant body. This leads to an increase in the prosthetic base because the hex dimension (2.7 mm) remains identical to that of the standard implant (Fig 2-23). This feature allows better stability of the prosthetic components and reduces forces applied to the abutment screws and/or prosthetic screws.

The 5- and 6-mm implants are, respectively, three and six times more resistant to fracture than standard implants (Fig 2-24). The neck-

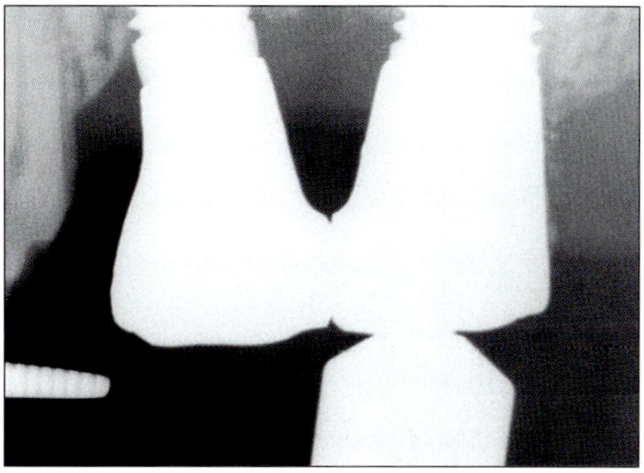

Fig 2-28 Radiographic control of prosthetic component adaptation.

supporting surface of the 5- and 6-mm implants is increased (122% and 281%, respectively) compared to a standard implant (Fig 2-25). This characteristic allows a better distribution of the occlusal loads.[20] According to Graves et al,[20] a force applied on the prosthetic screw undergoes a 20% decrease with a 5-mm-diameter implant and a 33% decrease with a 6-mm-diameter implant (Fig 2-26). These implants are indicated for single molar replacement. An emergence profile similar to that of a posterior tooth may be obtained

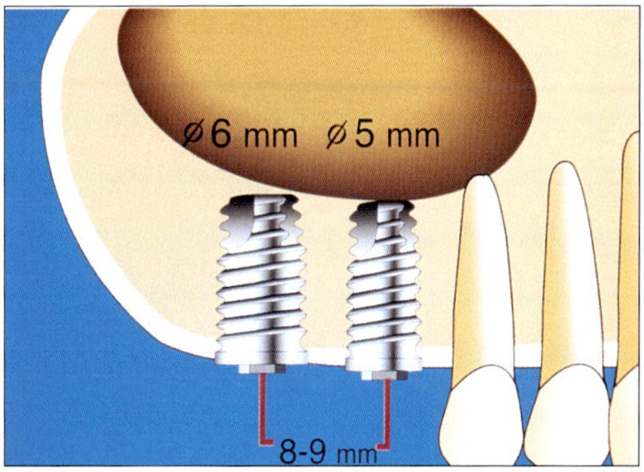

Fig 2-29 The distance between the center of two implants must be adapted to the implant diameter.

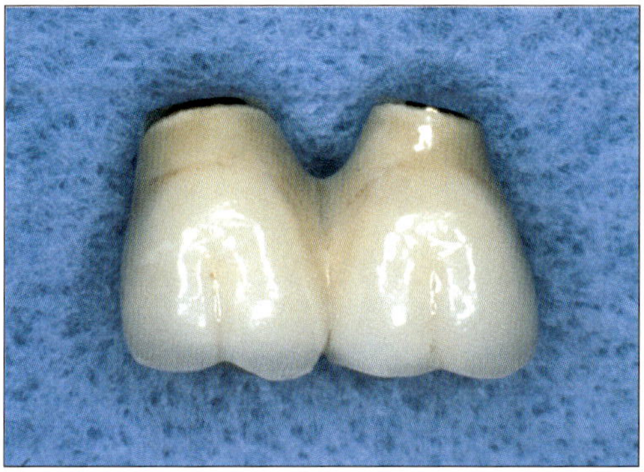

Fig 2-30 Respect of the distance between the center of two implants allows proper embrasures.

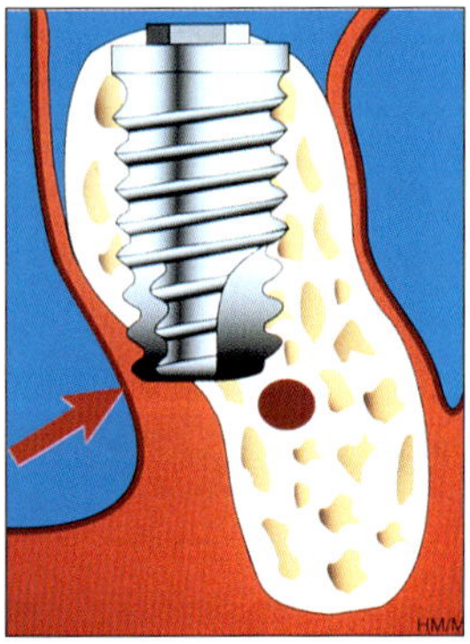

Fig 2-31 Perforation of the lingual cortical layer using a large-diameter implant.

because of the neck's width. The esthetic outcome is thus optimized. The similarity between the implant and the prosthetic perimeters allows achievement of a more natural crown anatomy (Figs 2-27 and 2-28).

In 1996, Nobel Biocare proposed a new large implant in two diameters: 5 and 5.5 mm (Wide Platform). Different from the first large-diameter Brånemark implant, this one presents a smooth neck of 5.1 mm and a larger hex (3.4-mm diameter, compared to 2.7 mm for the standard implant). Resistance to fracture of a 5-mm implant is three times greater than that of the 3.75-mm implant.

1. Specifications

The new large-diameter implants unquestionably allow better control of biomechanical risks in the posterior regions and in single missing molar treatment. Problems of screw loosening and fracture of prosthetic parts also are under better control. Positioning in the mesiodistal aspect is specific. A distance of at least 8 mm between the centers of the two large-diameter implants is essential (Figs 2-29 and 2-30). In the buccolingual aspect, the buccal bony defects, as well as the lingual concavities, must be anticipated. Fenestrations and dehiscences may occur using large-diameter implants (Fig 2-31).

2. Biomechanical advantages

The biomechanical advantages are:

- better distribution of occlusal forces
- better primary stability of the implant
- optimization of the prosthetic emergence profile
- better prosthetic stability

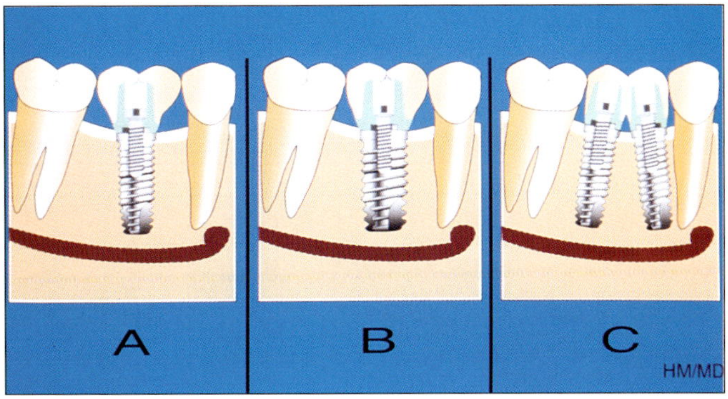

Fig 2-32 Implant options for a single missing molar: a = standard implant; b = large-diameter implant; c = two standard implants.

–reduced risk of screw loosening and abutment screw fracture
–reduced risk for implant fracture

D. Single molar tooth replacement: Which treatment choice?

The treatment choice for molar replacement is based on three criteria (Fig 2-32):

–anchoring surface
–mesiodistal space
–residual ridge width

The mesiodistal diameter of a molar is larger than that of a standard implant (Table 2-4). Moreover, intensity of the chewing forces in the posterior regions must be accurately assessed. For molar crowns fabricated on a standard implant, misfit and occlusal overload may lead to screw loosening, screw fracture, or even implant fracture.[23,26]

Two treatment options may be considered:

–placing two implants (if there is sufficient mesiodistal distance) (Figs 2-33 to 2-37)
–placing one large-diameter implant (Figs 2-38 to 2-41).

Balshi et al[27] report results over 3 years using one or two standard implants (Brånemark system) to treat single missing molar cases. Twenty-two sites were treated using one implant, and 25 sites were treated using two implants. The number of implants to be placed (one or two) was decided according to the available mesiodistal space. In order to treat a space greater than or equal to 12 mm, two implants were placed. Over 3 years, the cumulative success rate was 98.6%. Prosthetic complications were numerous for the crowns fabricated on single-unit implants (48%) compared to the group using two implants (8%).

Table 2-4 Mean measurements (mm) of the posterior teeth

Tooth	Cervical mesiodistal diameter	Cervical buccolingual diameter
Maxillary first premolar	5.0	8.0
Maxillary second premolar	5.0	8.0
Maxillary first molar	8.0	10.0
Maxillary second molar	8.0	9.0
Mandibular first premolar	5.0	7.0
Mandibular second premolar	5.0	8.0
Mandibular first molar	8.5	9.0
Mandibular second molar	8.0	9.0

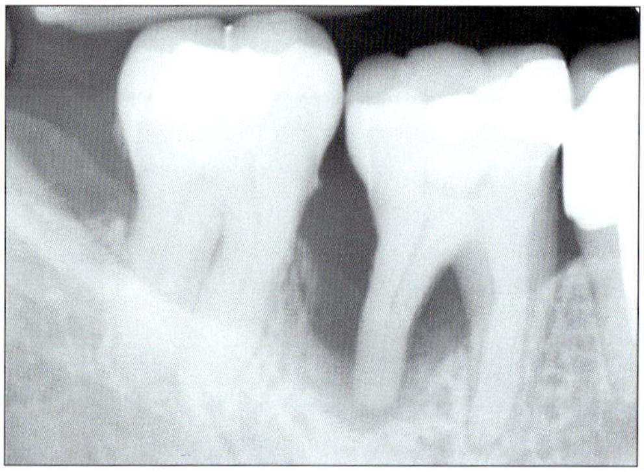

Fig 2-33 Periapical radiograph demonstrating a terminal periodontal defect on the mandibular right first molar.

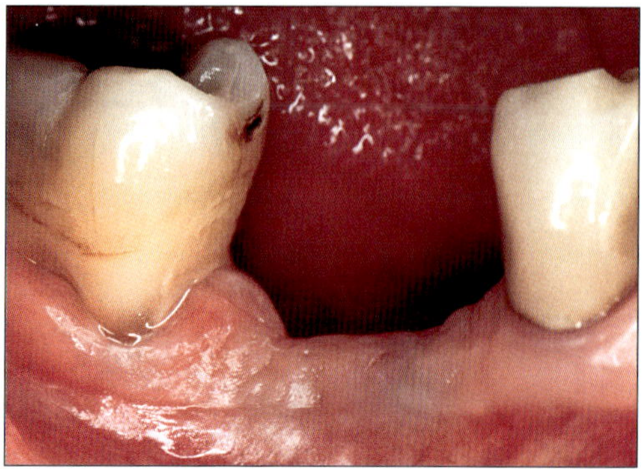

Fig 2-34 Clinical view following extraction of the first molar.

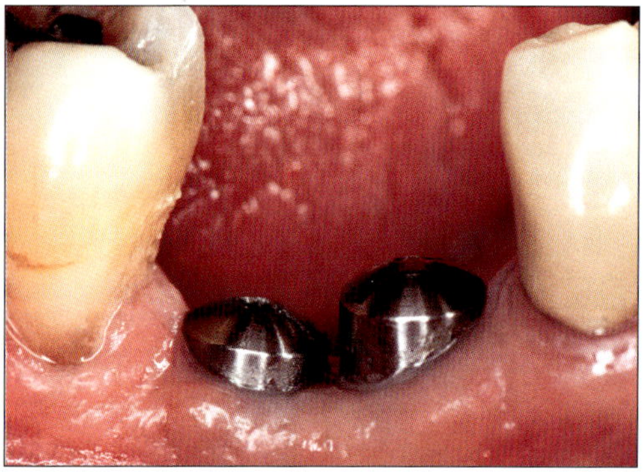

Fig 2-35 Soft tissue aspect following placement of the healing abutments.

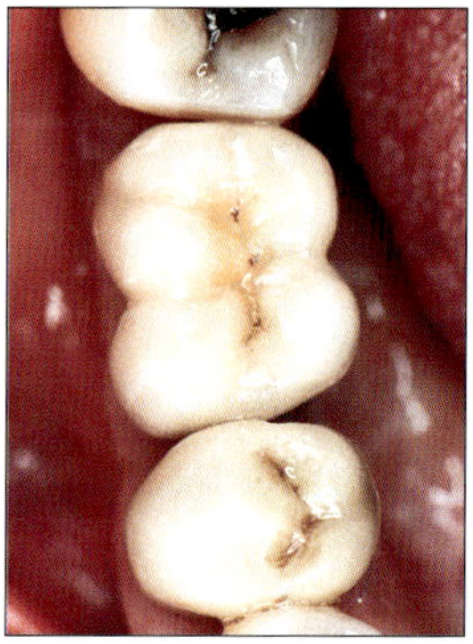

Fig 2-36a Occlusal view of the prosthesis.

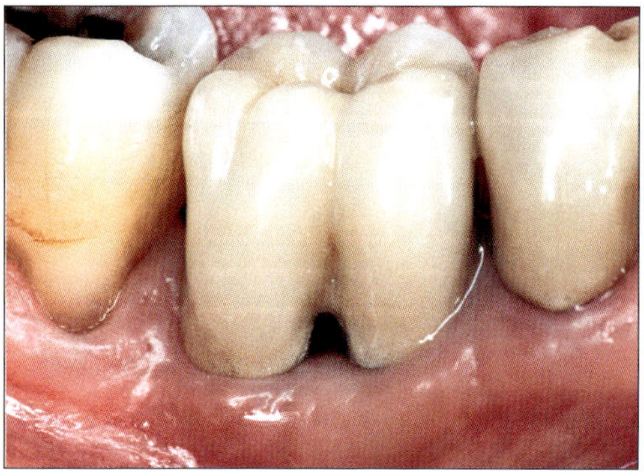

Fig 2-36b Final prosthetic work (Dr C. Raygot).

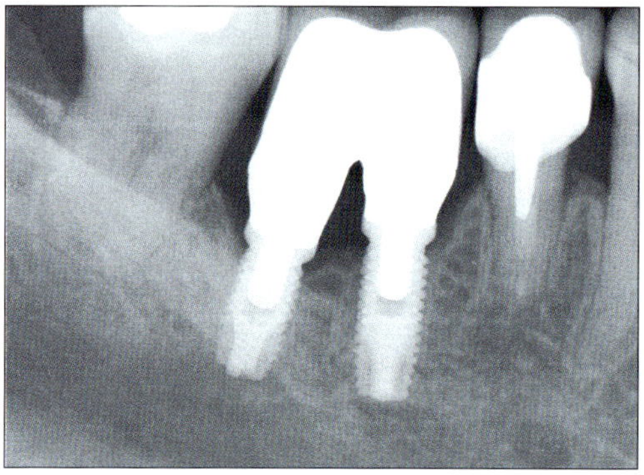

Fig 2-37 Periapical radiograph of the two 3i implants following 6 months of loading.

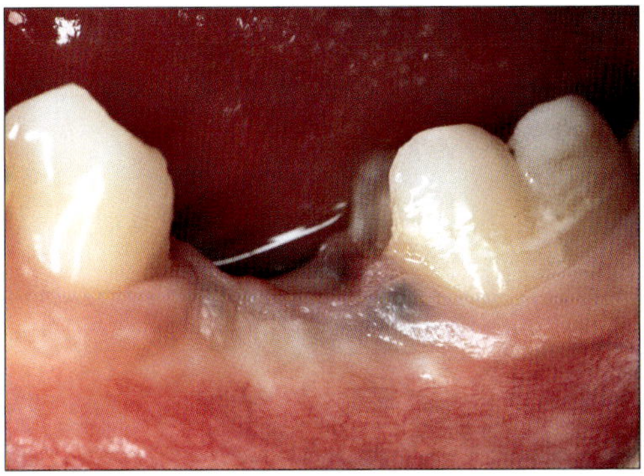

Fig 2-38 Single missing mandibular left first molar.

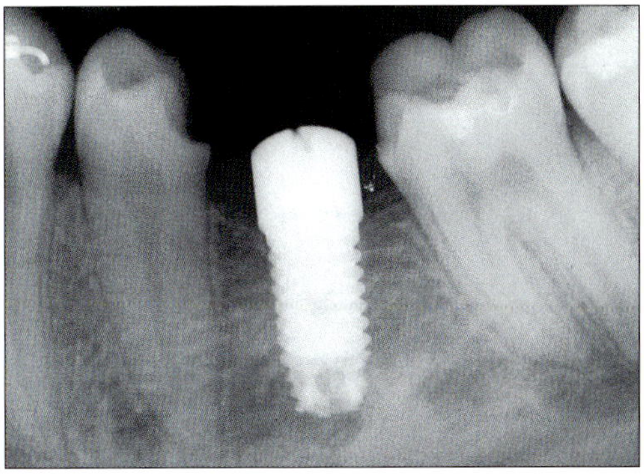

Fig 2-39 Stage-two radiograph of a 5-mm-diameter 3i implant following healing abutment placement.

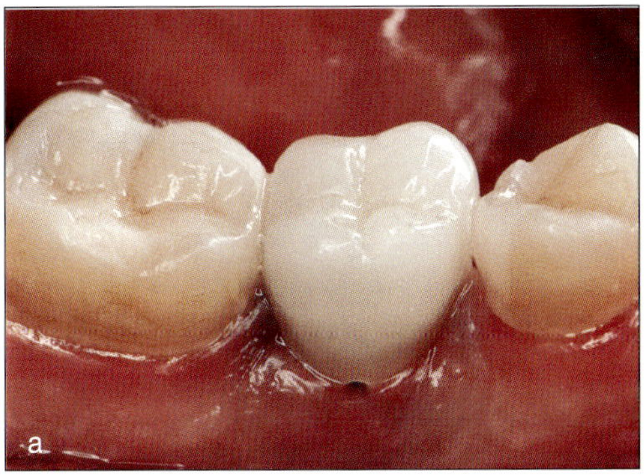

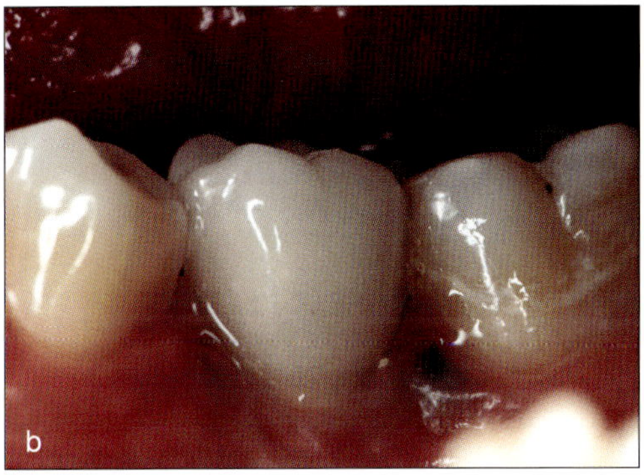

Figs 2-40a and 2-40b Final prosthetic work (Dr S. Neyret).

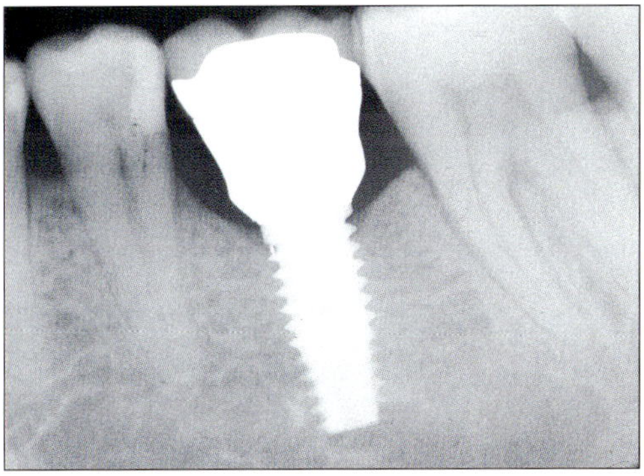

Fig 2-41 Radiograph following 2 years of loading.

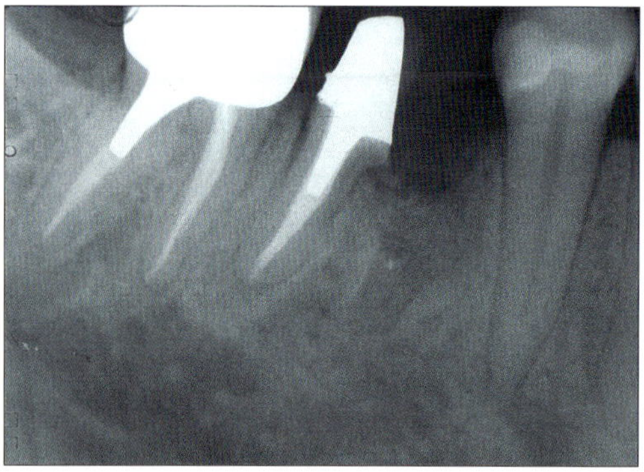

Fig 2-42 Radiograph prior to distal root extraction of mandibular right first molar.

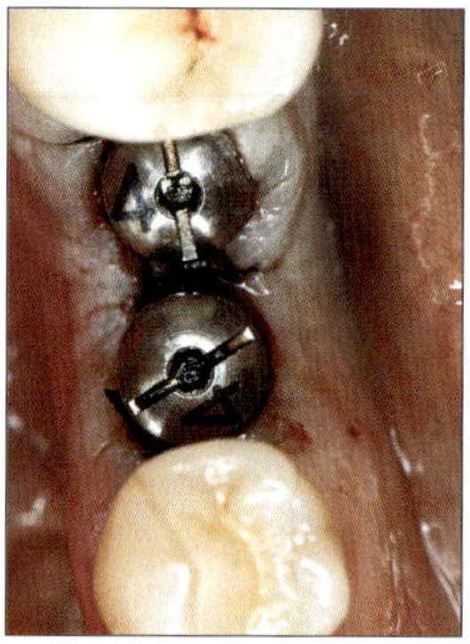

Fig 2-43 Stage-two clinical view following placement of two healing abutments.

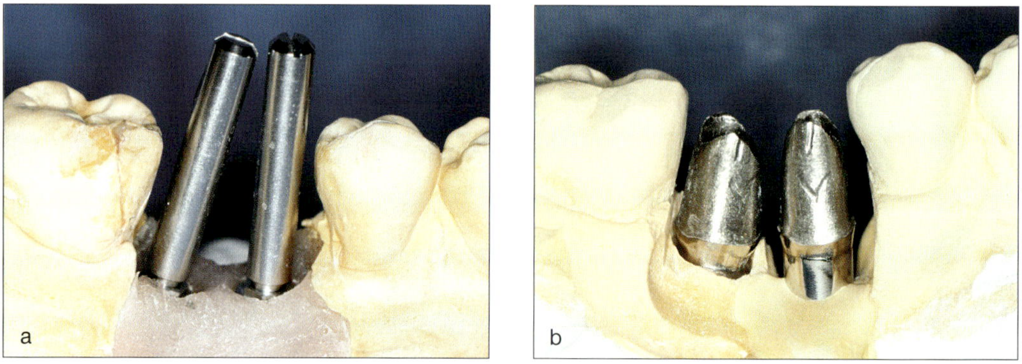

Figs 2-44a and 2-44b Working cast: a = note the convergence of the implant axes; b = placement of two perfectly adjusted UCLA gold abutments.

1. Biomechanical advantages

According to Balshi et al,[27] using two implants to replace a single missing molar reduces occlusal stresses and prosthetic complications. Indeed, implant anchorage is dramatically increased, and biomechanical forces are better distributed. However, greater bone loss is frequently observed between the two standard implants.

2. Disadvantages

Positioning the implants close to each other may compromise the prosthetic achievement and the peri-implant tissue longevity. According to Dawood,[28] the disadvantages of using two implants are an often-limited edentulous mesiodistal space and an unfavorable morphology and esthetic outcome for the final restoration (Figs 2-42 to 2-47).

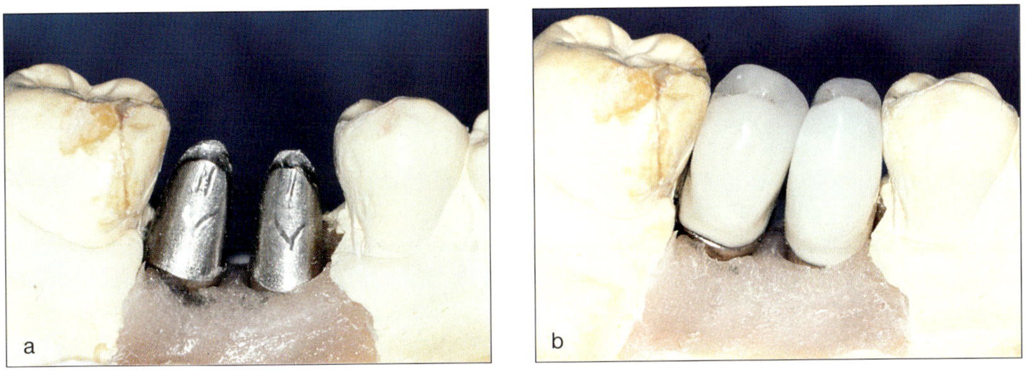

Figs 2-45a and 2-45b Working casts: a = view of the abutments with the soft tissue analogue; b = view of the final prosthetic work.

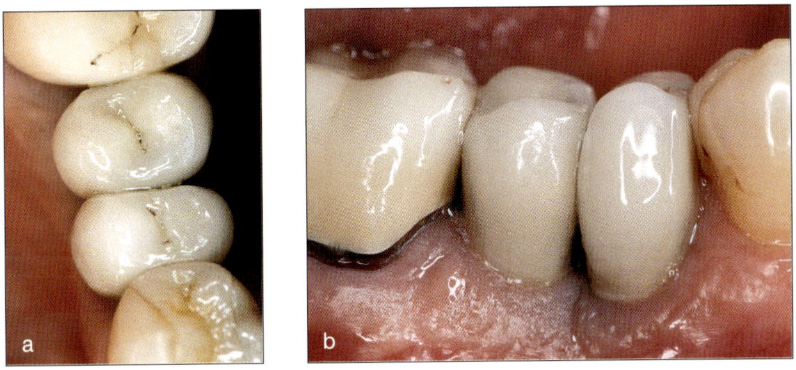

Figs 2-46a and 2-46b Prosthetic work: a = occlusal view; note the mesiodistal diameter. b = buccal view; note the insufficient embrasure (prosthetic work, Dr P. Raygot).

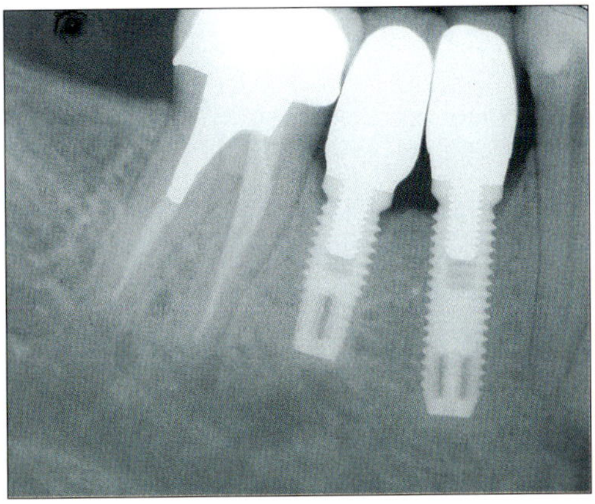

Fig 2-47 Radiograph of the two 3i implants following 1 year of loading. Note the proximity between the distal implant and the mandibular right second molar.

III. Implant diameter selection

Implant diameter selection depends on the type of edentulism, residual bone volume, available prosthetic space, emergence profile, and occlusal pattern. During the past 10 years, the development of new surgical and prosthodontic components has allowed optimization of the functional and esthetic results. Different implant diameters have been proposed since the end of the 1980s. To date, few studies have been published concerning such use of different implant diameters. However, satisfactory results have been reported in the short and mid term. The various parameters guiding implant diameter selection will be presented.

A. Indications for different implant diameters

Today, most implant systems market different types of implant diameters. They can be grouped as small-diameter implants (less than or equal to 3.4 mm), standard implants (3.75 to 4 mm), and large-diameter implants (greater than or equal to 4.5 mm) (Table 2-5).

The idea behind different implant diameters is to adapt the implant to the available bone volume. However, all the clinical parameters must be assessed for proper selection: bone quality and quantity, edentulous site, available prosthetic space, and occlusal pattern. Selecting a diameter for the implant body and neck depends on the surgical and prosthetic imperatives. From a surgical point of view, optimal use of the available bone volume and primary stabilization of the implant must be achieved. From a prosthetic point of view, an emergence profile adapted to the future prosthetic tooth and adequate force distribution are sought.

The standard implant, developed in the 1960s and marketed in the early 1980s, is the reference implant; its long-term reliability has been largely demonstrated. This implant may be used in most situations for which implant treatment is indicated.

The small-diameter implant is indicated in specific clinical situations:

Table 2-5 Implant diameters (mm) of different systems

	Standard implant		Small-diameter implant		Large-diameter implant	
System	**Body**	**Collar**	**Body**	**Collar**	**Body**	**Collar**
Frialit-2	3.8	3.8			4.5 5.5 6.5	4.5 4.5 6.5
ITI	3.5 4.1 4.1	4.8 4.8 4.1	3.3 3.3	4.8 3.5	4.8 5.5 6.5	4.8 4.5 6.5
Nobel Biocare	3.75 4.0	4.1 4.1	3.3	3.5	5.0 5.5	5.1 5.1
Screw-Vent	3.8	3.5	3.3	3.5	4.7	4.5
Steri-Oss	3.8 3.8	3.8 4.1	3.25	3.25	4.5 4.5 6.0	4.1 5.0 6.0
3i	3.75 4.0	4.1 4.1	3.25 3.25	3.4 4.1	5.0 6.0	5.0 6.0

Fig 2-48 Oblique CT scan showing sufficient bone volume for placing a standard implant.

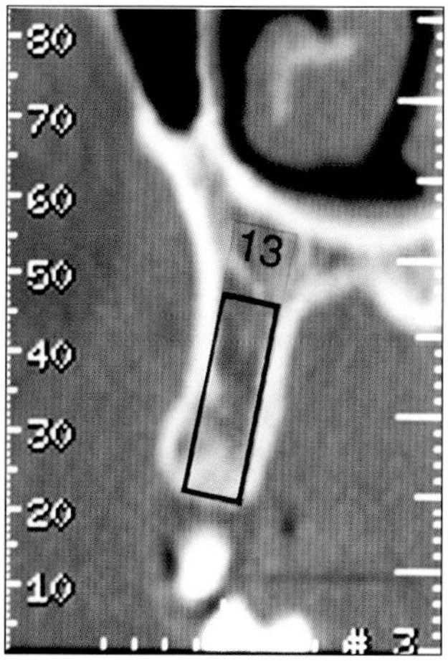

Fig 2-49 Oblique CT scan showing a thin alveolar ridge. A small-diameter implant is indicated.

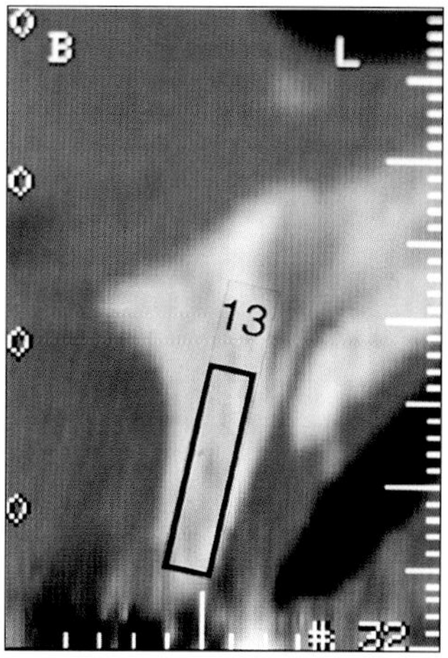

—reduced inter-root space
—thin alveolar ridge
—limited cervical prosthetic diameter

The large-diameter implant was developed for specific bone and prosthetic situations:

—poor bone quality
—insufficient ridge height
—immediate replacement of a nonosseointegrated implant
—immediate replacement of a fractured implant
—immediate implant placement following tooth extraction
—single missing molar

B. Implant diameter selection

Implant diameter selection depends on the following parameters: residual bone volume, bone quality, anchoring surface, anatomy of the replaced tooth, available mesiodistal space, prosthetic emergence profile, and biomechanical factors.

1. Residual bone volume

Placement of a standard implant requires a minimum bone volume in the three dimensions of space. Ideally, the whole implant surface should be surrounded by at least 1 mm of bone. In the mesiodistal and buccolingual aspects, the distance must be greater than or equal to 7 mm (Fig 2-48). Placing a standard implant in borderline anatomic and/or biomechanical conditions increases the risk for complications and implant failures.

A small-diameter implant may be selected for a thin alveolar ridge (Fig 2-49). In some cases, the use of bone reconstruction techniques (grafting, GBR) or widening of the prosthetic mesiodistal and/or bone space (orthodontics) may be considered. However, the occlusal pattern and biomechanical stresses must be assessed. In this case, the risk for implant fracture is increased.

Concerning the posterior regions, bone height is frequently insufficient and combined with a ridge width greater than or equal to 8 mm. Anatomic structures (sinus and inferior dental nerve) often limit the indications for short implants. Several studies have shown a

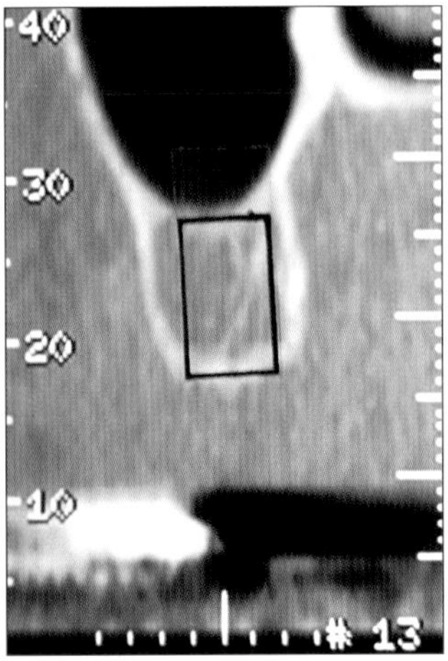

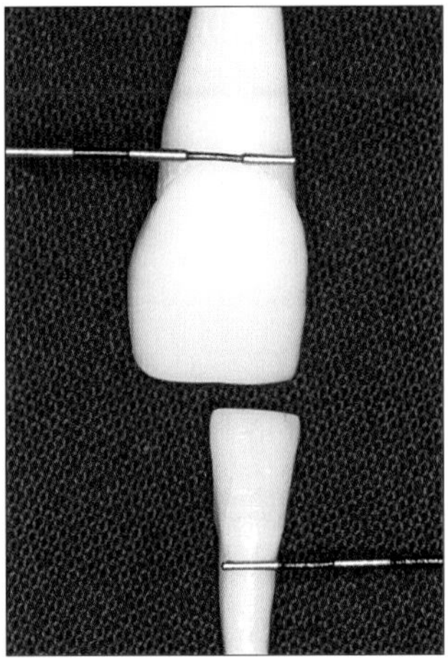

Fig 2-50 Oblique CT scan showing sufficient bone volume for placing a large-diameter implant.

Fig 2-51 The mesiodistal diameter of the replaced tooth is a determining factor in selecting implant diameter.

higher failure rate with standard-diameter implants shorter than 10 mm. Wide implants offer an anchoring surface larger than that of standard implants. The length decrease is compensated for by the increase of the implant diameter. In some cases, the use of wide implants may avoid the need for invasive surgical techniques such as bone grafting, sinus lift and grafting procedures, and mandibular nerve repositioning.

2. *Bone quality*

During stage-one surgery, primary stability of the implant is essential. Implants of 3.75- or 4.0-mm diameter do not offer a good primary stability in low-density bone. Several papers in the literature report high failure rates using standard implants in poor-quality bone. In 1991, Jaffin and Berman[29] reported a 35% failure rate at 5 years postsurgery for 102 standard implants placed in type IV bone. Johns et al[30] also observed a 28% failure rate at 5 years for 57 standard implants placed in poor-quality bone. The use of a large implant body and neck allows better bicortical stabilization (Fig 2-50).

The use of small-diameter implants is not recommended in the presence of poor-density bone. If clinical imperatives (bone or prosthetics) indicate the use of a small-diameter implant, the diameter decrease must be compensated for by an increase of implant length and by different surface properties.

3. *Anchoring surface and tooth anatomy*

When selecting implant diameter, the reference anchoring surface is the root surface of the replaced tooth (Fig 2-51). However, this varies according to the patient. Several authors have assessed this anchoring surface (Table 2-6). Le Gall and Saadoun[31] suggest a mean root surface size based upon the studies carried out by Marseiller[32] and Jepsen.[33] Manufacturers offer different implant diameters to anticipate the future prosthetic crown (Figs 2-52 and 2-53). The anchoring surface will depend on implant form, threading anatomy, and implant surface properties. Most systems advocate the following indications: standard implants to replace maxillary incisors, canines, and premolars; small-diameter im-

Table 2-6 Mean anchoring root surface (root length × mesiodistal cervical diameter; in mm^2)

Tooth	Mean anchoring surface for maxillary teeth	Mean anchoring surface for mandibular teeth
Central incisor	237	132
Lateral incisor	180	152
Canine	283	250
First premolar	191	207
Second premolar	233	217
First molar	311	352
Second molar	274	328

Table 2-7 Mean implant surface anchorage (length × implant diameter)

Implant diameter (mm)	Implant length (mm)	Implant anchorage surface (mm^2)
3.75	10	157
3.75	13	210
5.0	10	194
5.0	13	257
6.0	10	243
6.0	13	323

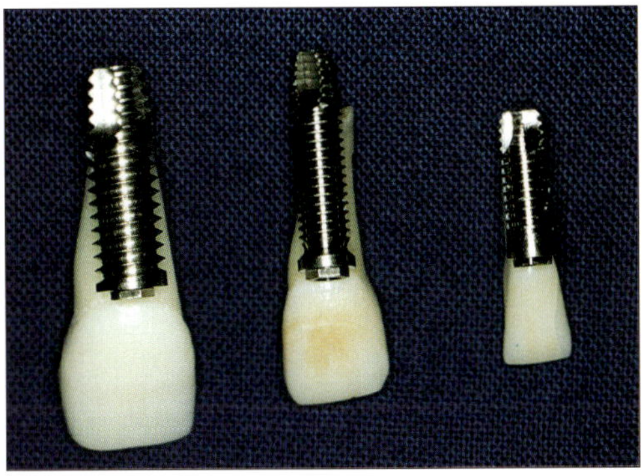

Fig 2-52 Tooth morphology and implant diameter selection. Left: 3i large-diameter implant for a maxillary central incisor. Center: 3i standard implant for a maxillary lateral incisor. Right: small-diameter 3i implant (3.4-mm collar) for a mandibular lateral incisor.

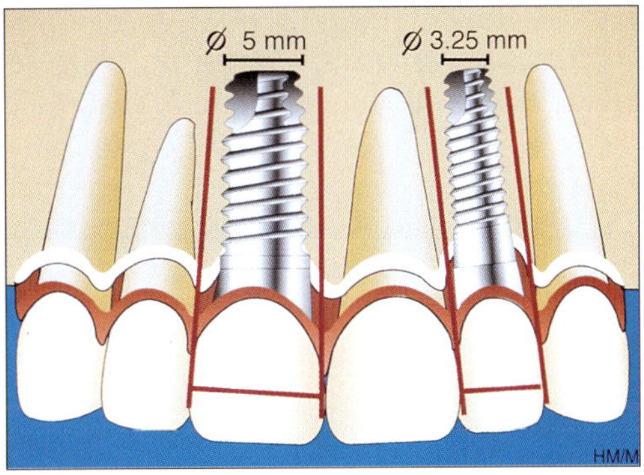

Fig 2-53 Implant diameter selection in relation to the future prosthetic tooth.

plants to replace some maxillary lateral incisors; and large-diameter implants to replace molars.

The treatment option for molar replacement is based on three criteria:

—anchoring surface
—mesiodistal space
—residual alveolar ridge

The mesiodistal diameter and the perimeter of a molar are largely oversized compared to those of a standard implant. Moreover, the impact of chewing forces on the posterior region must be taken into account. For molar crowns fabricated on a standard implant, inaccuracy and occlusal overload may generate screw loosening, prosthetic screw fractures, or even implant fractures. Two treatment options are recommended: either the use of two implants when enough mesiodistal space is available, or the placement of a large-diameter implant. Large-diameter implants provide an anchoring surface similar to that of a molar (Table 2-7). Bahat and Handelsman[23] published the clinical results of different implant treatment choices for posterior edentulous cases. The four treatment options assessed (ie, one large-diameter implant, two large-diameter implants, one large-diameter implant combined with a standard implant, or two standard implants) produced short-term success rates of more than 96%. The authors, however, give no information concerning the prosthetic follow-up.

4. Available mesiodistal space

Ideally, the number of standard implants recommended for treating an edentulous case must be similar to the number of lost roots. However, the available mesiodistal space and the proximity of anatomic structures often limit this number. For completely edentulous cases, the residual bone volume and the prosthetic design determine the number and type of implants. In the partially edentulous patient, the number of standard implants is traditionally selected according to the available mesiodistal space. The formula (X – 1 mm/7) allows establishment of the number of implants to be placed, X being the ideal distance between the centers of two standard implants. However, in this formula, two factors are not taken into consideration: emergence profile and tooth morphology.

In the presence of a large ridge in the partially edentulous patient, implant number and diameter should be determined according to the number and type of teeth to be replaced and the available mesiodistal space. In the posterior regions, the replacement of premolars using standard implants and molars using large-diameter implants allows better management of problems related to emergence profile, prosthetic morphology, and occlusion.

In the mandibular region (four incisors), the use of standard implants leads to an emergence profile discrepancy. The available mesiodistal space limits the placement of standard implants. It is impossible to place one implant per tooth, because the implant neck diameter (4.1 mm) is frequently greater than the cervical tooth diameter. Two treatment options may then be considered: either two standard implants are placed near the canines, or three to four small-diameter implants are used (Figs 2-54 and 2-55).

5. Emergence profile

The use of an implant diameter adapted to the cervical diameter of the replaced tooth allows an acceptable esthetic result and an appropriate emergence profile (Fig 2-56). In the cervical aspect, the mesiodistal diameter of the implant must be slightly less than that of the future prosthetic tooth in the apicocoronal direction with no adjacent teeth. At that level, the root diameter is inevitably less than that at the cementoenamel junction (Fig 2-57). In the anterior regions, the anatomy of the contralateral tooth must be precisely assessed in order to obtain a more natural emergence profile.

The mesiodistal prosthetic space available for the mandibular incisors, and sometimes for the maxillary lateral incisors, is less than 4.5 mm. With a standard implant neck diameter (4.1 mm), it is often impossible to achieve an acceptable esthetic result (Figs 2-58 and 2-59).

For the posterior teeth or the maxillary central incisors, a more adapted emergence profile may be obtained using wide-neck implants. The parallel between implant and prosthetic parameters allows a more natural crown anatomy. The esthetic result of large crowns is optimized with a widened implant neck (Figs 2-60 to 2-62). According to the mean values of cervical diameters assessed by Wheeler,[10] the following use may be advised: small-diameter implants for mandibu-

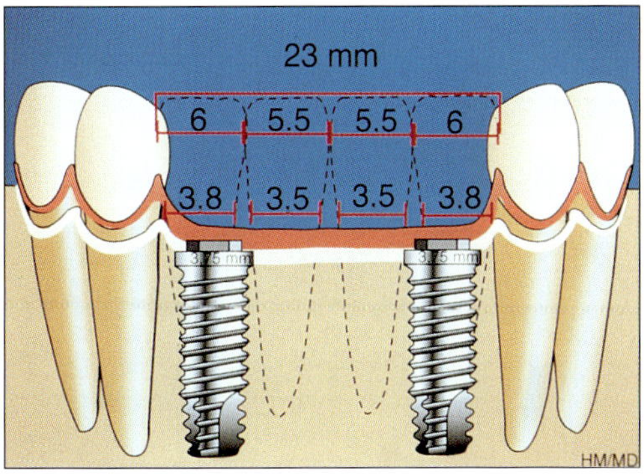

Fig 2-54 Selecting two standard implants to replace four mandibular incisors leads to an inadequate emergence profile.

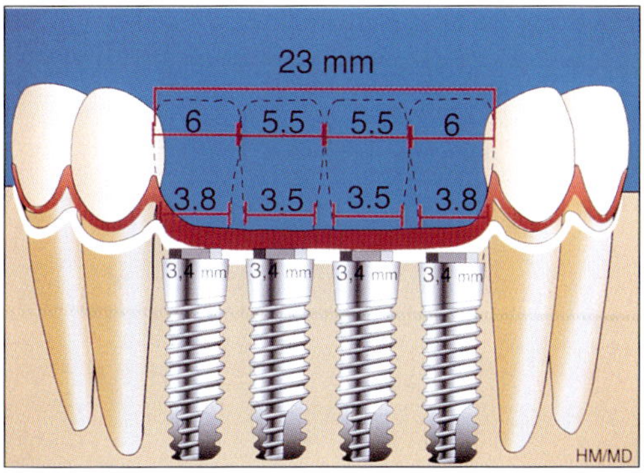

Fig 2-55 Selecting small-diameter implants (reduced neck) to replace four mandibular incisors allows a good esthetic result.

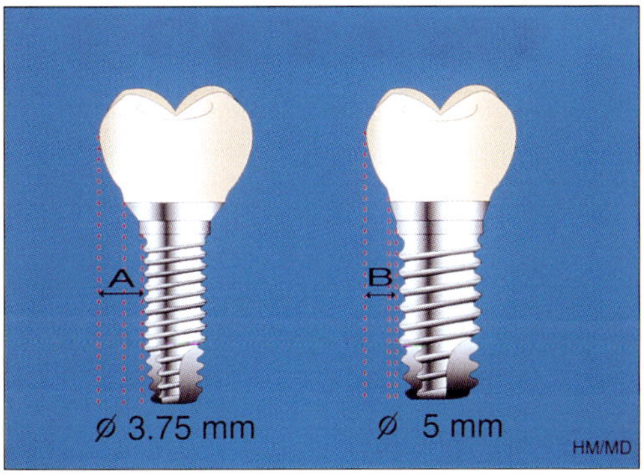

Fig 2-56 The large-diameter implant offers a more appropriate emergence profile for posterior teeth.

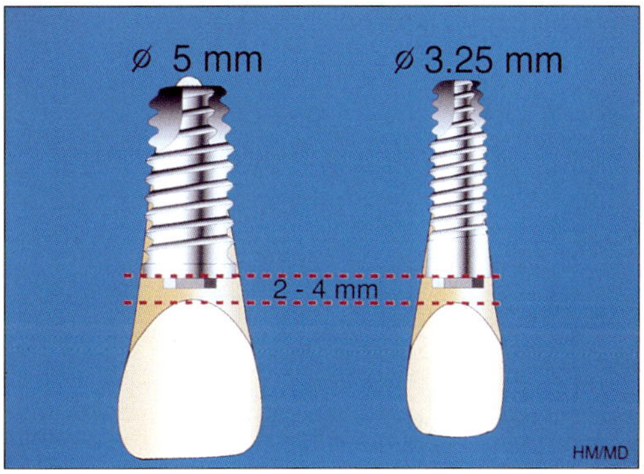

Fig 2-57 The new implant diameters allow a more adapted implant selection.

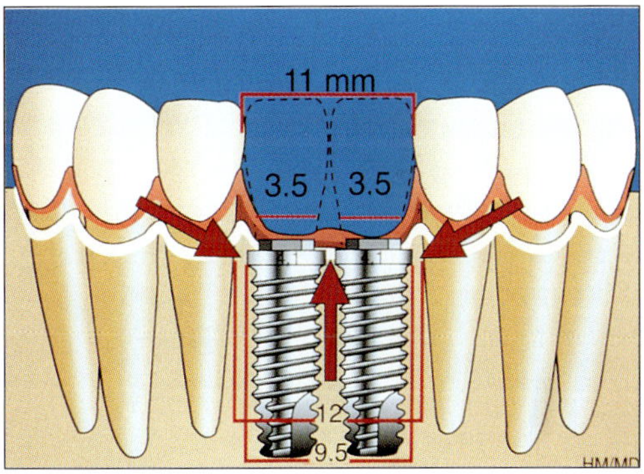

Fig 2-58 Placing two standard implants to replace two mandibular central incisors is incompatible with a good esthetic result.

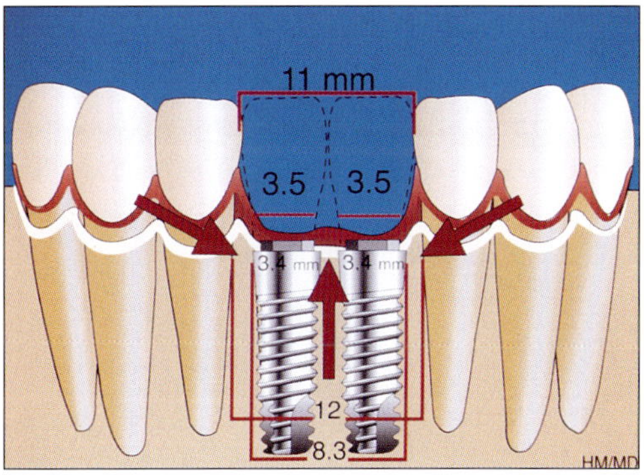

Fig 2-59 Placing two small-diameter implants to replace two mandibular central incisors allows a good esthetic result.

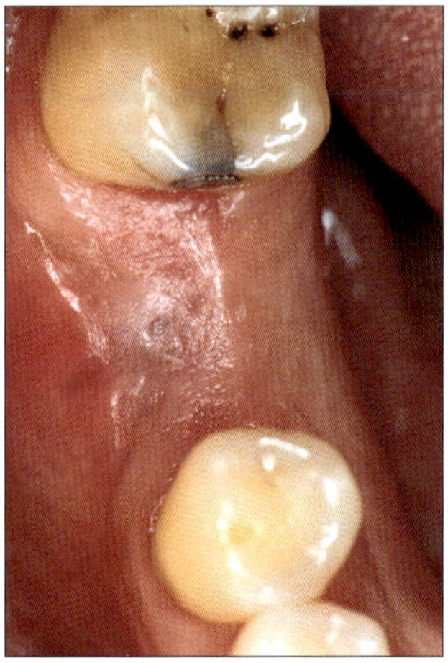

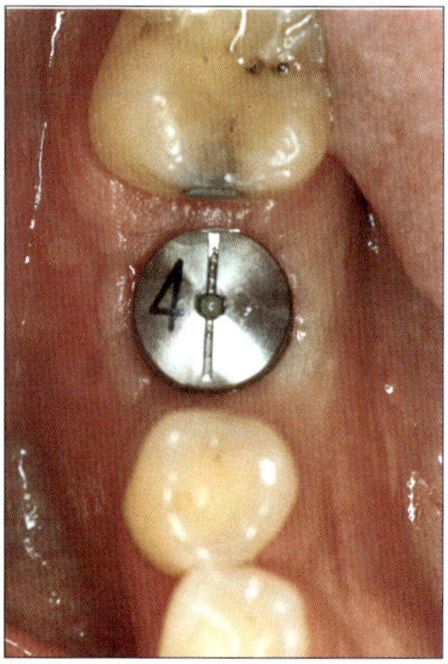

Fig 2-60 Clinical view of a single missing mandibular right first molar prior to stage-two surgery.

Fig 2-61 Placing a 3i large-diameter healing abutment.

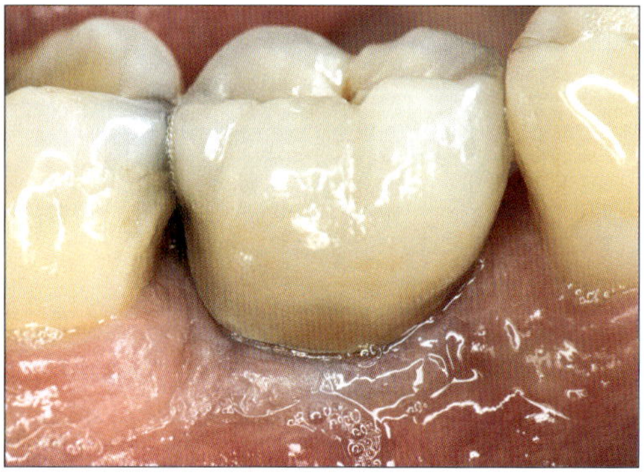

Fig 2-62 Final prosthetic result. Note the good emergence profile.

lar incisors and premolars, standard implants for maxillary incisors and premolars, and large-diameter implants to replace molars (Tables 2-8 and 2-9). However, other factors must be considered (anatomic structures, residual bone quality and type, available prosthetic space) in order to select the appropriate implant diameter.

6. *Biomechanical behavior*

Tooth position on the arch, occlusal pattern, and parafunction are the main biomechanical factors to be assessed in order to select implant diameter (Figs 2-63 and 2-64). Before considering the use of this type of implant, occlusal forces must be adequately assessed. This implant is contraindicated for canine and molar replacement. The 20% decrease of the implant diameter (from 3.75 to 3 mm) leads to a reduced resistance to fracture of about 50%. For Forsmalm,[11] resistance to fracture using 3.3-mm implants is 25% less than with a standard implant. Some systems offer small-diameter implants machined in different types of alloys in order to increase resistance to fracture.

Problems related to screw loosening and fracture of prosthetic parts using the standard implant have been reported in the litera-

Table 2-8 Mean measurements for maxillary teeth and recommended implant diameter

Maxillary tooth	Mesiodistal cervical diameter (mm)	Buccolingual cervical diameter (mm)	Recommended implant diameter
Central incisor	7.0	6.0	Standard or large
Lateral incisor	5.0	5.0	Standard or small
Canine	5.5	7.0	Standard or large
First premolar	5.0	8.0	Standard
Second premolar	5.0	8.0	Standard
First molar	8.0	10.0	Large
Second molar	8.0	9.0	Large

Table 2-9 Mean measurements for mandibular teeth and recommended implant diameter

Maxillary tooth	Mesiodistal cervical diameter (mm)	Buccolingual cervical diameter (mm)	Recommended implant diameter
Central incisor	3.5	5.5	Small
Lateral incisor	4.0	5.5	Small
Canine	5.0	6.5	Standard
First premolar	5.0	7.0	Standard
Second premolar	5.0	8.0	Standard
First molar	8.5	9.0	Large
Second molar	8.0	9.0	Large

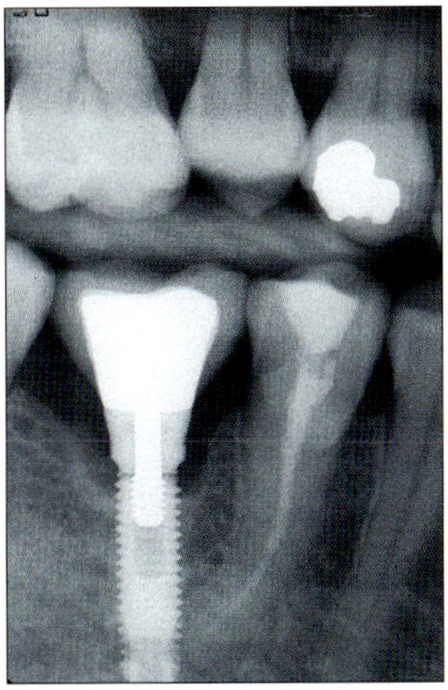

Fig 2-63 Radiograph showing the fracture of a standard implant located at the mandibular right first molar.

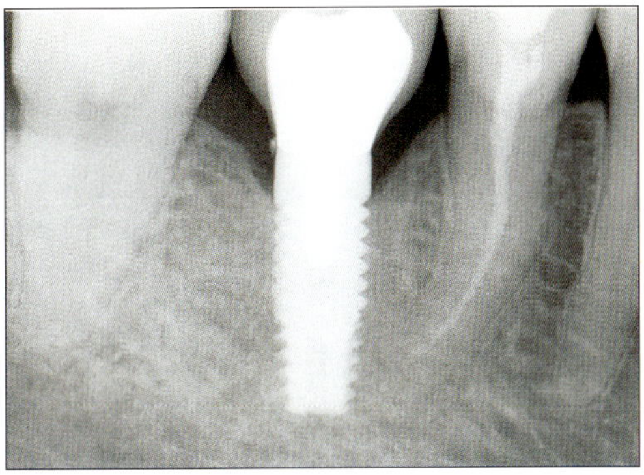

Fig 2-64 The fractured implant was removed and immediately replaced by a large-diameter 3i implant.

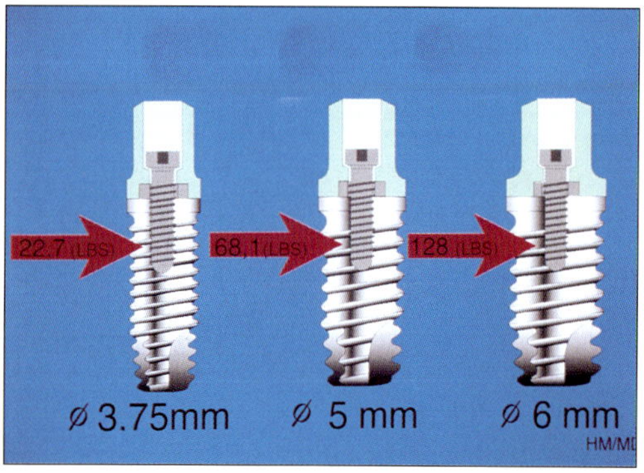

Fig 2-65 The fracture threshold is considerably increased with large-diameter implants.

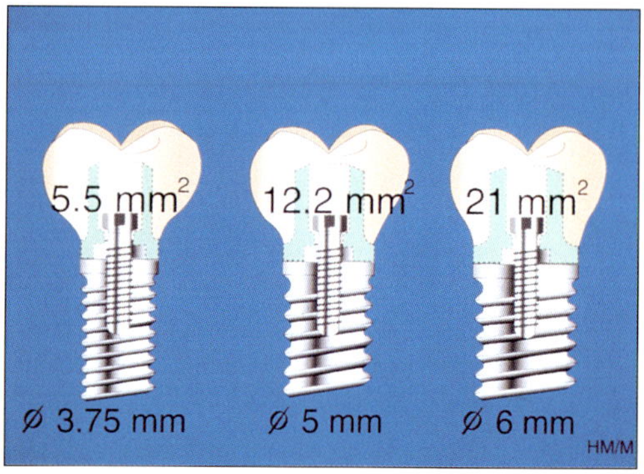

Fig 2-66 Increase of the prosthetic base surface area allows a better distribution of the occlusal forces.

ture.[26,34,35] Large-diameter implants unquestionably limit biomechanical complications when treating posterior regions and single missing molar situations (Fig 2-65). Balshi et al[27] reported similar implant results over 3 years using one or two standard implants (Brånemark system) when treating single missing molar cases. However, numerous prosthetic complications were observed for crowns placed on standard implants (48%) compared to the group using two implants (8%). According to these authors, occlusal stresses and prosthetic complications are limited when placing two implants.

A wide-diameter implant must have a large neck. This increase of the prosthetic base allows a better stability for the prosthetic components and reduces forces applied on the prosthetic screws (Fig 2-66).[36] Five- and 6-mm-diameter implants (3i) are, respectively, three and six times more resistant to fracture than standard implants. The prosthetic base surface area for 5- and 6-mm implants is increased by 122% and 281%, respectively, compared to standard implants. This characteristic allows a better distribution of the occlusal stresses.[20] The force applied on the prosthetic screw decreases by 20% using a 5-mm-diameter implant and by 33% using a 6-mm-diameter implant.[20]

The standard-diameter implant remains the reference. Small- and large-diameter implants extend the implant treatment options, thus optimizing the final outcome for specific clinical situations. The short-term clinical follow-up using the new implant diameters is very satisfactory.

Different issues still need to be clarified:

- mean or long-term fracture risk for small-diameter implants
- tissue behavior around small- and large-diameter implants
- bone longevity around large-diameter implants
- the best choice to support occlusal loads in the posterior regions
- the proper implant diameter to use in types I and IV bone

References

1. Davarpanah M, Martínez H. L'implant de petit diamètre. Inf Dent 1998;41:3333–3337.
2. Dexter Barber H, Seckinger R. The role of the small-diameter dental implant: A preliminary report on the Miniplant System. Compendium 1994;15:390–392.
3. Jornéus P. Developing the narrow platform. Nobel Biocare Global Forum 1996;10:3.
4. Block MS, Kent JN. Cylindrical HA-coated implants–8-year observations. Compend Contin Educ Dent 1993;14(suppl):5526–5532.
5. Spiekermann H, Jansen VK, Ritcher EJ. A 10-year follow-up study of IMZ and TPS implants in the edentulous mandible using bar-retained overdentures. Int J Oral Maxillofac Implants 1995;10:231–243.
6. Saadoun A, Le Gall MG. An 8-year compilation of clinical results obtained with Steri-Oss endosseous implants. Compendium 1996;17:669–688.
7. Sethi A, Harding S, Sochor P. Initial results of the Osteo Ti implant system in general dental practice. Eur J Prosthodont Restorative Dent 1996;4:21–28.
8. Lazzara RJ, Siddiqui AA, Binon P, et al. Retrospective multicenter analysis of 3i endosseous dental implants placed over a five-year period. Clin Oral Implants Res 1996;7:73–83.
9. Buser D, Mericske-Stern R, Bernard JP, et al. Long-term evaluation of non-submerged ITI implants. Clin Oral Implants Res 1997;8:161–172.
10. Wheeler R. Dental Anatomy, Physiology and Occlusion. Philadelphia: WB Saunders, 1974:520.
11. Forsmalm G. Evaluating implant post strength. Nobel Biocare Global Forum 1996;10:5.
12. Matsushita Y, Kitoh M, Mizuta K, Ikeda H, Suetsugu T. Two-dimensional analysis of hydroxyapatite implants: Diameter effects on stress distribution. J Oral Implantol 1990;16:6–11.
13. Rieger MR, Adams WK, Kinzel GL. A finite element survey of eleven endosseous implants. J Prosthet Dent 1990;63:457–465.
14. Block MS, Delgado A, Fontenot MG. The effect of diameter and length of hydroxylapatite-coated dental implants on ultimate pullout force in dog alveolar bone. J Oral Maxillofac Surg 1990;48:174–178.
15. Sendax VI. Réponse tissulaire de la crête osseuse aux implants de 4 mm revêtus d'HA comparés à ceux de 3.25 mm de diamètre. Personal communication, 1992.
16. Davarpanah M, Martínez H, Tecucianu JF, Etienne D, Askari N, Kebir M. Les implants de large diamètre. Implant 1995;1:289–299.
17. Davarpanah M, Martínez H, Kebir M, Tecucianu JF. Les implants de gros diamètre: Évolution des concepts. Implant 1998;4:249–258.
18. Jornéus L. Developing the wide platform. Nobel Biocare Global Forum 1996;10:4.
19. Langer B, Langer L, Herrmann I, Erug M. The wide fixture: A solution for special bone situations and rescue for the compromised implant. Part 1. Int J Oral Maxillofac Implants 1993;8:400–408.
20. Graves SL, Jansen CE, Siddiqui AA, Beaty KD. Wide diameter implants: Indications, considerations and preliminary results over a two-year period. Aust Prosthodont J 1994;8:31–37.
21. Barrachina M, Calvo AJA, Calvo JA, Arias A. Implantes de 5 milimetros: A proposito de 84 implantes. Av Odontoestomatol 1994;10:633–640.
22. Barrachina M, Neira AC, Calvo JA. Greater diameter implants after four years of experience. Nobel Biocare Global Forum 1996;10:8–9.
23. Bahat O, Handelsman M. Use of wide implants and double implants in the posterior jaw: A clinical report. Int J Oral Maxillofac Implants 1996;11:379–386.
24. Davarpanah M, Martínez H. L'implant large: Indications, avantages et réflexions. Implant 1998;4: 275–277.
25. Lazzara RJ. Criteria for implant selection: Surgical and prosthetic considerations. Pract Periodontics Aesthet Dent 1994;6:55–62.
26. Balshi T. An analysis and management of fractured implants: A clinical report. Int J Oral Maxillofac Implants 1996;11:372–378.
27. Balshi T, Hernandez R, Pryslak M, Rangert B. A comparative study of one implant versus two replacing a single molar. Int J Oral Maxillofac Implants 1996; 11:400–408.
28. Dawood A. The implant-supported single molar replacement. Careful pre-operative evaluation is the key to success. Nobel Biocare Global Forum 1996; 10:6.
29. Jaffin RA, Berman CL. The excessive loss of Brånemark fixtures in type IV bone. A 5 year analysis. J Periodontol 1991;62:2–4.
30. Johns RB, Jemt T, Heath MR, et al. A multicenter study of overdentures supported by Brånemark implants. Int J Oral Maxillofac Implants 1992;7: 513–522.
31. Le Gall MG, Saadoun AP. Quelle surface portante pour un implant? J Parodontol 1993;12:317–332.
32. Marseiller E. Les dents humaines: Morphologie. Paris: Gauthiers-Villars, 1958.
33. Jepsen A. Root surface measurement and method for X-ray determination of root surface area. Acta Odontol Scand 1963;21:35–46.
34. Morgan MJ, James DF, Pilliar RM. Fractures of the fixture component of an osseointegrated implant. Int J Oral Maxillofac Implants 1993;8:409–414.

35. Rangert B, Krogh P, Langer B, van Roekel N. Bending overload and implant fracture: A retrospective clinical analysis. Int J Oral Maxillofac Implants 1995;10: 326–334.

36. Sullivan DY. Wide implant for wide teeth. Dent Econ 1994;March:82–83.

CHAPTER 3

Surgical Approach

M. Davarpanah/H. Martínez/R. Lazzara/J.-F. Tecucianu/D. Etienne

I. Stage-one surgery

A. Patient preparation

The patient must be prepared as follows:

- –premedication (antibiotics, anti-inflammatories, and possible prescription of anxiolytics), chlorhexidine mouthwash, and local preanesthesia are performed
- –patient must wear a cap, a nonsterile disposable gown, and overshoes before entering the operatory
- –the perioral region is cleaned (by the operating assistant) using an antiseptic solution (chlorhexidine, Betadine)
- –patient's body and the upper part of the head are covered with sterile sheets
- –a sterile mask covers the face

The preformed surgical template must be sterilized (quaternary ammonia, autoclave).

B. Surgical protocol

1. Patient premedication

Premedication is recommended, for example, using benzodiazepines (anxiolytic) 1 hour before surgery, and possibly the day before. The oral environment is particularly septic. Antibiotic therapy is indicated prior to implant placement; it must be started 1 hour before surgery and continued for 6 days. The use of a chlorhexidine mouthwash (0.12% or 2%) before surgery for 1 minute considerably reduces the number of bacteria.

2. Anesthesia

Implant placement is most often performed under local anesthesia. Before the patient enters the operatory, local and block infiltrations are performed. The anesthetic is selected according to the anesthesia technique and the expected surgery duration.

C. Implant technique

1. Incisions and flap elevation

Several types of incisions have been described. In 1985, Brånemark et al[1] recommended for edentulous jaws a curved incision line that inclines toward the ridge (between the mental foramina in the mandible and medial to the first molars in the maxilla). The postoperative sequelae of this type of incision are often difficult (edema, pain).

Today, it is recommended to make a primary incision line on top of the ridge or incline (in keratinized tissue). This incision line is continued with secondary buccal and/or lingual releasing incisions respecting the marginal gingiva of the adjacent teeth (Fig 3-1). A mucoperiosteal flap is reflected using an elevator. Following bone ridge exposure, the lin-

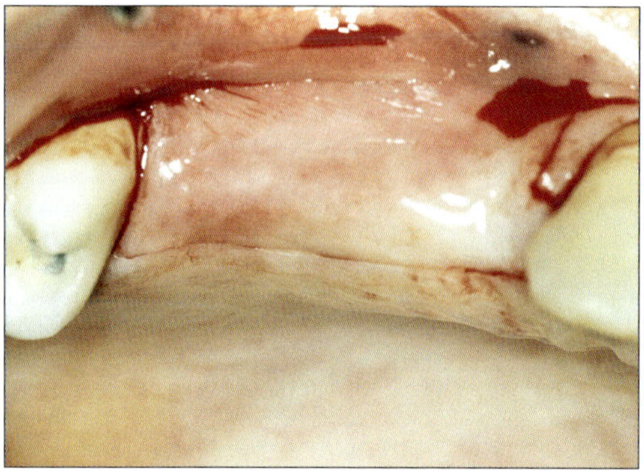

Fig 3-1 Incision line moved toward the palatal aspect.

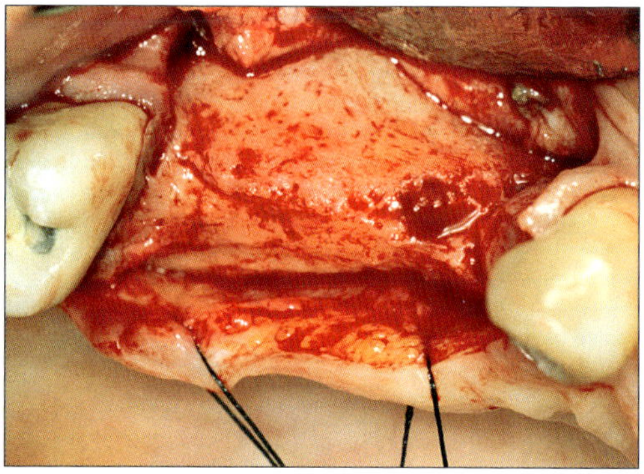

Fig 3-2 Flap reflection allowing good visualization of the alveolar crest. Note the preservation of the papilla distal to the canine.

gual or palatal flap is reflected and secured using sutures anchored around the teeth collars or on the contralateral ridge (Fig 3-2). Granulation tissue adherent to bone is removed using bone forceps. The bone surface must be as regular and flat as possible before starting the implant site preparation. Management is essential to avoid extensive postoperative side effects (pain, edema, hematoma).

2. *Implant site preparation*

Profuse saline irrigation avoids bone heating during the overall bone preparation.

a. *Cortical bone perforation*

The surgeon must place the surgical template prior to the initial drilling. Using a high-speed pilot twist drill (2,000 rpm) and constant irrigation, the marginal compact bone layer is penetrated at the previously determined emergence point of the implant site (Fig 3-3).

- A minimum space of 7 mm must be observed between the center of the two implant sites (diameter 3.75 or 4 mm).
- The bone chips must be constantly removed from the different rotating instruments to avoid bone heating.
- Peri-implant bone necrosis may occur following temperature elevation over 47°C for more than 1 minute.

b. *Implant site depth*

A 2-mm graded twist drill is used at high speed in order to reach the previously determined implant site depth (Fig 3-4). The preparation direction must be checked in the three dimensions of space using the surgical template and a direction indicator. A millimeter-graduated gauge allows checking of the drilling depth. Successive vertical (removal) movements must be applied in order for the working end of the twist drill to be regularly irrigated. During implant placement, the direction of the different sites compared to the surgical template is checked using direction indicators (Fig 3-5).

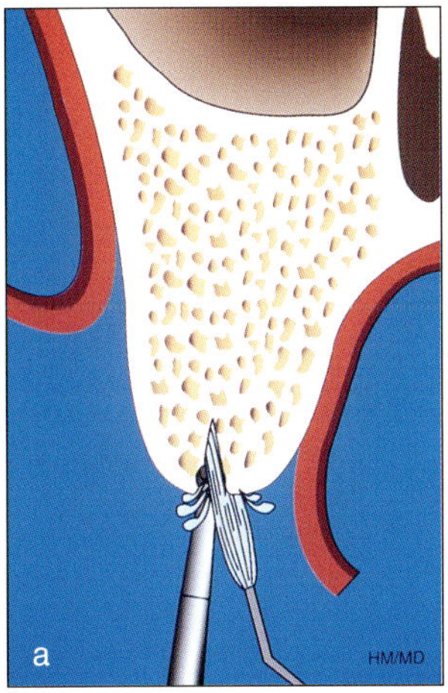

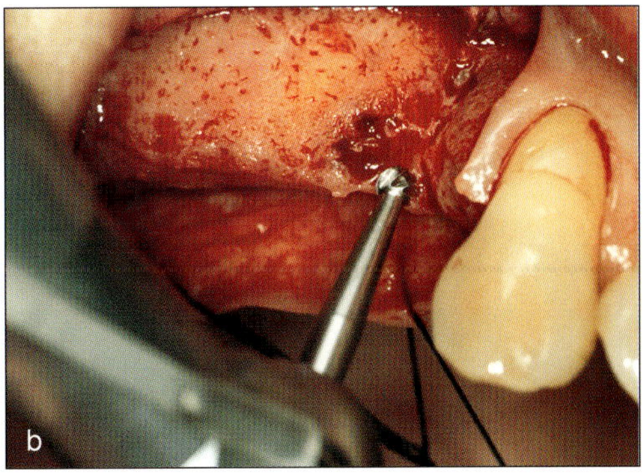

Figs 3-3a and 3-3b The pilot drill locates the implant emergence site. Profuse irrigation is essential during all surgical phases.

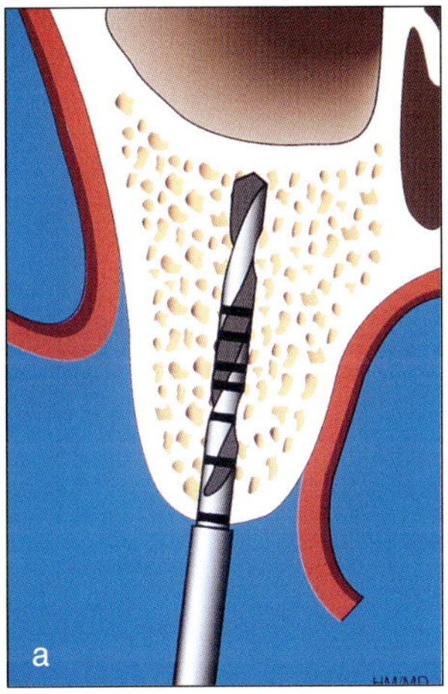

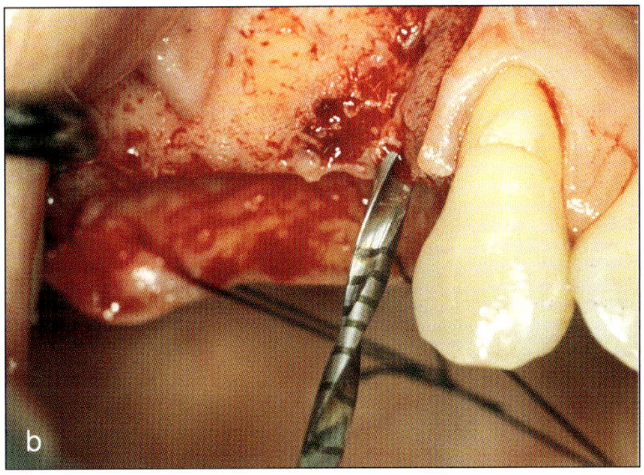

Figs 3-4a and 3-4b The 2-mm twist drill is inserted down to the anticipated depth for the implant site.

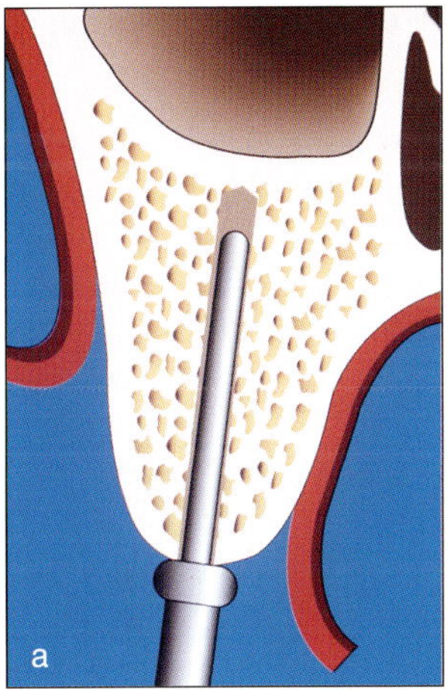

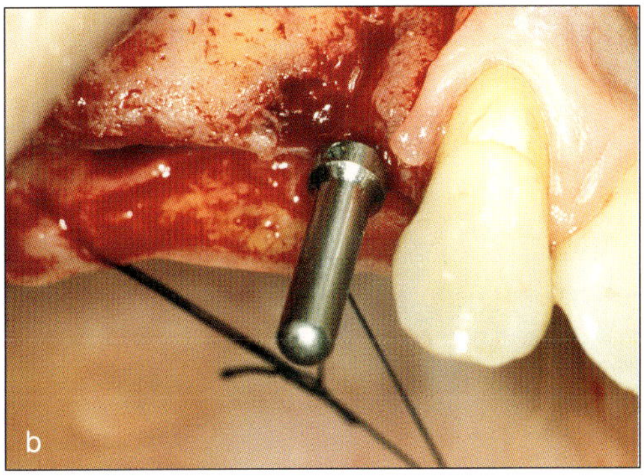

Figs 3-5a and 3-5b The direction indicator checks the implant axis.

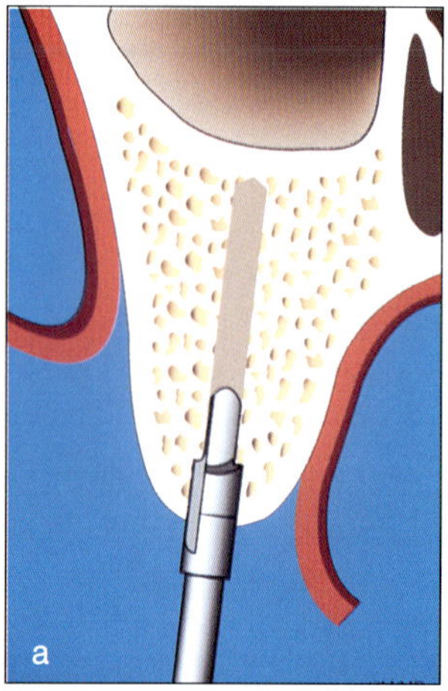

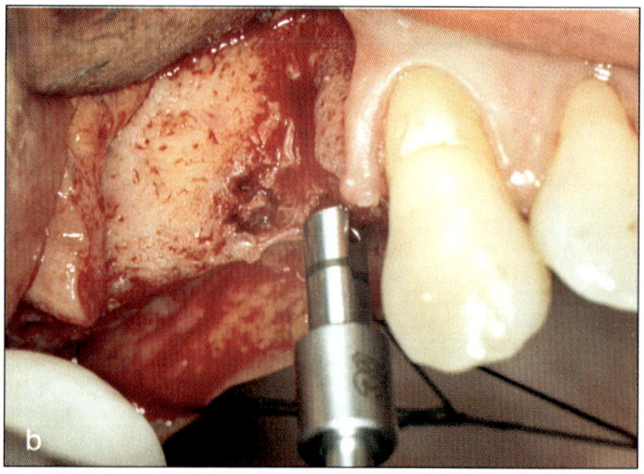

Figs 3-6a and 3-6b The intermediate twist drill allows widening of the site diameter to 2 to 3 mm.

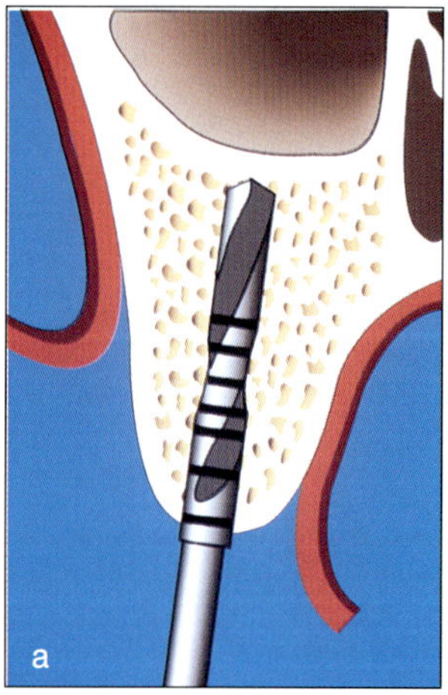

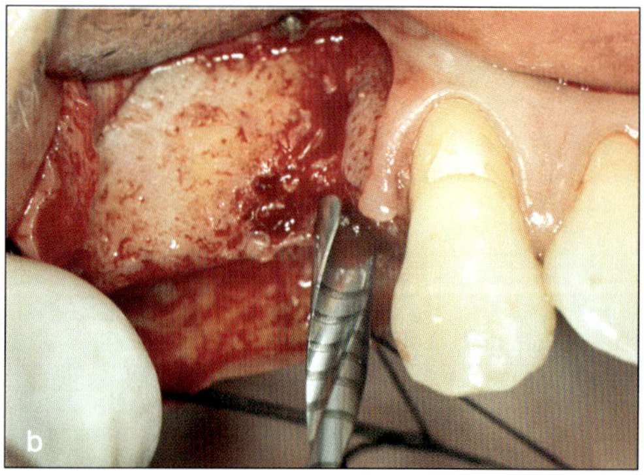

Figs 3-7a and 3-7b The 3-mm twist drill allows enlargement to the total height of the implant site.

—The twist drill is 1 mm longer than the selected implant. A safety margin of at least 2 mm above the mandibular nerve canal must be observed.
—Protect the back of the patient's throat with gauze or connect the direction indicators when using them in the oral cavity.

c. *Intermediate 2- to 3-mm drilling*

An intermediate twist drill with a nonworking end is inserted in the 2-mm graded preparation. This drill allows enlargement of the cavity to 3 mm. The active part of the twist drill perforates the marginal compact bone layer (Fig 3-6). The drilling direction must always be noted.

d. *Drilling at 3 mm*

A 3-mm graded twist drill allows enlargement of the preparation to its total height (Fig 3-7). A graded gauge will allow checking of the drilling depth. A larger twist drill (3.15 or 3.25 mm) is sometimes indicated for very hard

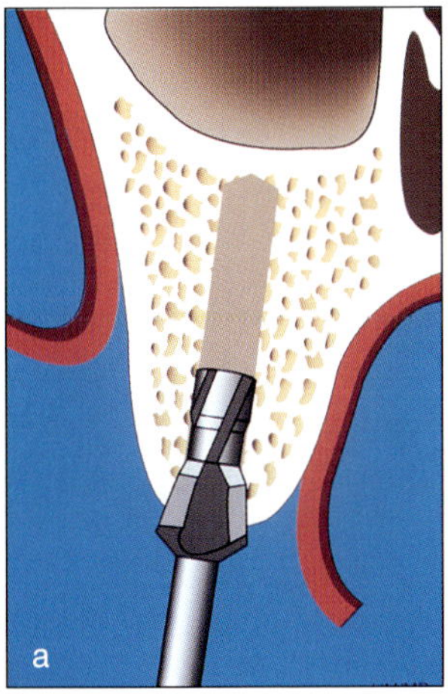

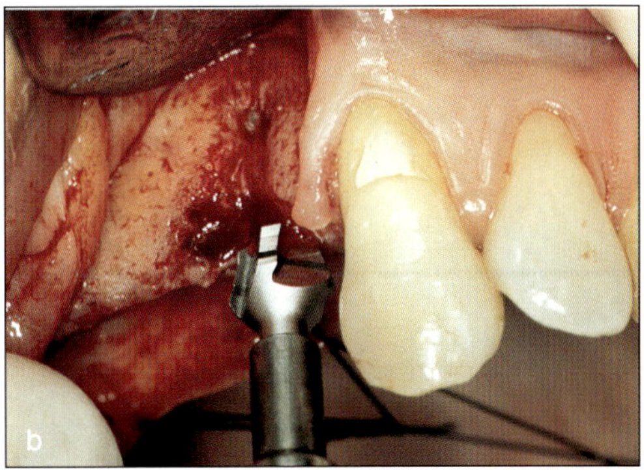

Figs 3-8a and 3-8b The countersink drill prepares the marginal compact bone layer for the placement of the implant neck.

bone. When placing a standard implant in type III or IV bone, the 3-mm twist drill should be used minimally.

e. Countersinking

The marginal entry to the preparation site is countersunk using a conical twist drill in order to allow the implant and the cover screw to be completely submerged. Countersinking must remain within the marginal compact bone layer. The groove of the direction indicator offers the same diameter as the implant neck. Submerging of the implant may thus be visualized (Fig 3-8).

—Too-extensive countersinking in poor quality bone may compromise the primary stability of the implant.
—In the posterior regions and/or when soft tissues are very thick, a modified surgical protocol recommends avoiding use of the conical twist drill. The wearing of a removable denture is contraindicated. This modified protocol increases the primary stability at the implant neck, which remains in a supracortical position. Stage-two implant surgery is also facilitated.

f. Tapping

Most of the new implants are self-tapping. Tapping is only indicated in dense bone. The preparation is performed using a low-speed (15 to 20 rpm) contra-angle handpiece. For very dense bone, the threading is performed on the total height of the preparation site without exerting any pressure on the tap. The surgeon must make sure to preserve the direction of the preparation site and avoid damaging the threading during drill removal. When several implants are placed, the bone chips are removed from the tap before each use.

3. Implant positioning (standard)

The implant is positioned according the direction of the preparation site. Rotating speed must not be over 20 to 40 rpm. As soon as the first threads of the implant penetrate the site, the rest of the implant body must be allowed to freely follow the pretapped preparation without undue force (Fig 3-9). The implant is irrigated after submerging the first apical third. Submerging is performed up to the coronal limit of its body (Fig 3-10). The implant posi-

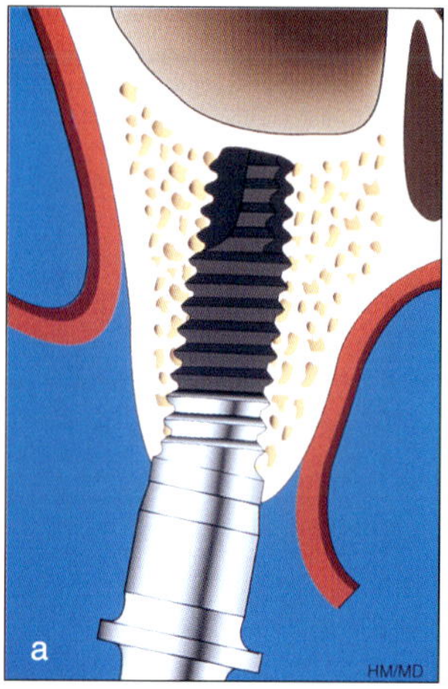

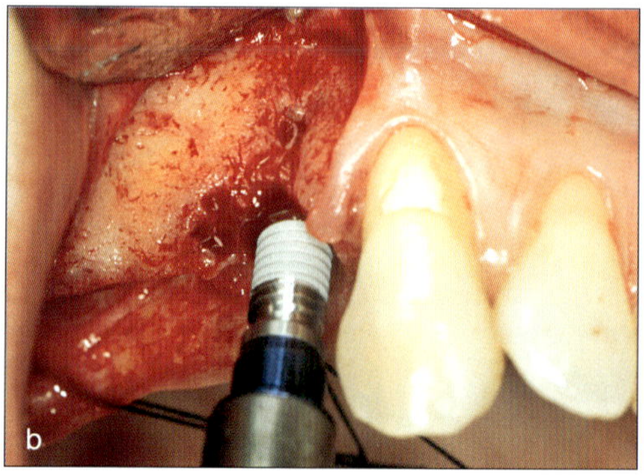

Figs 3-9a and 3-9b Placing a self-tapping implant (Osseotite).

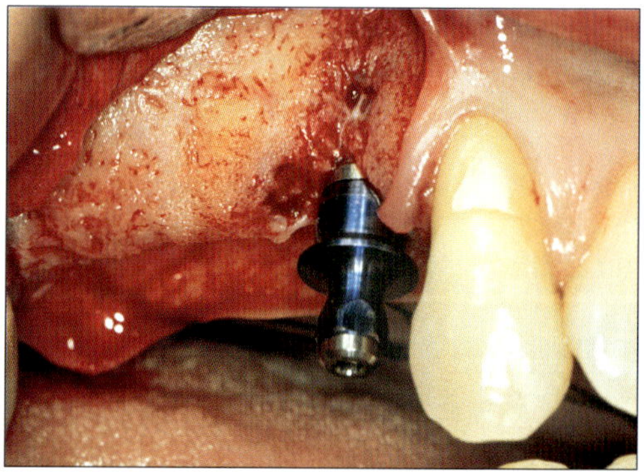

Fig 3-10 Clinical view of the implant with its premounted implant holder.

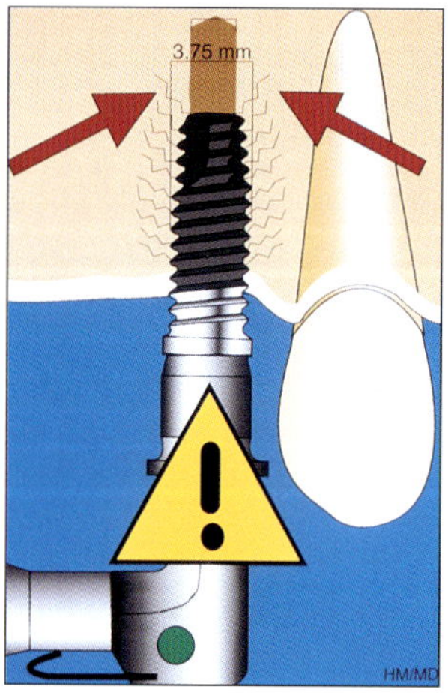

Fig 3-11 Excessive tightening on the implant may cause bone microfractures.

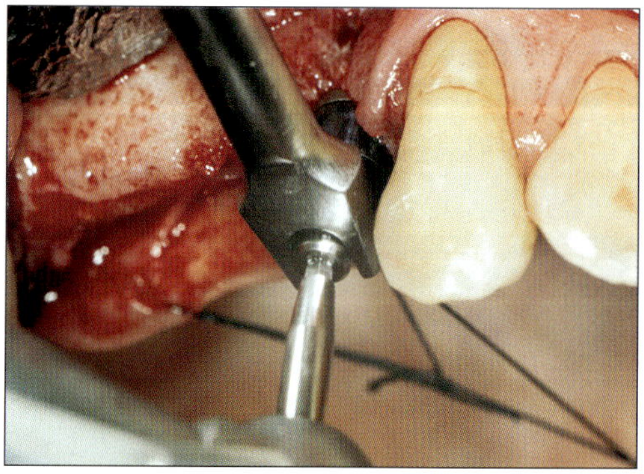

Fig 3-12 Unscrewing of the implant mount using a screwdriver mounted on a low-speed contra-angle handpiece.

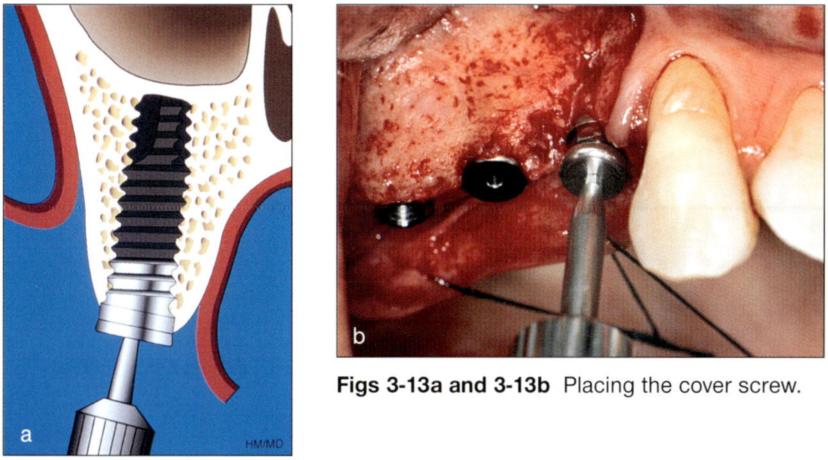

Figs 3-13a and 3-13b Placing the cover screw.

tioning is completed manually using a wrench. The surgeon must exert a vertical force using this wrench. Excessive tightening on the implant must be avoided because it may cause bone microfractures (Figs 3-11 and 3-12).

4. Placing the cover screw

The cover screw is placed using a screwdriver attached to a contra-angle handpiece. The tightening is performed using a low speed (15 to 20 rpm) (Fig 3-13a). The final tightening is performed manually using the adapted screwdriver (Fig 3-13b). It is recommended to rinse the implant hexagonal head (hex) before inserting the cover screw. The presence of blood may lead to some newly formed bone around the hex, thus rendering stage-two surgery more difficult.

5. Flap repositioning and suturing

The surgical site should be profusely irrigated and cleaned. All bone chips or soft tissue tags must be removed. The flap is carefully replaced, then compressed in order to obtain complete closure of the soft tissue flaps. Simple sutures allow hermetic closure. It is recommended to ask the patient to bite carefully on sterile gauze rolls.

II. Stage-two surgery

A. Surgical technique

Stage-two surgery, or placing implants in function, consists of implant exposure. Prior to stage-two surgery, periapical radiographs allow checking for the absence of radiolucency and/or bone defects around the implant (Fig 3-14).

1. Flap incision and elevation

A full-thickness flap is created on top of the crest. A slight reflection is also made, allowing direct access to the cover screws (Figs 3-15 and 3-16). A visual examination determines the bone overgrowth on the screws. An adapted trephine that fits into the center of the cover screw allows removal of all bone overgrowth. After complete exposure of the cover screws, they are removed using an adapted screwdriver.

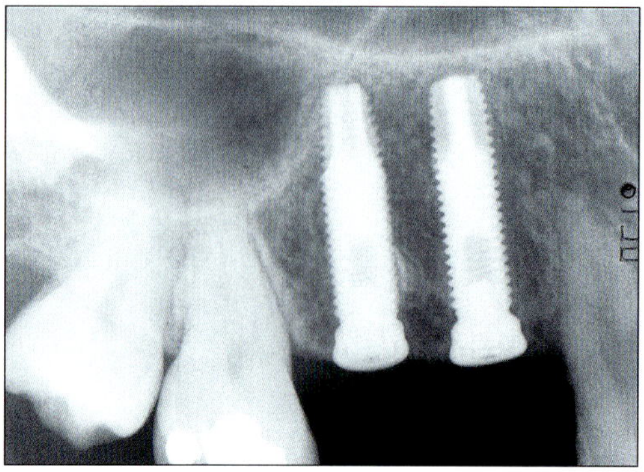

Fig 3-14 Control radiograph after 6 months of bone healing for two implants positioned to replace the maxillary right premolars. The two implants seem to be radiographically osseointegrated.

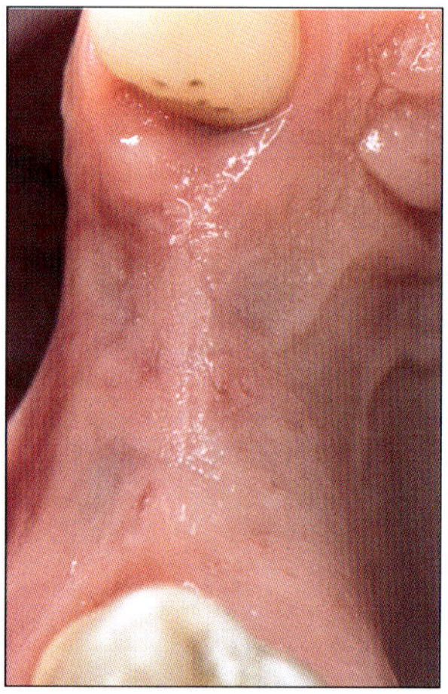

Fig 3-15 Clinical view of the alveolar crest prior to stage-two implant surgery.

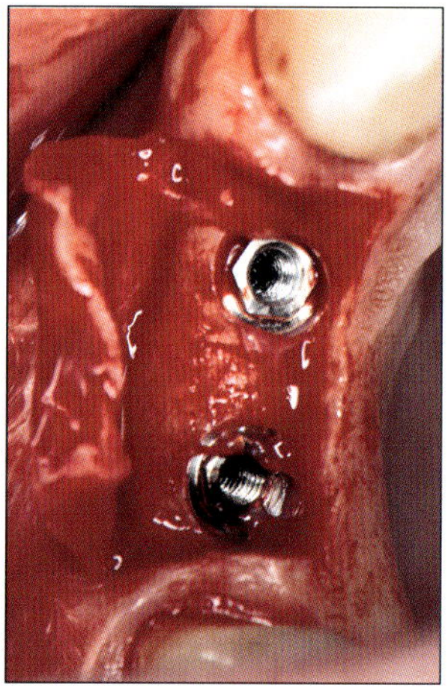

Fig 3-16 Clinical view after flap reflection and removal of the cover screws. Note the incision line moved toward the palatal aspect, thus preserving the papillae.

All soft and hard tissue fragments located on the implant hex or neck must be removed. Any scratching of the implant surface must be avoided. Selecting an appropriate trephine allows adaptation of the bone environment to the emergence profile of the abutment (Figs 3-17 to 3-20).

2. Healing abutment selection

A graded gauge or a periodontal probe allows determination of the thickness of the mucosa in order to select the abutment. The abutment must emerge from the mucosa by about 2 mm. The surgeon must check the abutment axis during its insertion in order to avoid damaging the internal threading of the implant.

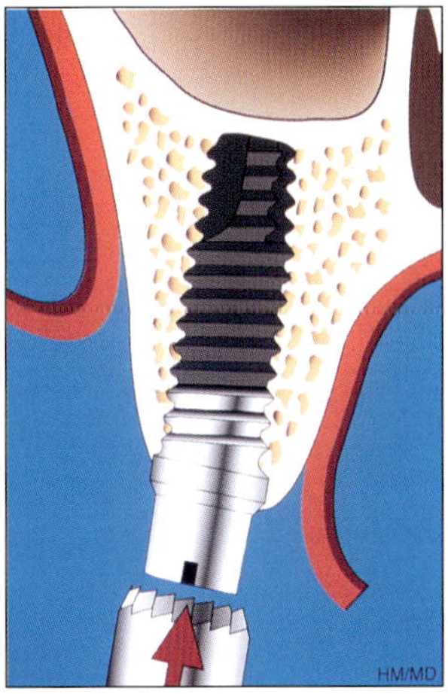

Fig 3-17 Diagram illustrating trephine adaptation on a guiding abutment screwed to the implant.

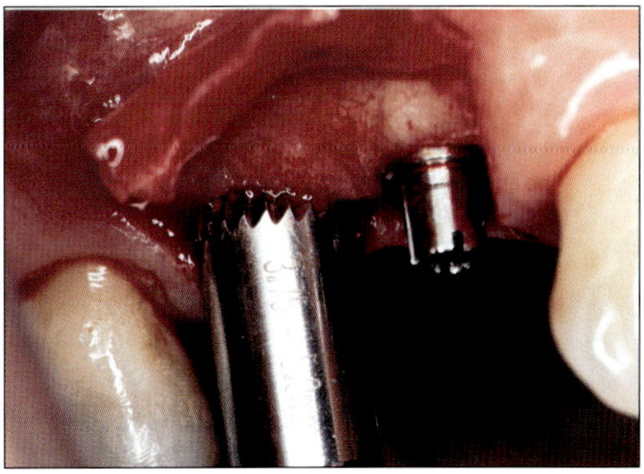

Fig 3-18 The trephine allows adaptation of the bone to the healing abutment. Trephines adapted to each healing abutment are available.

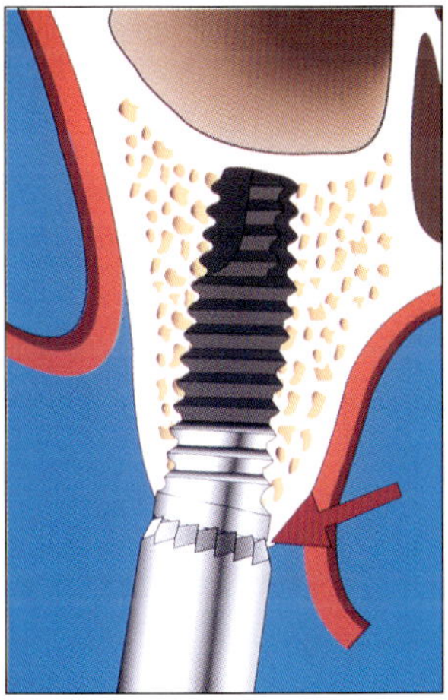

Fig 3-19 Diagram illustrating the osteoplasty performed with the trephine.

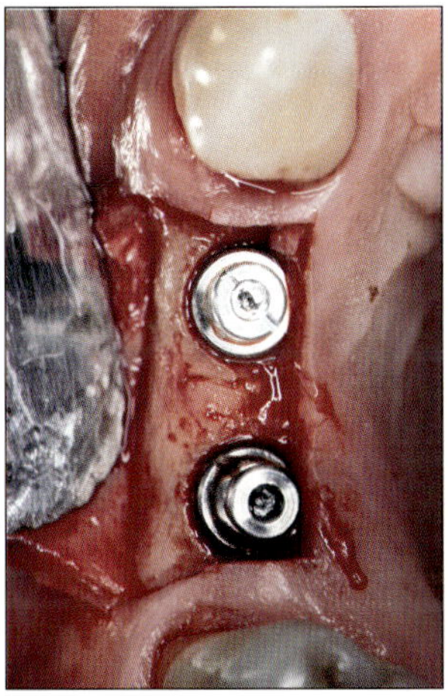

Fig 3-20 Occlusal view of guiding abutments screwed on the implants. Note the bone perfectly adapted to the emergence profile of the future abutment.

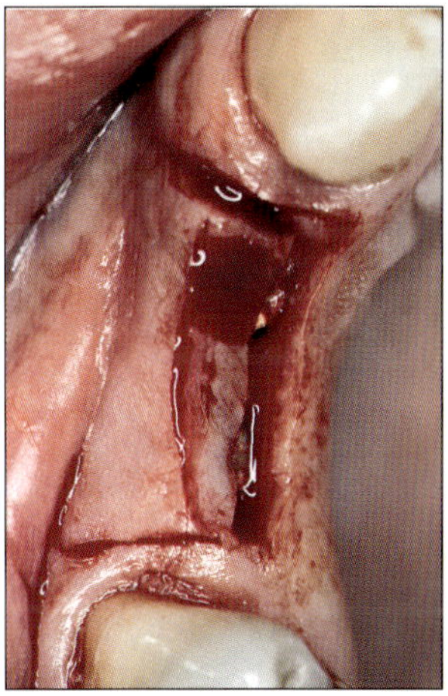

Fig 3-21 The most coronal part of the flap is de-epithelialized in order to perform optimal tissue management using a connective tissue graft (roll technique).

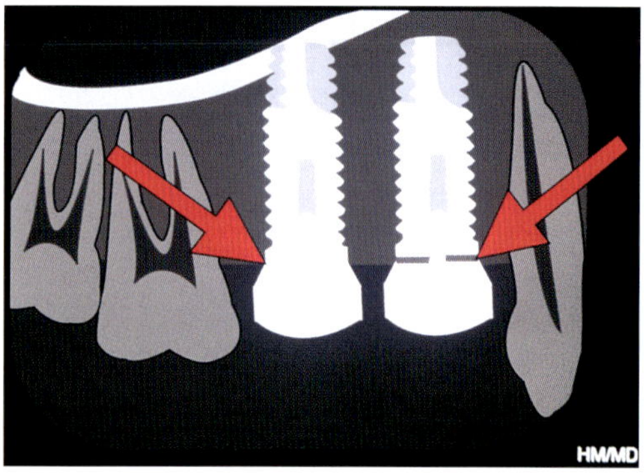

Fig 3-22 Diagram of a radiograph after placing the healing abutments. Note the gap on the mesial implant.

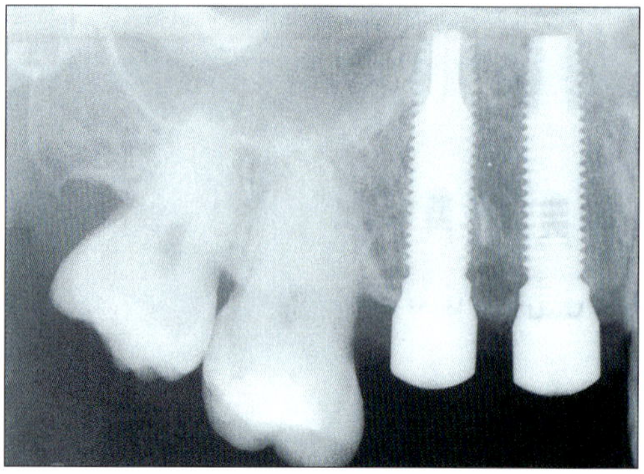

Fig 3-23 Radiograph showing perfect adaptation of the healing abutments on the implants.

—When no esthetic imperatives are required, it is advised to surgically reduce excessive soft tissue thickness. On the other hand, in some cases, the use of peri-implant mucogingival management procedures allows optimization of the esthetic outcome (Fig 3-21).

—No tissue must be interposed between the abutment and the implant during its placement. This can cause painful postoperative side effects or abscess formation.

3. Flap repositioning and suturing

The surgical site is profusely irrigated and cleaned. All soft and hard tissue fragments must be removed. The flap must be carefully adapted around the abutments. Simple sutures allow good flap closure.

B. Control of osseointegration

Any micromovement of the implant is suspect and truly indicates the absence of osseointegration. Peri-implant pain despite local anesthesia is also suspect. It may be related to the presence of soft tissue formation around the implant. Periapical radiographs allow checking for good fit of the healing abutments and the absence of radiolucency around the implant (Figs 3-22 to 3-25).

III. Peri-implant soft tissue management

The aim of second-stage surgery is to place the healing abutments or the final abutments over the implants. The development of surgical and prosthetic techniques aims to optimize the functional and esthetic result. Recent treatment approaches allow a more natural emergence profile.[2–7]

The goal of peri-implant soft tissue management is to improve the quality and the thickness of the peri-implant mucosa. Different types of mucogingival procedures may be indicated for peri-implant soft tissue management:

—apical positioning of the buccal flap
—lateral or coronal sliding flaps
—free gingival graft
—free gingival connective tissue graft
—gingivoplasty

We will describe the most recent techniques:

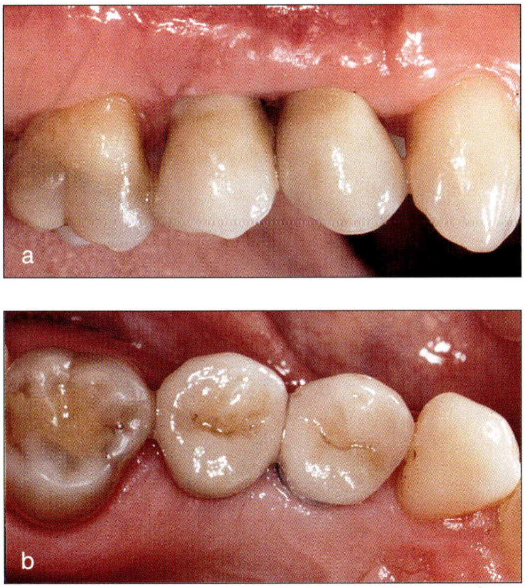

Fig 3-24a and 3-24b Occlusal and buccal views of the final prosthetic restorations.

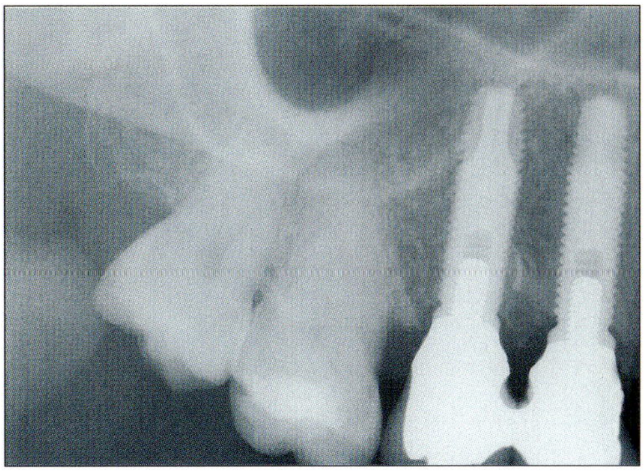

Fig 3-25 Control radiograph at 1 year.

—guided tissue healing
—papilla regeneration
—guided soft tissue regeneration
—positioning of the interdental contact points

On a natural abutment, the marginal limit of a crown is located 0.5 to 1 mm subgingival. For esthetic reasons, the implant-supported crown is often located 2 to 4 mm subgingival. The presence of keratinized tissue is therefore essential in order to obtain an esthetic and functional result.

A. Guided tissue healing

Three techniques are proposed:

—emergence profile system (EPS) concept
—impression taking at stage-one implant surgery
—using a provisional crown as an impression transfer coping

Recent technology innovations allow guidance of soft tissue healing. An improved esthetic result is obtained while preserving access for strict hygiene and maintenance care.[7–13]

1. Emergence profile concept

This technique is based on using the healing abutments and the impression transfer copings adapted to each implant diameter and to the future prosthetic crown. The aim of this approach is that the future prosthetic crown really mimic a natural tooth (Figs 3-26 and 3-27).

a. Technique

During second-stage surgery, a healing abutment corresponding to the emergence profile of the future prosthetic crown (5, 6, or 7.5 mm diameter) is placed. After 8 weeks of soft tissue healing, an impression transfer coping

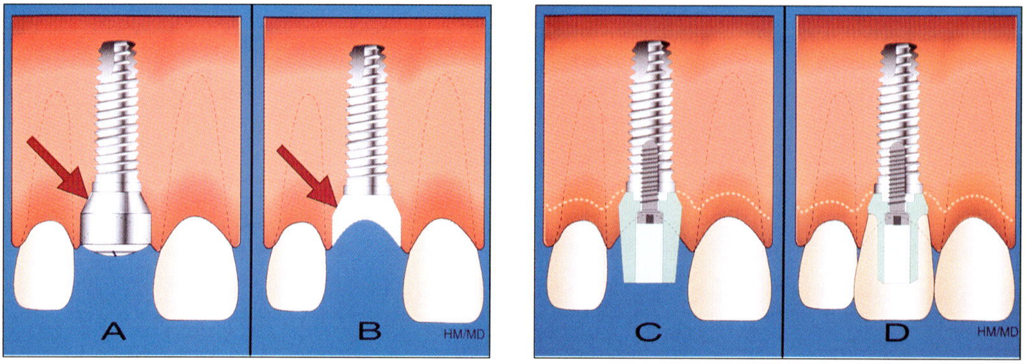

Fig 3-26 a = placement of a large healing abutment on a maxillary central incisor; b = soft tissues are trimmed according to the selected emergence profile; c = placement of the corresponding final abutment; d = fabrication of an anatomic crown.

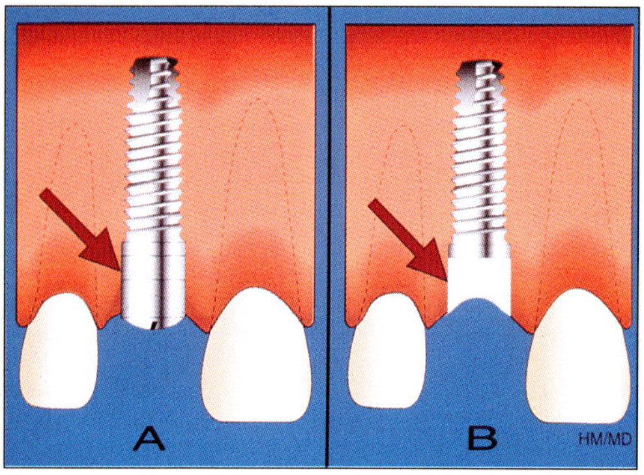

Fig 3-27 a = placement of a healing abutment with insufficient diameter on a maxillary central incisor; b = inappropriate emergence profile.

corresponding the selected abutment is positioned for impression taking. All the features of the peri-implant soft tissues are accurately reproduced on the working cast. The prosthetic crown is fabricated at the laboratory with ideal contours. The practitioner removes the healing abutment prior to final restoration placement (Figs 3-28 to 3-32).

b. Advantages

The emergence profile concept offers several advantages:

- This method avoids the laboratory technician having to grind down the working cast in an empiric manner in order to shape an emergence profile adapted to the prosthetic crown contours.
- Tissue expansion during healing allows improvement of the quality of the gingival margin.
- Placing the prosthetic crown does not require gingival tissue alterations.
- EPS allows avoidance of prosthetic overcontours.
- The EPS impression transfer copings allow registration of the implant external hex position and soft tissue anatomy.

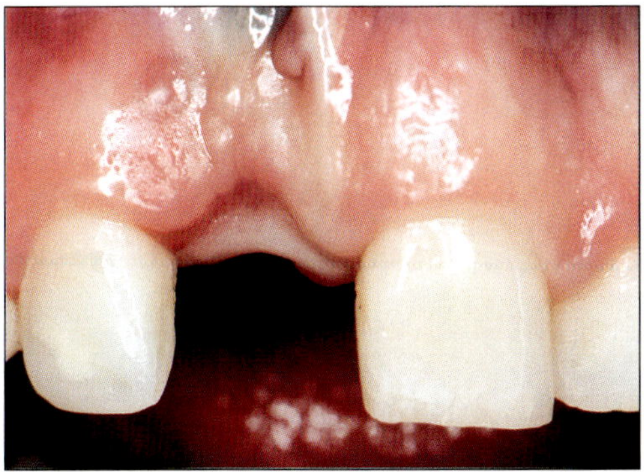

Fig 3-28 Clinical view of a single missing tooth, the maxillary right central incisor.

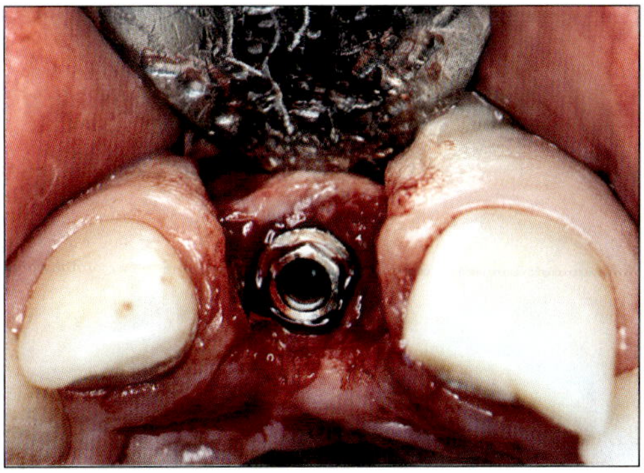

Fig 3-29 Occlusal view after bone regeneration of the tissue loss using a Gore-Tex membrane.

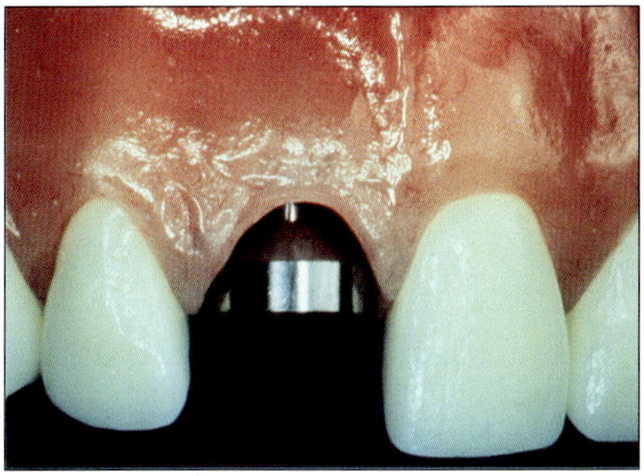

Fig 3-30 Study cast showing the mucosa healing around a large-diameter 3i implant.

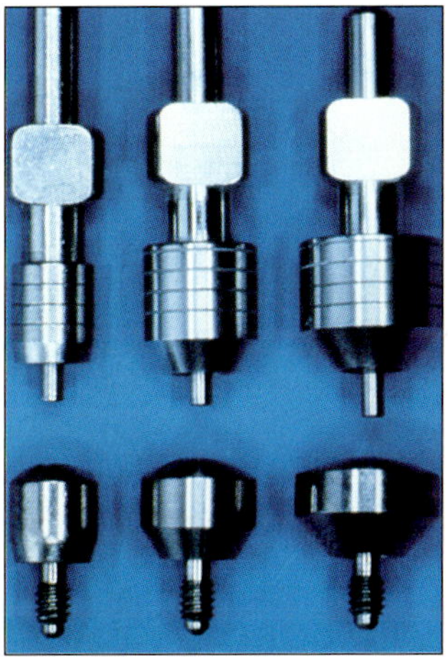

Fig 3-31 3i healing abutments of different diameters (5, 6, and 7.5 mm) with the corresponding transfer copings.

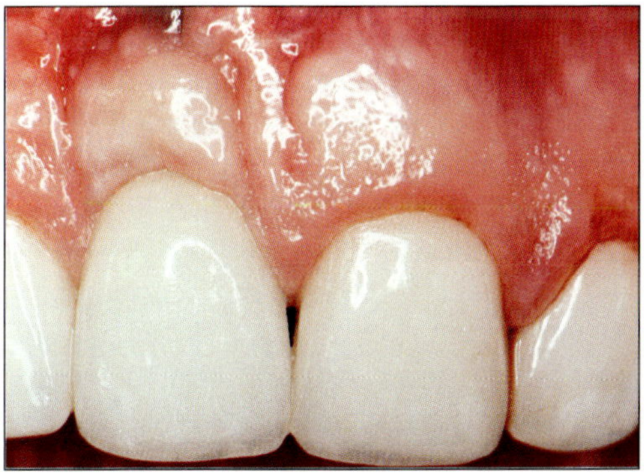

Fig 3-32 Clinical view of the final prosthetic restoration (restoration, Dr S. Neyret).

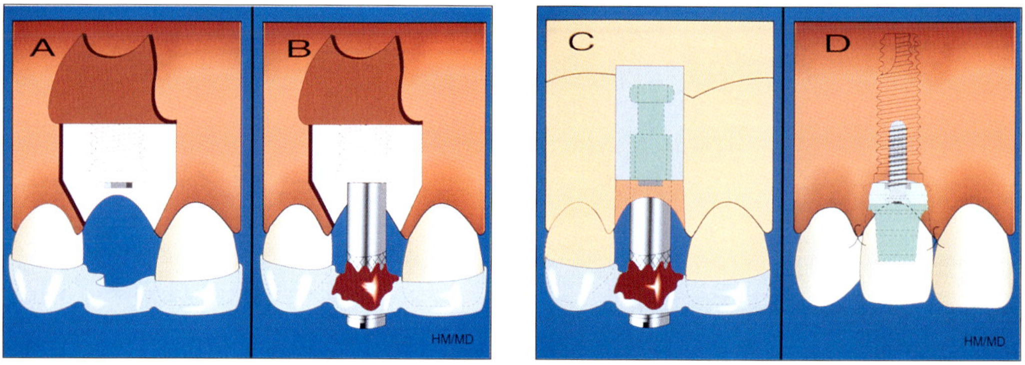

Fig 3-33 Impression taking at stage-one implant surgery: a = placing the implant using a surgical template; b = the impression transfer coping screwed on the implant head is splinted to the surgical guide with acrylic resin; c = the transfer coping is transferred to the working cast. The final prosthetic restoration is fabricated at the laboratory during the osseointegration period: d = the final crown is placed at stage-two implant surgery.

—The healing abutments are sometimes too wide and may lead to soft tissue compression against the adjacent tooth and/or implant.
—According to the extent of implant submerging, placement of the healing abutment requires an adjustment of the emergence profile to the bone level. We advise the use of a trephine adapted to each emergence profile.
—The emergence profile concept was recently refined. New anatomic healing abutments allow trimming of the peri-implant soft tissues according to each tooth.

2. *Stage-one implant surgery impression taking*

An implant positioning transfer or indicator placed on the implant head allows recording of its position using a modified surgical template (Fig 3-33).

a. *Indications*

The different indications for stage-one impression taking are:

—esthetic objectives: rapidly guiding soft tissue healing when connecting the implant abutment
—preparing the prosthetic stages at the laboratory during the osseointegration period for short-span prosthetic restorations
—reducing the number of appointments required for the final prosthetic work

b. *Technique*

Implant placement is performed according to the usual protocol. Once the implant is placed, the transfer coping is positioned over the head of the implant. It is splinted with acrylic resin to the surgical template that has been previously used for implant placement. If necessary, the surgical template may be modified around the transfer coping. Once the acrylic resin is set, the fixation screw of the transfer coping is removed. The surgical template and the transfer coping are then removed en bloc. Implant

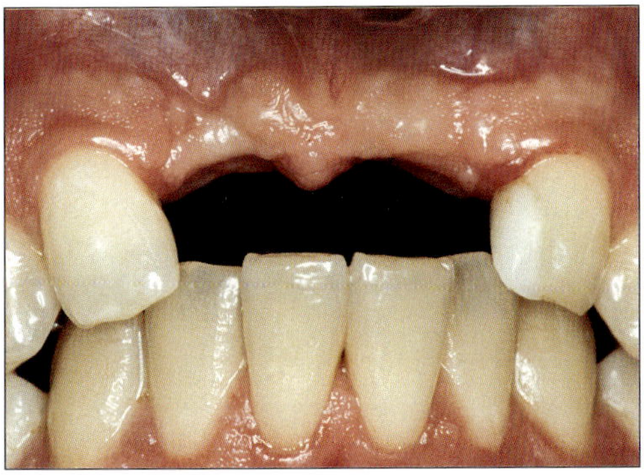

Fig 3-34 Clinical view of missing maxillary central incisors.

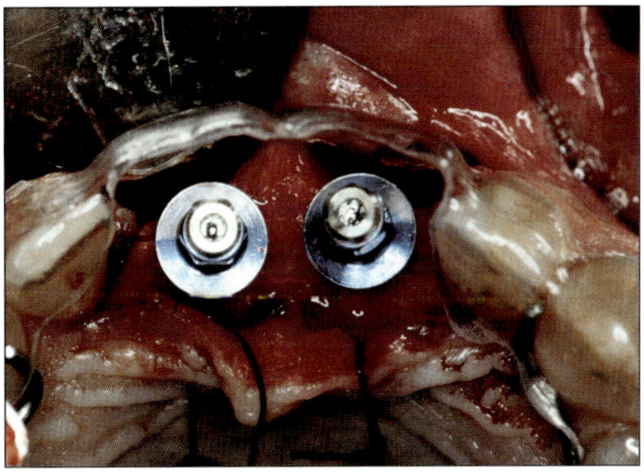

Fig 3-35 Placement of two implants using the surgical template.

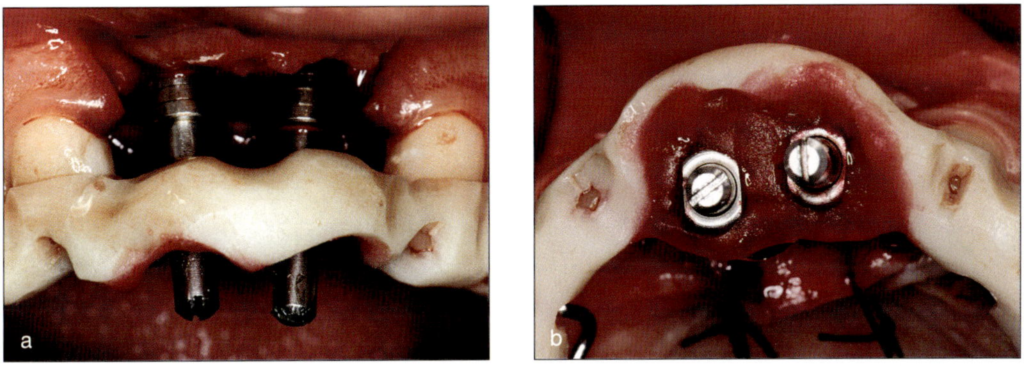

Figs 3-36a and 3-36b Positioning of the impression transfer copings splinted to the template.

surgery is then completed according to the standard protocol.

At the laboratory, the implant abutment analogue is positioned on the transfer coping. The working cast is modified in order to allow repositioning of the surgical template splinted to a transfer coping and to the analogue. The analogue is then connected to the working cast using plaster. The final implant position is thus registered. During the osseointegration period, the prosthetic restoration is fabricated at the laboratory. The provisional restoration is placed as soon as the implant abutment is connected. Soft tissue healing is thus guided around the restoration (Figs 3-34 to 3-42). Mucogingival surgery may be required during or after implant abutment connection in order to improve the esthetic result.

c. *Advantages*

Impression taking at stage-one surgery offers some advantages:

- soft tissue management to receive an ideally contoured prosthetic restoration
- reduced chairside time
- prosthetic restoration fabricated during osseointegration

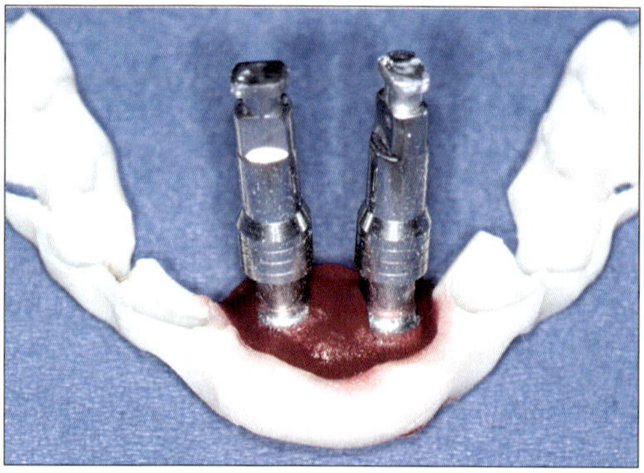

Fig 3-37 Placement of the implant analogues on the transfer copings.

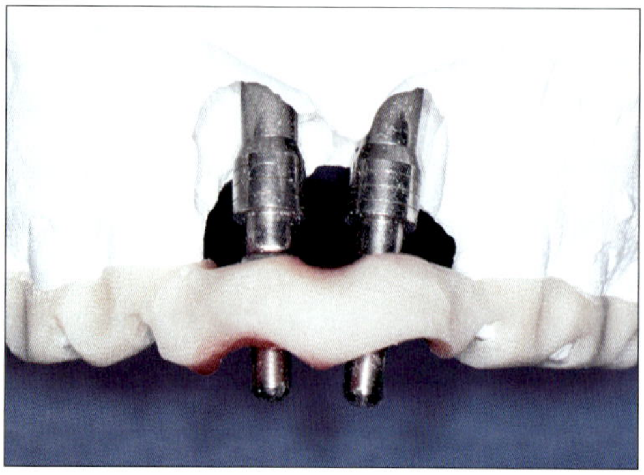

Fig 3-38 The whole device (guide/transfer coping/analogues) is transferred to the working casts.

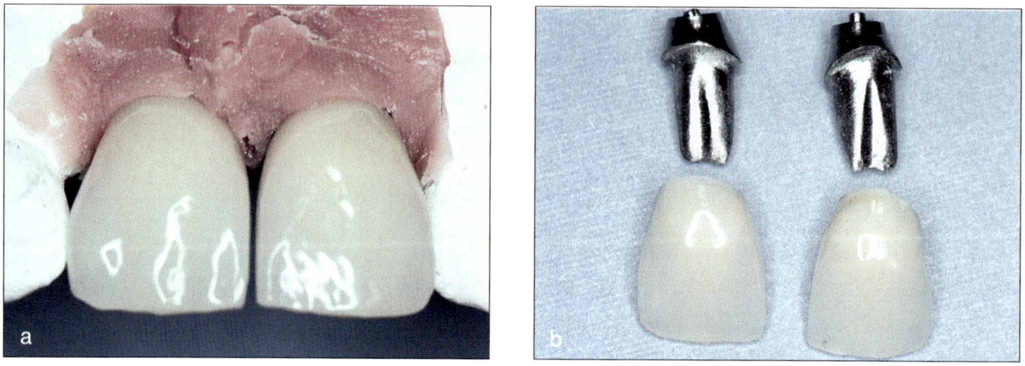

Fig 3-39a and 3-39b Final prosthetic restorations are fabricated at the laboratory during the osseointegration period.

d. Disadvantages

The disadvantages of this technique are:

—lengthened first-stage surgery
—compromise concerning surgical asepsis

3. Using a provisional restoration as an impression transfer coping

The principle of this technique is to guide the soft tissue healing around a provisional restoration fabricated during stage-two implant surgery. This provisional restoration is used as an impression transfer coping, allowing an accurate registration of the peri-implant soft tissues (Fig 3-43).

a. Indications

Indications for the provisional restoration are:

—single missing tooth situation
—short-span partially edentulous situation

b. Technique

A provisional restoration fabricated during the

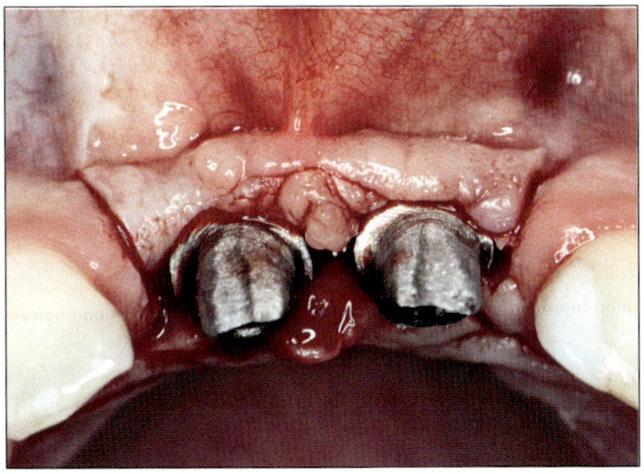

Fig 3-40 The gold UCLA abutments are tightened on the implants at 32 N.

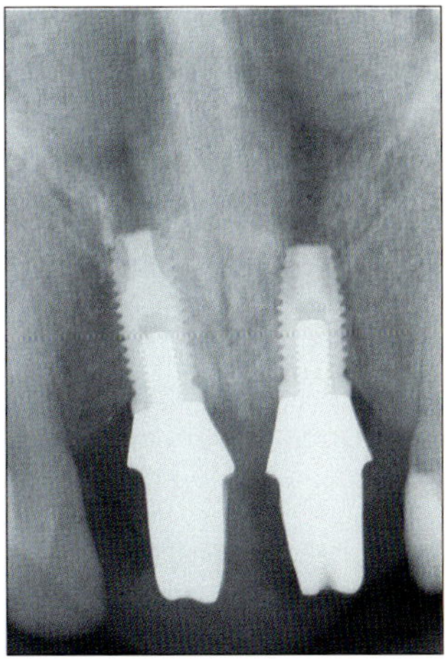

Fig 3-41 Radiographic control of the abutment positioning. Note the absence of gap.

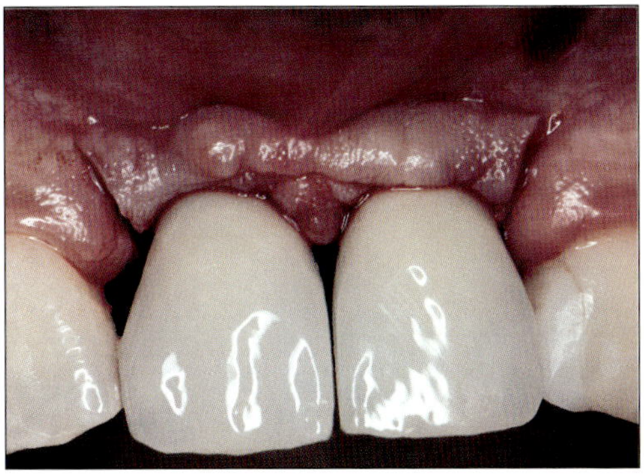

Fig 3-42 Placement of the porcelain crowns at the end of stage-two surgery (restoration, Dr P. Raygot).

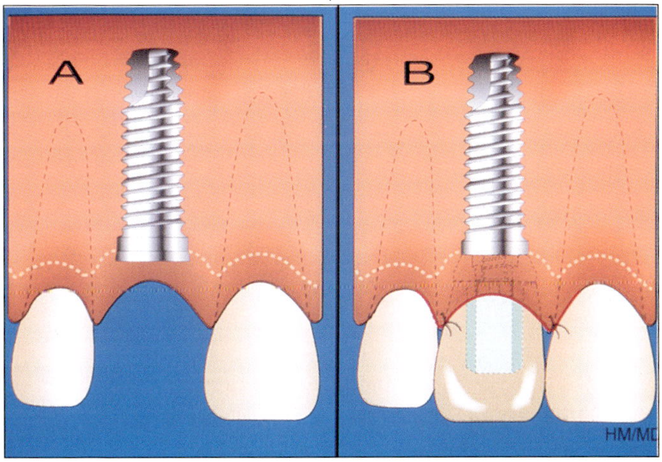

Fig 3-43 Using a provisional crown as a transfer coping: a = implant replacing a central incisor prior to stage-two implant surgery; b = a provisional crown is fabricated at stage-two implant surgery. This provisional crown will be used as an impression transfer coping.

second stage of implant surgery, or a little after, will guide the soft tissue healing. Two provisional restorations are required. The first is used to guide tissue healing during the first 6 to 8 weeks. The second is modified and used as an impression transfer coping. The laboratory technician may fabricate the final restoration on the working cast. The technician thus has an accurate record of the peri-implant soft tissues. Once the restoration is completed, the clinician removes the provisional and inserts the final prosthesis within a stable mucosa.

c. Advantages

The advantages offered by this technique are threefold:

—The laboratory technician may achieve the final restoration with perfectly determined and stable soft tissue contours.
—Chairside time during the final restoration placement is reduced.
—No tissue management is required.

d. Disadvantages

Several disadvantages should be mentioned:

—lengthened working time during phase-two implant surgery
—fabrication of two provisional restorations

B. Papilla regeneration

In 1992, Palacci[14] described a surgical technique to regenerate papillae during stage-two implant surgery. Vertical incisions are performed at least 3 mm mesial and distal to the implant. These incisions are connected with a horizontal incision on the lingual or buccal aspect. A full-thickness flap is reflected, thus giving access to the cover screws. These screws are replaced by titanium healing abutments (which exceed the soft tissue level by at least 2 mm). The buccal flap shows a 3- to 5-mm tissue excess.

A semilunar incision around each implant allows shaping of the marginal mucosa around each abutment. This incision extends to the adjacent abutment. It allows a 90-degree rotation of the created pedicle. This pedicle will fill the interimplant space (of about 3 mm) and allows creation a papilla. The flap is sutured using periosteal sutures. The pedicles must be secured and maintained using tension-free sutures.

—Sufficient quantity and thickness of keratinized tissue are required.
—Great care must be taken to avoid excessive tension on the pedicles. An excessive handling may lead to papilla necrosis and compromise the final result.

C. Guided soft tissue regeneration

In 1995, Salama et al[15] suggested using guided soft tissue regeneration to optimize the esthetic result in the anterior segments. This alveolar ridge augmentation technique allows new formation of interdental papillae (Fig 3-44).

1. Indications

Indications for guided soft tissue regeneration concern alveolar bone tissue loss (apicocoronal direction) in the anterior maxilla.

2. Contraindications

This technique presents several contraindications:

—extensive bone resorption
—presence of very thin mucosa
—insufficient quantity of keratinized tissue

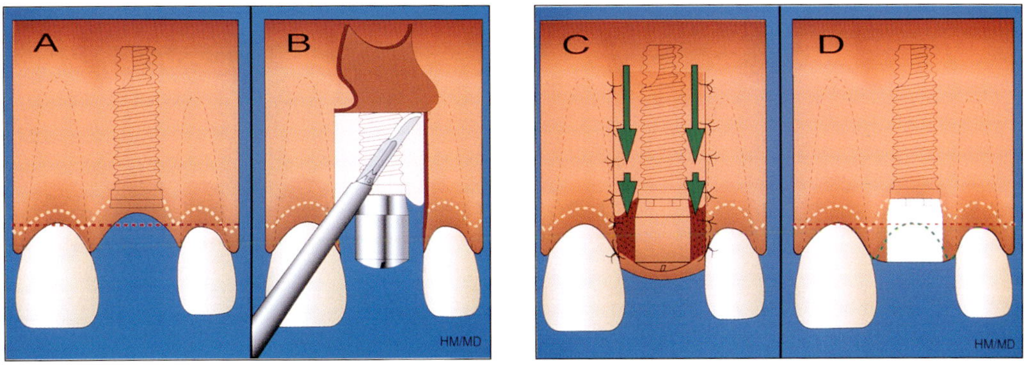

Fig 3-44 Guided soft tissue regeneration: a = placement of an implant replacing a central incisor with alveolar bone loss; b = placement of the healing abutment at stage-two surgery; c = coronal flap translation to achieve primary closure over the healing abutment; d = new soft tissue formation around the abutment enhances a natural esthetic result.

3. Technique

A Z-shaped incision is performed on the palatal aspect. A partial-thickness flap is elevated 3 to 4 mm. The flap is completed in full thickness. This type of flap allows healing by primary intention.

Flap reflection allows access to the cover screw. It is removed and replaced by a healing abutment. The height of this abutment must correspond to the tissue loss. A limited space between the bone and the healing abutment is thus created after primary closure of the site. This space is initially filled with a blood clot prior to the new formation of a thicker soft tissue volume. After complete soft tissue healing (8 to 12 weeks), implant abutment connection may be considered.

4. Modification

In the presence of extensive tissue loss, a free gingival connective tissue graft may be combined with this technique.

5. Considerations

The use of this technique increases the number of surgical procedures and delays the implant abutment connection for several weeks. Primary closure of the flap is sometimes difficult to achieve. This proposition is not documented by sufficient clinical follow-up: What will become of this newly formed soft tissue? There is a risk for subsequent recession (soft tissues must be supported by underlying bone).

D. Positioning of the interdental contact point and papilla regeneration

Proper evaluation of the distance between the alveolar ridge and the prosthetic contact point is essential to obtain new interdental papillae. The papillae are supported by the underlying alveolar bone. New formation of the papilla will depend on the interproximal alveolar ridge–interdental contact point distance.[16] Tarnow et al[16] reported a study on 288 teeth. Complete papilla regeneration may be

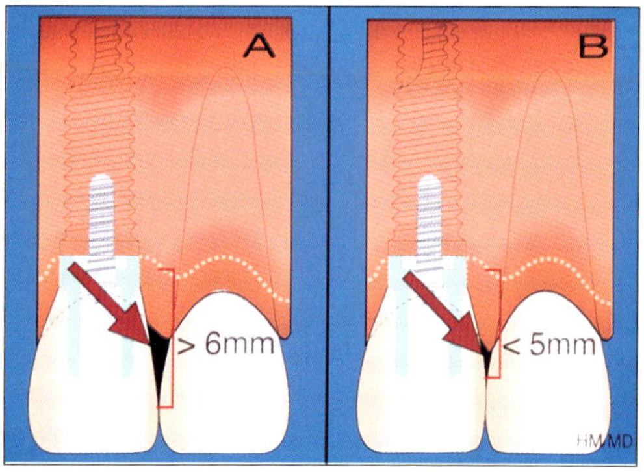

Fig 3-45 a = alveolar ridge-prosthetic contact point distance greater than 6 mm; new papilla formation cannot be complete. b = alveolar ridge-prosthetic contact point distance less than 5 mm; papilla regeneration can be complete.

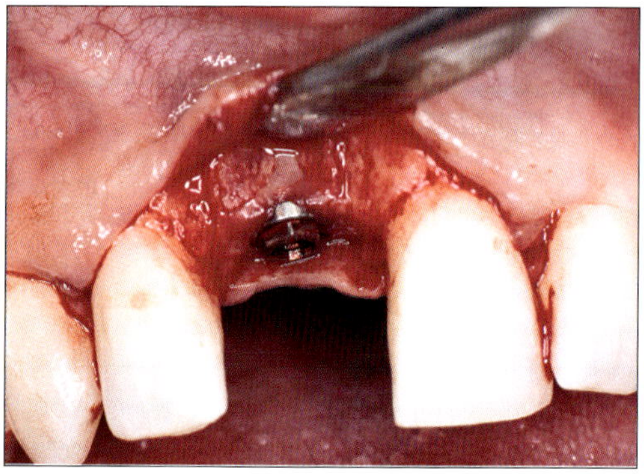

Fig 3-46 Clinical view at stage-two surgery after 8 months of bone healing. Note the crestal bone level.

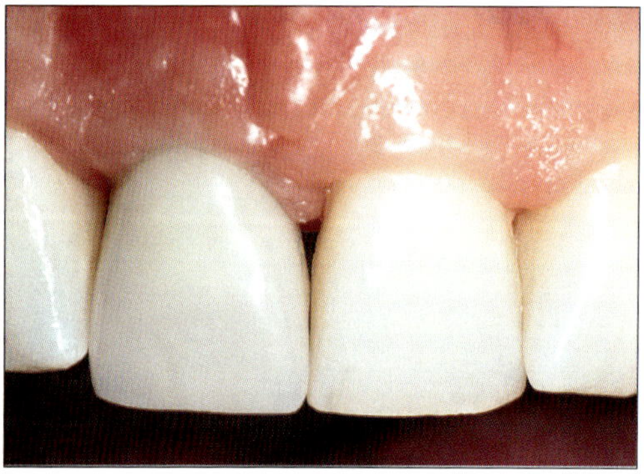

Fig 3-47 Clinical view 3 months after placing a provisional restoration on the maxillary right central incisor.

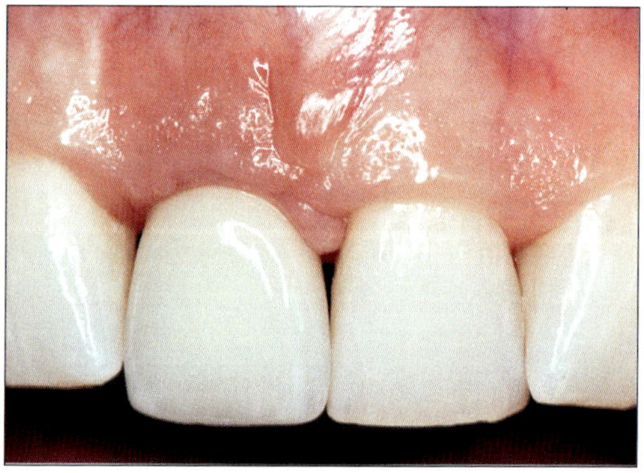

Fig 3-48 Clinical view 1 year after placing the final restoration.

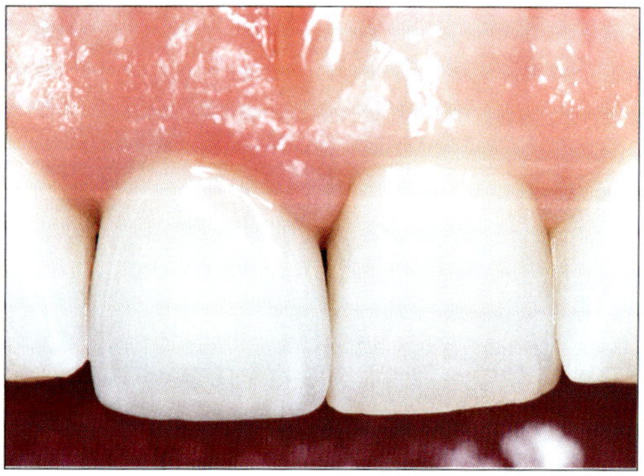

Fig 3-49 Clinical view at 2 years. Note the complete papilla regeneration (restoration, Dr E. Cohen).

achieved if the interdental contact point distance is less than or equal to 5 mm. When the distance is 6 mm, the papilla regenerates in 56% of the cases.[16] In the presence of an alveolar ridge–contact point distance greater than 7 mm, papilla regeneration occurs only 27% of the time. The quality of the provisional restoration is also very important. It must rapidly exert a lateral pressure on the soft tissues after implant abutment connection.

In the presence of ideal interdental contact points, peri-implant papilla regeneration may be achieved (Fig 3-45).[17] The alveolar ridge–contact point distance must be less than or equal to 5 mm. It is therefore essential to optimally position the interdental contact point during temporization (Figs 3-46 to 3-49). Even if these results may be applied to dental implants, it is important to mention that Tarnow et al's study[16] was performed on natural teeth. The available clinical follow-up around implants is very short.

References

1. Brånemark P-I, Zarb GA, Albrektsson T. Tissue-Integrated Prostheses. Chicago: Quintessence, 1985.
2. Bahat O. Interrelations of soft and hard tissues for osseointegrated implants. Compend Contin Educ Dent 1996;17: 1161–1170.
3. Bichacho N, Landsberg CJ. A modified surgical/prosthetic approach for an optimal single implant-supported crown. Part II–The cervical contouring concept. Pract Periodontics Aesthet Dent 1994;6:35–41.
4. Daftary F. Natural esthetics with implant prostheses. J Esthet Dent 1995;7:9–17.
5. Gelb D, Lazzara R. Hierarchy of objectives in implant placement to maximize esthetics: Use of pre-angled abutments. Int J Periodontics Restorative Dent 1993;13:277–282.
6. Israelson H, Plemons JM. Dental implants, regenerative techniques and periodontal plastic surgery to restore maxillary anterior esthetics. Int J Oral Maxillofac Implants 1993;8:555–561.
7. Neale D, Chee W. Development of implant soft tissue emergence profile: A technique. J Prosthet Dent 1994;71:364–368.
8. Garber DA. The esthetic dental implant: Letting the restoration be the guide. J Am Dent Assoc 1995;126:319–325.
9. Grunder U, Spielman HP, Gaberthuel T. Implant-supported single tooth replacement in the aesthetic region: A complex challenge. Pract Periodontics Aesthet Dent 1996;8:830–842.
10. Jansen CE, Weisgold A. Presurgical treatment planning for the anterior single-tooth implant restoration. Compend Contin Educ Dent 1995;16:745–762.
11. Lazzara RJ. Managing the soft tissue margin: The key to implant esthetics. Pract Periodontics Aesthet Dent 1993;5:1–12.
12. Salama H, Salama M, Li TF, Garber D, Adar P. Treatment planning 2000: An esthetically oriented revision of the original implant protocol. J Esthet Dent 1997;9:55–67.
13. Spielman HP. Influence of implant position on the aesthetics of the restoration. Pract Periodontics Aesthet Dent 1996;8:897–904.
14. Palacci P. Aménagement des tissus peri-implantaires: Intérêt de la régénération des papilles. Réal Clin 1992;3:381–387.
15. Salama H, Salama M, Li TF, Garber D, Adar P. Developing optimal peri-implant papillae within the esthetic zone: Guided soft tissue augmentation. J Esthet Dent 1995;7:125–129.
16. Tarnow DP, Wagner AW, Fletcher P. The effect of the distance from the contact point to the crest of bone on the presence or absence of the interproximal dental papilla. J Periodontol 1992;63:995–996.
17. Tarnow DP. Personal communication. 3i Congress, Orlando, FL, 1997.

CHAPTER 4

Implant-Supported Prostheses

E. Hazan/C. Jansen/H. Martínez/M. Davarpanah/P. Raygot/C. Raygot

I. Impression taking in implant prosthodontics

Implant prosthodontics must allow the patient to recover an acceptable chewing function and an esthetic result. In order to achieve this goal, the prosthetic fabrication stages are similar to those of conventional tooth-supported prosthodontics.

In conventional fixed prosthodontics, impressions allow transfer of all information related to the tooth preparations to the laboratory. An accurate replica of the treatment procedure must be obtained intraorally. The same approach is considered for implant prosthodontics.

The aim of this chapter is to describe impression materials, and to analyze the different techniques and approaches to perform reliable, reproducible, and clinically realistic outcomes.

A. Basic concepts

Whatever prosthetic restoration is considered, the methodology used to transfer the intraoral information to the prosthodontic laboratory must follow the same steps: impression taking, master cast pouring, and prosthetic fabrication.

The prosthetic treatment is most often performed after implant exposure and placement of the healing abutments (stage-two surgery). However, some clinicians recommend impression taking at stage-one implant surgery.[1-3] This approach allows fabrication of the prosthetic restoration during the osseointegration period.

B. Prosthetic principles

In tooth-supported fixed prosthodontics, the marginal tooth-prosthesis junction must be as thin as possible and the prosthetic fit perfect. The dimensional changes that occur all along the technologic chain must therefore be compensated for. This chain involves various components and materials: preparation form and contour, impression materials, impression tray, working cast, die spacer, wax pattern, investment material, metal, and cosmetic material.

In implant-supported prosthodontics, the main difficulty is to obtain a passive adaptation of the prosthetic components over the implants.[4,5] It is impossible for the suprastructure to bend beyond its elastic limit. The occlusal forces risk compromising the osseointegration process.[6] Misfitting metal frameworks over the implants and excessive occlusal forces (bruxism) are frequent causes of complications (screw loosening and fracture of the different components).[7-9]

Fabrication of metal frameworks to fit passively over the implants is essential for treatment success. From a clinical point of view, it is difficult to control the potential distortions that may occur during the different prosthetic steps required to achieve the master cast and to control the errors related to the analogue transfer.[6] Radiographic control is essential. The patient must not feel any tension or pain while the screws are placed and tightened on the framework.

C. Impression materials

The impression materials currently used in implant prosthodontics are elastomers. An elastomer is composed of large molecules or polymers linked together by bridges to form a three-dimensional mesh. The elastic bending allows the polymers to distort up to a certain limit and then come back to their initial dimensions. The bridges linking the polymer chains determine the physical characteristics of rigidity and the elastic behavior of the material.

Four types of elastomers are available: the sulfide polymers, the condensation-polymerizing silicones, the addition-polymerizing silicones (polyvinyl siloxane), and the polyethers. The current classification of elastomers established by the American Dental Association is based on some elastic properties and on the dimensional changes.

The characteristics to keep in mind in relation to these materials are:

—Setting time: As a general rule, the setting times recommended by the manufacturers are too short. Waiting an additional amount of time compared to the recommended setting time improves the likelihood of success.
—Registration accuracy: The current impression materials offer great precision in recording reproducible details; it is therefore important to handle them appropriately.
—Permanent bending (distortion): The distortion that occurs during impression removal is minimal if the impression is removed rapidly.

Among the four types of elastomers, the polyvinyl siloxane, or addition silicone, offers the best clinical qualities:

—the best elastic properties
—the lowest permanent bending (0.07%)
—remarkable dimensional stability (dimensional change at 24 hours 0.06%)

—The main disadvantage of these materials is their hydrophobic nature. It is recommended to eliminate all moisture traces prior to impression taking.
—The risk for cytotoxicity when impressions are taken directly on the bone at stage-one surgery must be remembered. A study on five different types of impression materials has demonstrated the risk for cell inhibition. All impression materials present some toxicity.[10] Given that polyethers are currently used in implant prosthodontics, it would be wise to avoid using this material at stage-one implant surgery.

D. Impression techniques

Two impression techniques have been described for implant-supported prosthodontics: the direct (pickup) technique and the indirect technique (Figs 4-1 to 4-9).[11,12]

1. Pickup impressions

An impression screwed-retained transfer coping and a perforated impression custom tray are used. Brånemark et al[4] recommend splinting the impression transfer copings intraorally using silk thread and acrylic resin (Duralay). Carr[13] suggests the use of square transfer copings to avoid any rotation.

The shrinking percentage of the acrylic resin during setting (7.9%) at 24 hours, with 80% of this shrinking occurring in the first 20 minutes, leads to a significant risk of bend-

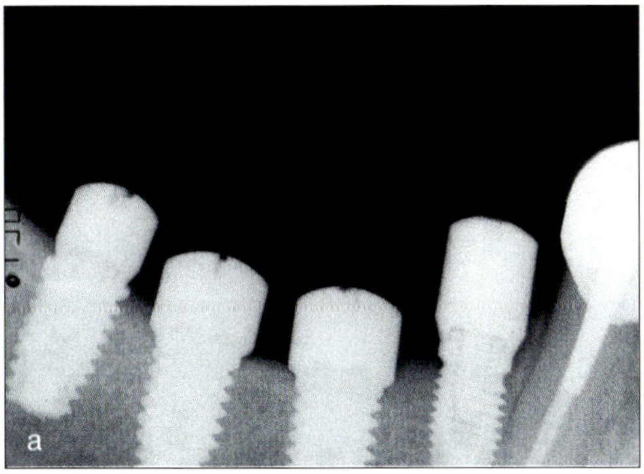

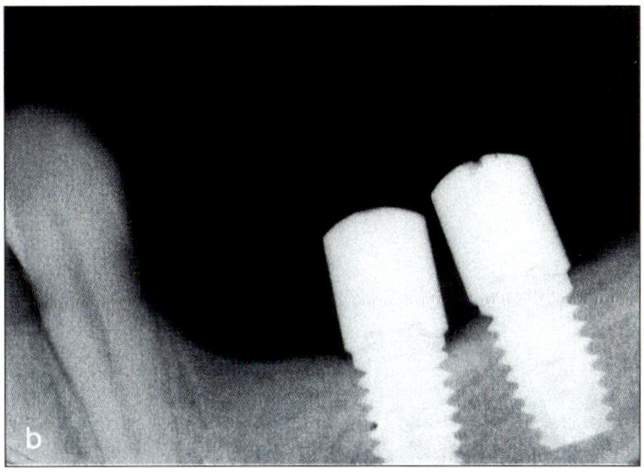

Figs 4-1a and 4-1b Radiographs after placement of the healing abutments. Four 3i implants were placed on the patient's right, and three on the left. The mesial implant on the left was lost during the osseointegration period.

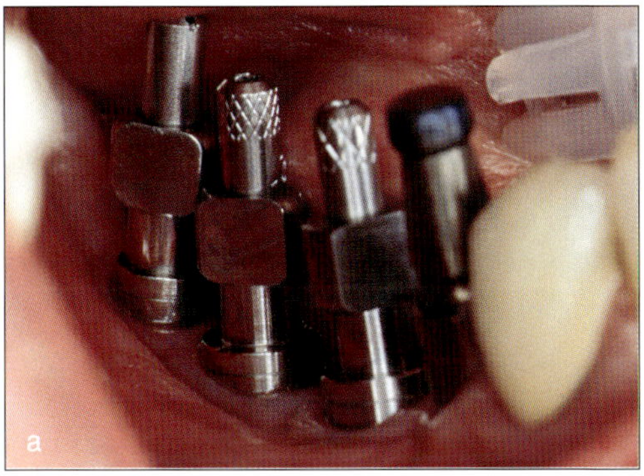

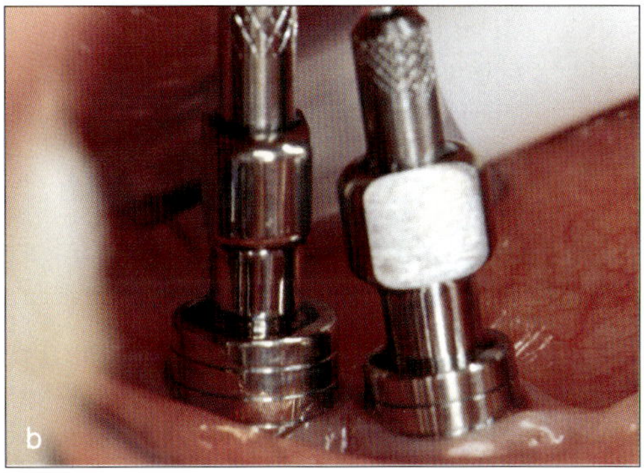

Figs 4-2a and 4-2b Clinical views of the positioned impression transfer copings.

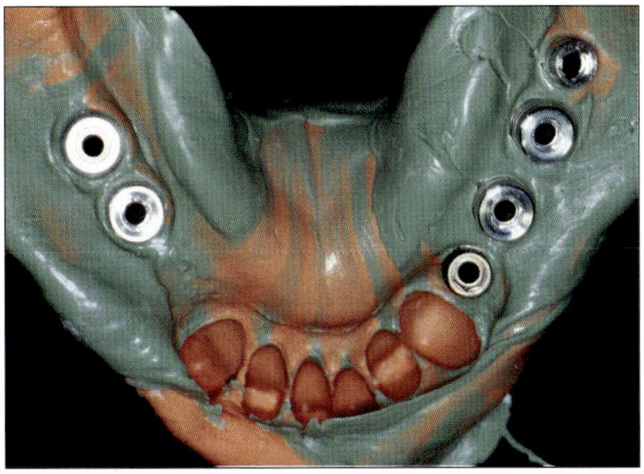

Fig 4-3 Overview of the impression with polyvinyl siloxane.

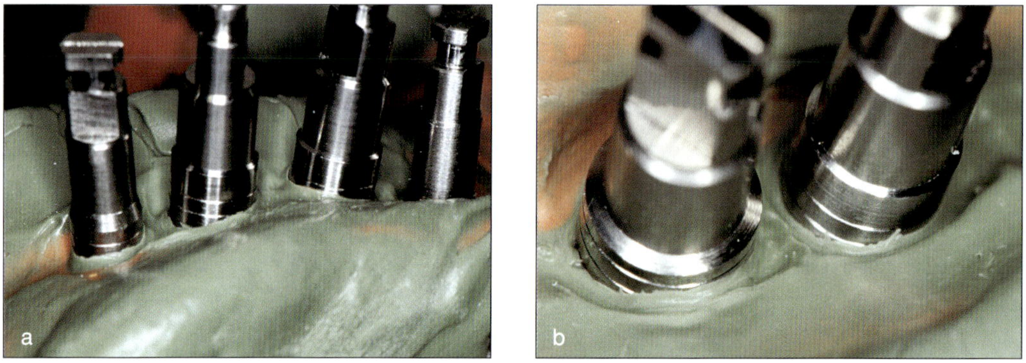

Figs 4-4a and 4-4b Implant abutment analogues positioned on the transfer copings.

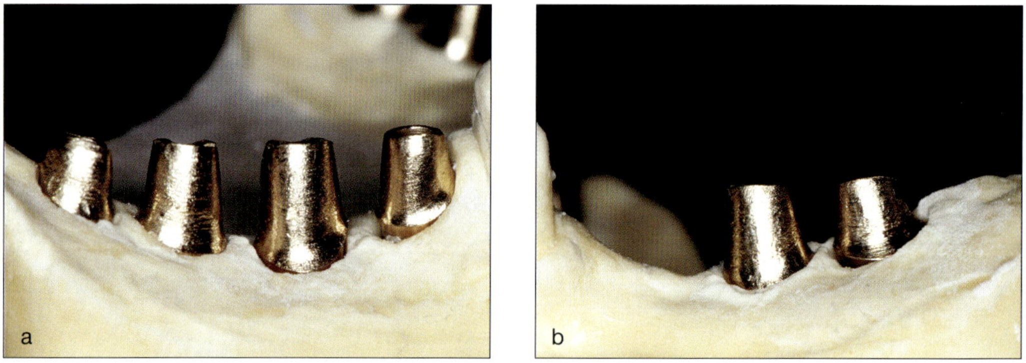

Figs 4-5a and 4-5b Buccal right and left views of UCLA gold inlay cores.

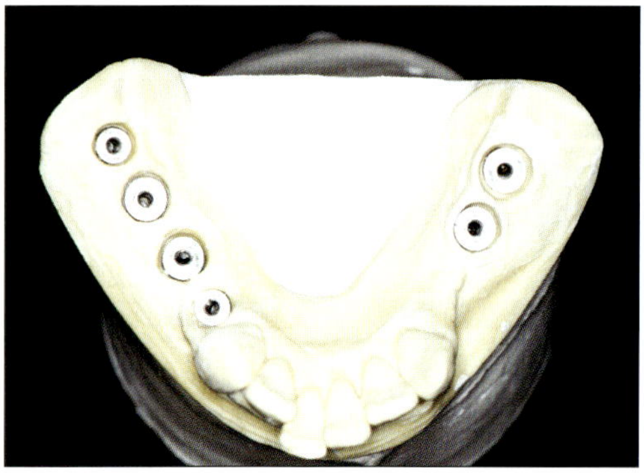

Fig 4-6 Occlusal view of the working cast.

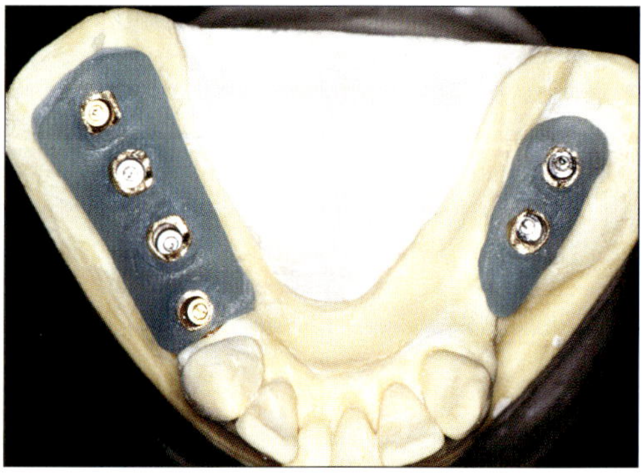

Fig 4-7 Occlusal view of the inlay cores with their acrylic resin guiding matrices, allowing an easy positioning in the mouth.

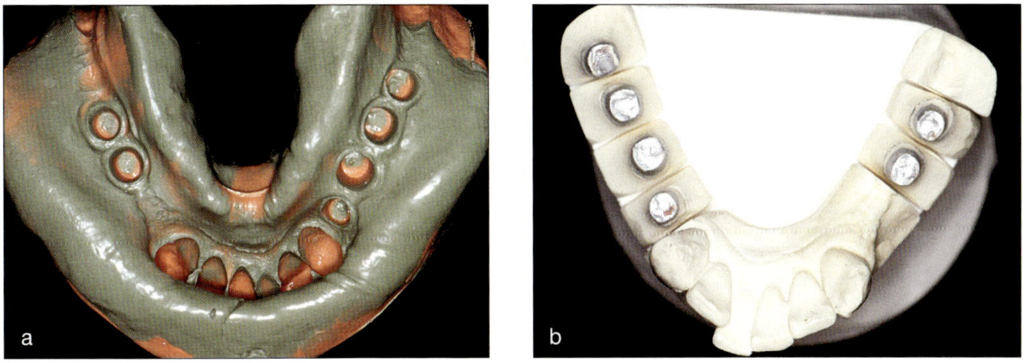

Figs 4-8a and 4-8b Occlusal view of the final impression and working cast.

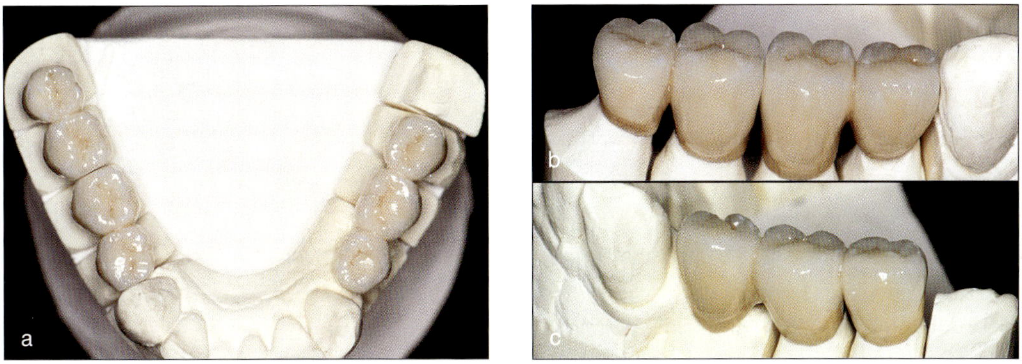

Figs 4-9a to 4-9c Occlusal and buccal views of the porcelain-fused-to-metal fixed partial dentures (restoration, Dr E. Hazan; lab, A. Rohart).

ing.[14] It is therefore recommended to limit the amount of acrylic resin. Assif et al[15] suggest the use of an acrylic resin block formed at least 24 hours prior to the procedure in order to limit distortion. However, other authors have found no significant difference in accuracy using three different techniques.[16,17]

2. *Indirect impressions*

Conical screw transfer copings are placed over the implants. They are then repositioned inside the impression. In this case, the use of a stock impression tray may be considered. For these two techniques, the different handlings may lead to errors in transfer coping positioning. In 1991, Carr[13] compared the accuracy of casts obtained using both impression techniques. This author considers the direct, or pickup, technique more accurate than the indirect technique.

Considerations:

- no consensus has been established for one particular type of impression material
- among the four types of elastomers, the polyvinyl siloxane, or addition silicone, offers the best clinical qualities

II. Screw-retained and cemented prostheses

The preimplant analysis allows the choice between the different prosthetic options. The available bone volume, occlusion, prosthetic imperatives, and the patient's esthetic demands guide the prosthetic choice.[18–23] An implant-supported, screw-retained prosthesis is defined as a restoration screwed onto intermediate abutments, which are in turn screwed onto the implants. An implant-supported cemented prosthesis is defined as a restoration cemented on intermediate inlay cores, which are screwed onto the implants.

A. Principles for implant-supported prosthodontics

Whatever the type of prosthetic anchorage (screw retained or cemented), passive fit of the different components is essential. The insertion of the prosthetic framework must not create any stress. These stresses may generate different prosthetic complications (screw loosening, fractures) or compromise osseointegration.

From a biomechanical point of view, distribution of forces must occur ideally according to the implant axis. However, in the presence of extensive bone loss, or in the anterior maxillary region, it is sometimes difficult to respect this principle.

The cervical limit of an implant-supported prosthesis must be located a maximum of 2 to 3 mm subgingival. The intermediate components adapting on the implant must be machined or cast onto a machined metal base. Good adaptation of these components on the implant collar, as well as perfect polishing of their transmucosal parts, is necessary to maintain soft tissue health.

B. Advantages and disadvantages

1. *Screw-retained prostheses (Figs 4-10 to 4-22)*

a. *Advantages*

The advantages of a screw-retained prosthesis are:

—easy retrievability of the prosthesis
—connections using the machined intermediate abutments
—no need for a luting agent

In the presence of significant soft tissue thickness, the use of an intermediate abutment moves the working surface of the laboratory technician coronally.

b. *Disadvantages*

Esthetics:

—modified occlusal anatomy
—anatomic emergence profile sometimes difficult to achieve
—emergence of the screws on the occlusal surfaces

Function:

—modified occlusal morphology
—difficult occlusal adjustment

Biomechanics:

—less resistance to screw loosening; the torque is 10 Ncm for the gold prosthetic screw and 20 Ncm for the titanium abutment screw
—less resistance to screw fracture
—porcelain fracture risk in the presence of a crown with a reduced occlusal table (premolar), or when the screw is located near the occlusal edge

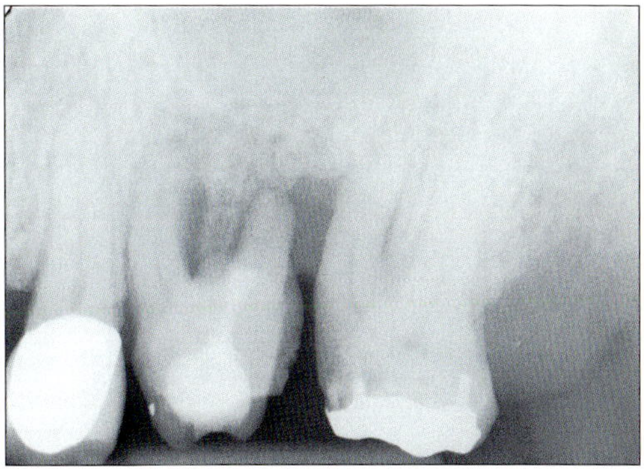

Fig 4-10 Presurgical radiograph showing an endodontic-periodontal involvement that is terminal on the maxillary left first molar and advanced on the buccal roots of the second molar. Extraction of the first molar and root amputation of the buccal roots of the second molar are indicated, with delayed placement of two 3i implants in order to replace the teeth.

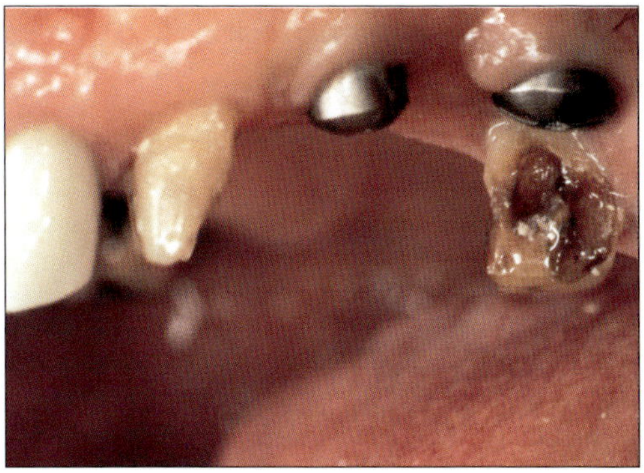

Fig 4-11 Clinical view 6 weeks after exposure of the 3i implants replacing the first and second molars.

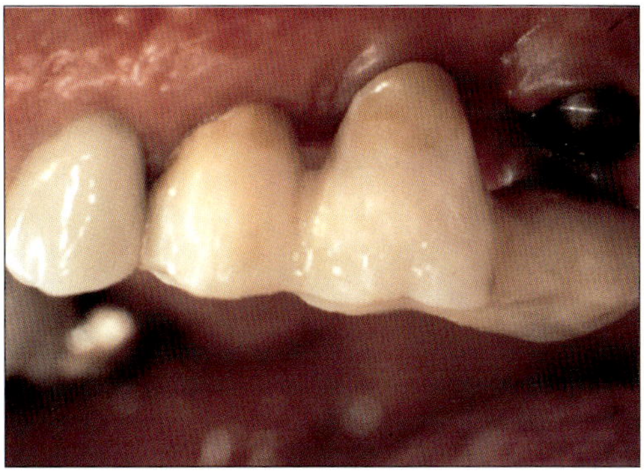

Fig 4-12 Provisional fixed partial denture extending from the second premolar to the palatal root of the second molar.

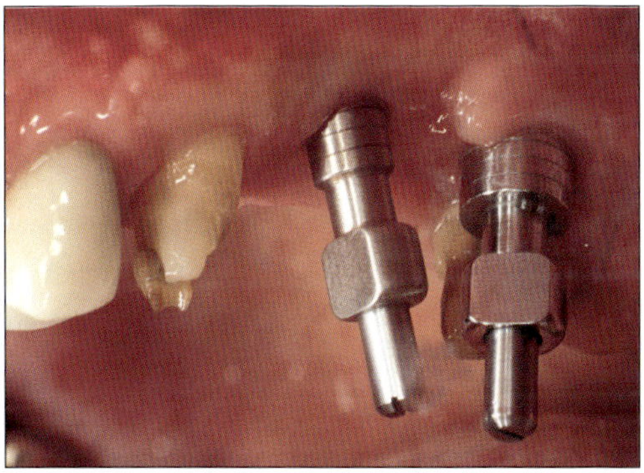

Fig 4-13 Clinical view of the impression transfer copings at intraoral try-in. A standard-diameter transfer coping is on the mesial implant, and a 6-mm-diameter transfer coping is on the large-diameter implant replacing the second molar.

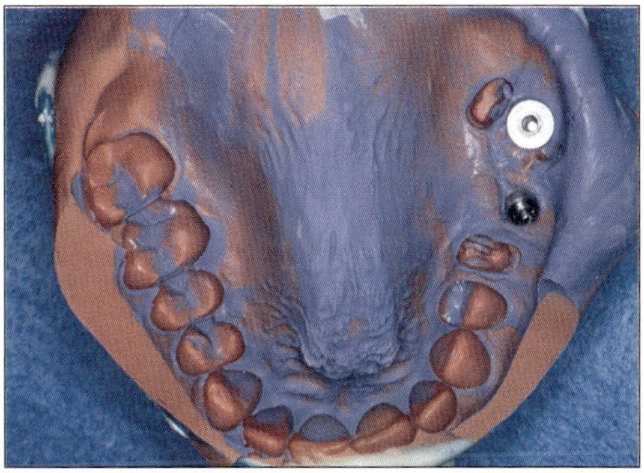

Fig 4-14 Occlusal view of the impression.

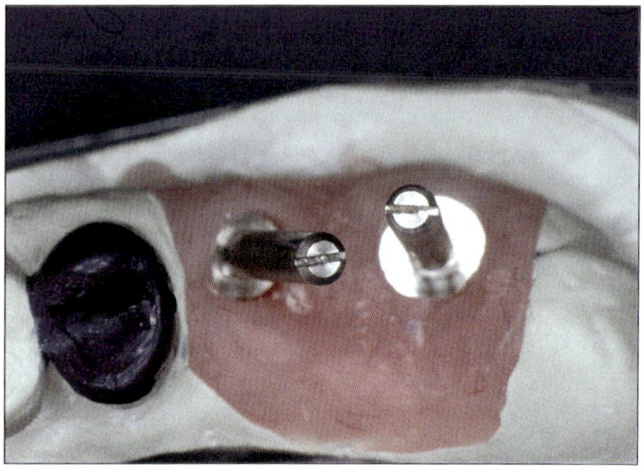

Fig 4-15 Die showing the analogues located in the first and second molar positions.

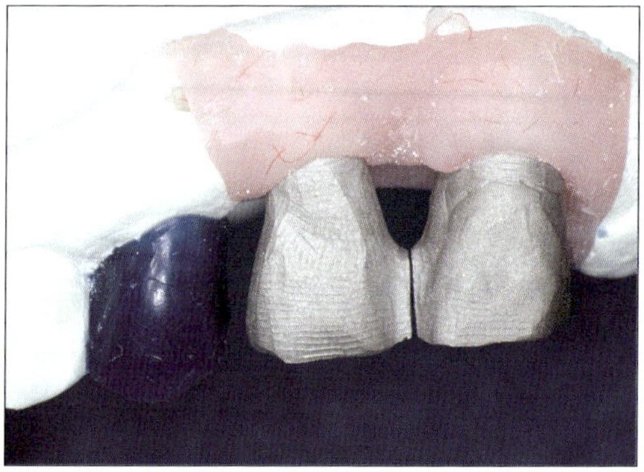

Fig 4-16 Laboratory view of the frameworks replacing the first and second molars.

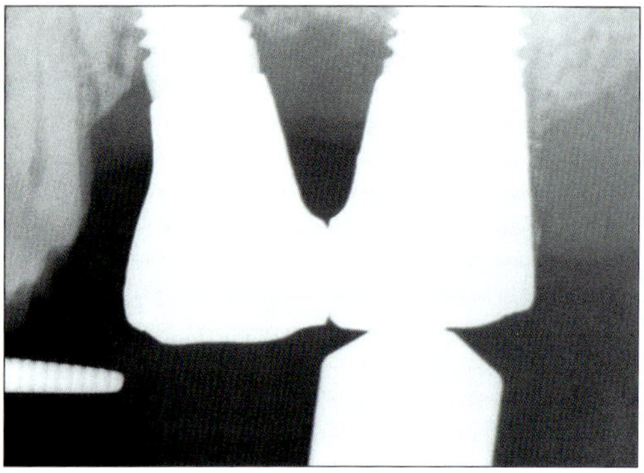

Fig 4-17 Radiographic control of framework fit.

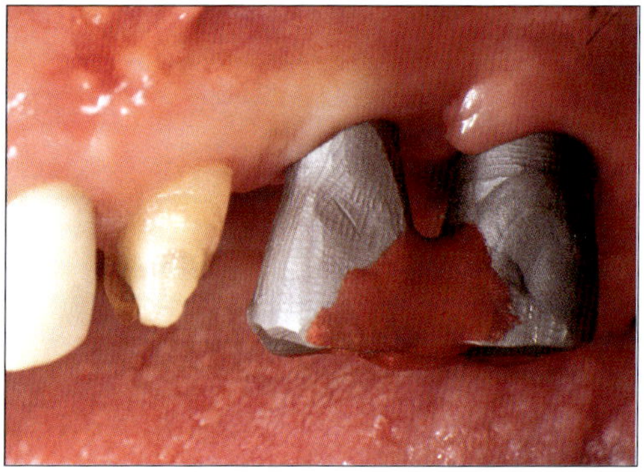

Fig 4-18 Duralay index for primary soldering.

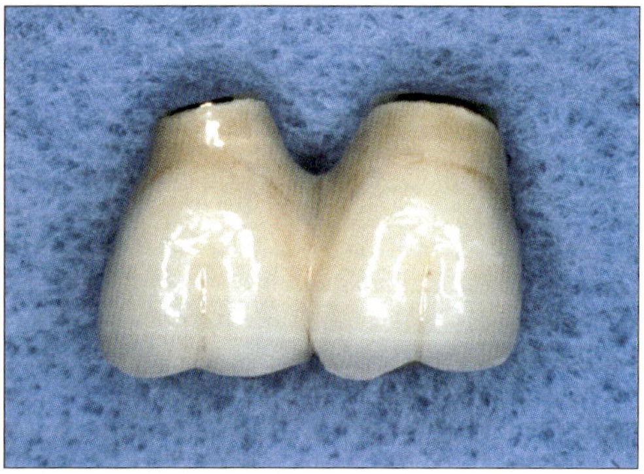

Fig 4-19 Buccal view of the porcelain-fused-to-metal crowns.

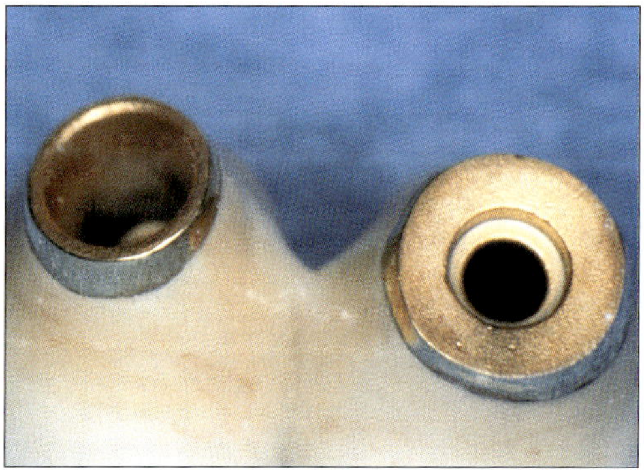

Fig 4-20 Interfacial view of the two splinted crowns: a gold UCLA abutment is used distally for the large-diameter implant, and a mesial conical abutment is on the standard implant.

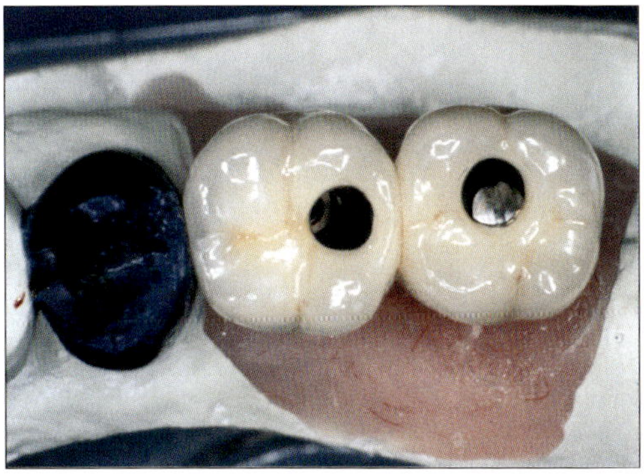

Fig 4-21 Occlusal view of the splinted crowns at the laboratory. Note the occlusal emergence of the screws.

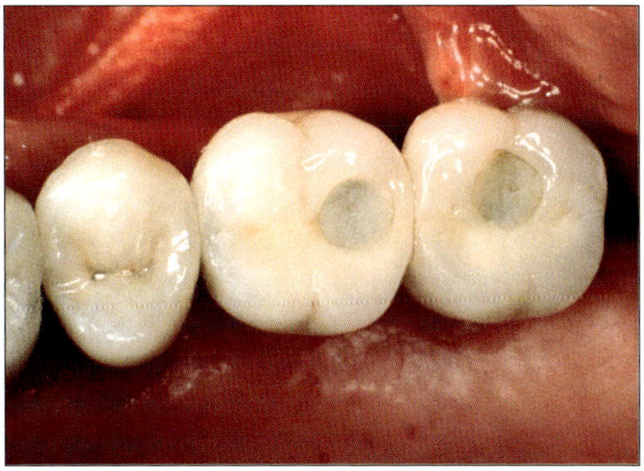

Fig 4-22 Intraoral clinical view after obturation of the access holes (restoration, Dr C. Jansen).

Technique:

–difficult control of passivity: during framework try-in, the screwing may generate distortion and give the illusion of a passive fit
–difficult to perform in the presence of a limited prosthetic space
–performance is rendered delicate by the number of screws and the screwing accuracy; the passivity is possible owing to the second-stage soldering
–difficulty fabricating a provisional restoration
–increased chairside working time

Restoration of a single-unit implant using a screw-retained prosthesis is not advised if the torque is less than 32 Ncm. Intermediate components screwed at 20 Ncm are therefore contraindicated for single-unit restorations.

2. *Cemented prostheses (Figs 4-23 to 4-34)*

a. *Advantages*

Esthetics:

–respect of the prosthetic occlusal surface anatomy
–anatomic emergence profile

Biomechanics and function:

–cementation facilitates a passive adaptation of the framework
–significant resistance to screw loosening torque ranging from 32 to 45 Ncm
–high resistance to screw fracture
–facilitated occlusal adjustment

Technique:

–laboratory technique close to that of conventional prostheses (parallel inlay cores on which a framework is cemented)
–possibility of visual checking for lingual or palatal adjustment
–provisional restoration simple to fabricate

b. *Disadvantages*

The disadvantages of a cemented prosthesis are:

–retrievability is difficult
–risk for subgingival cement excess

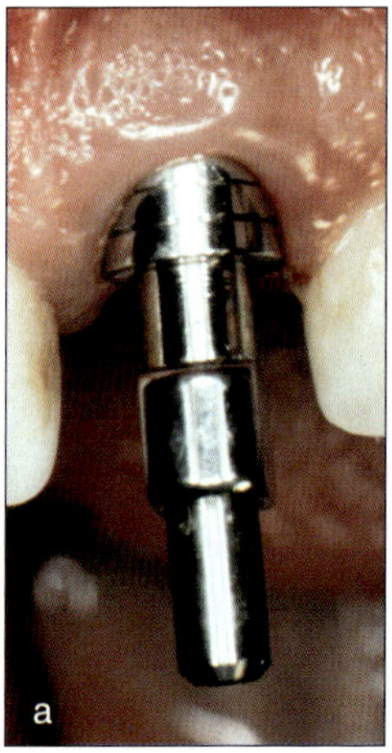

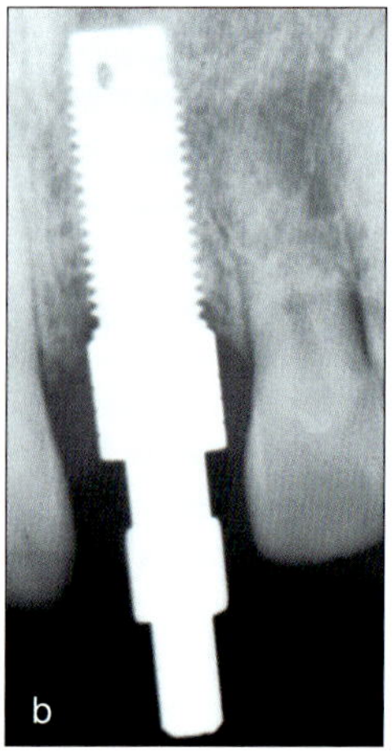

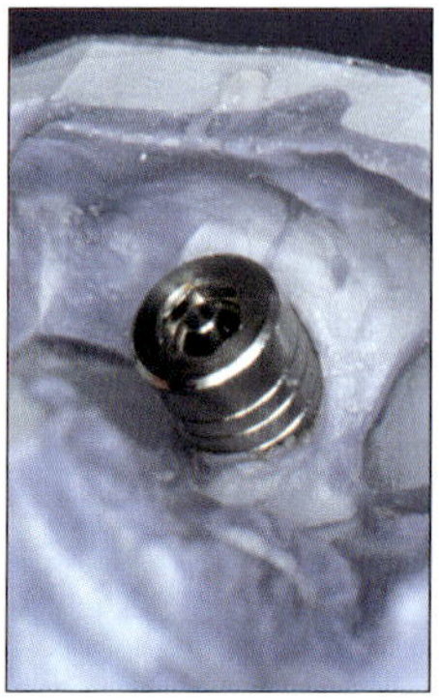

Figs 4-23a and 4-23b Clinical view and radiographic control of the intraoral transfer. Note the fit of the impression transfer coping on the implant head.

Fig 4-24 View of the impression transfer coping inside the impression.

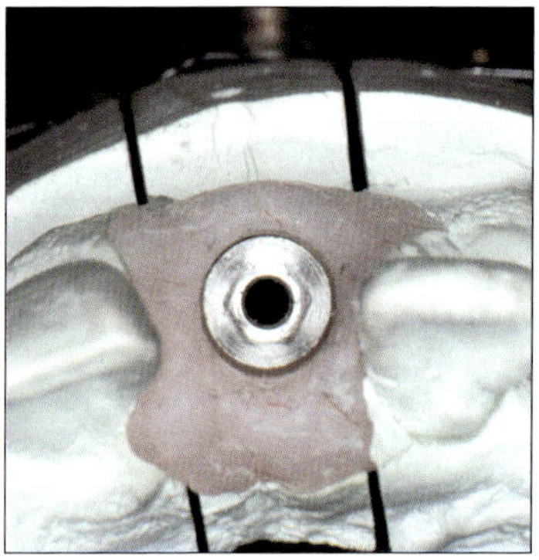

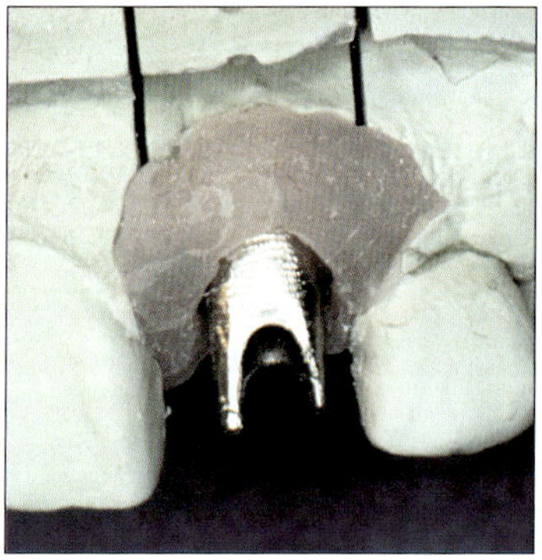

Fig 4-25 Die with the implant analogue. Note the resin soft tissue analogue.

Fig 4-26 Inlay core with the soft tissue analogue on the die.

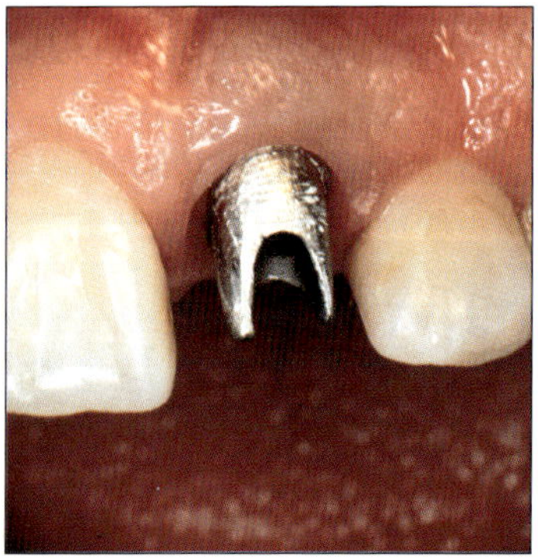

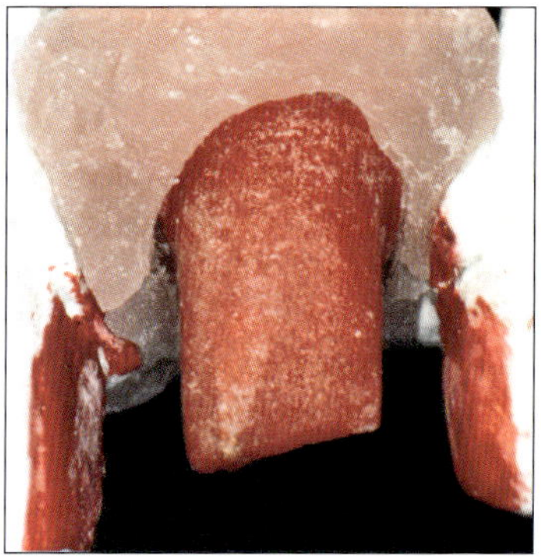

Fig 4-27 Buccal view of the intraoral inlay core.

Fig 4-28 Resin pattern of the future metal framework.

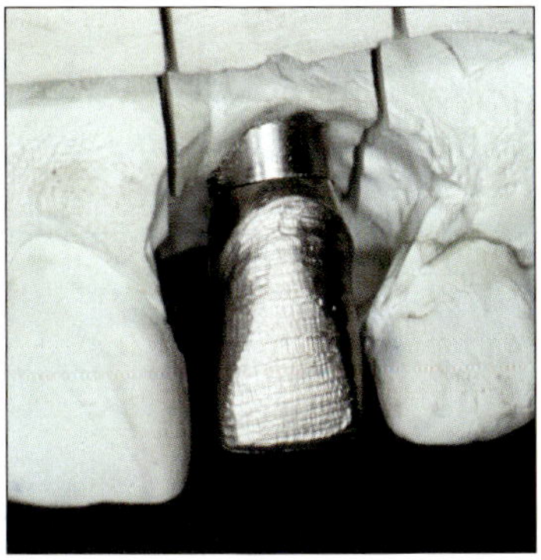

Fig 4-29 View of the framework positioned on the inlay core.

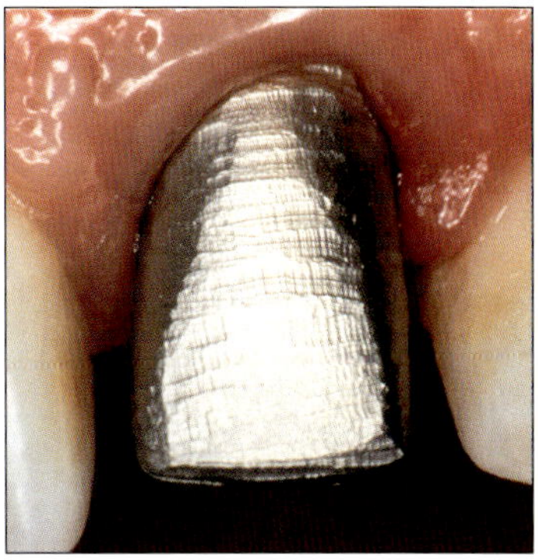

Fig 4-30 Intraoral try-in and control of the framework.

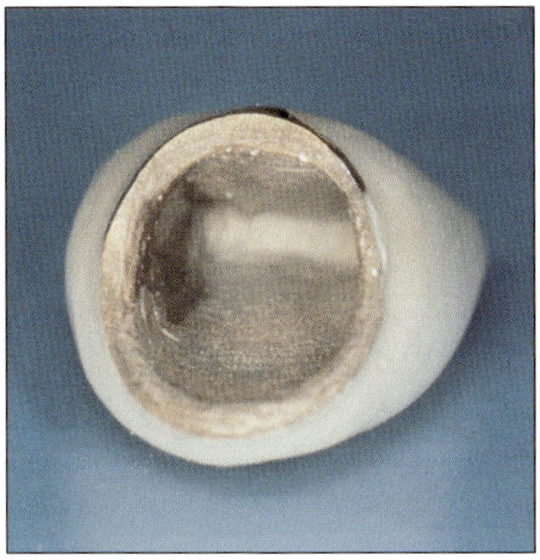

Fig 4-31 View of the porcelain-fused-to-metal interface.

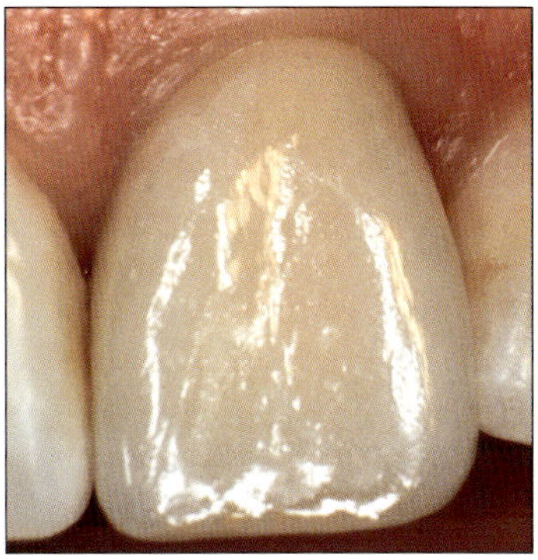

Fig 4-32 Intraoral try-in of the crown.

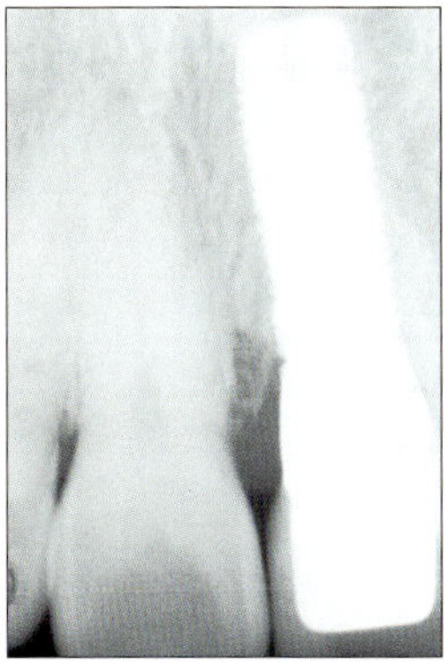

Fig 4-33 Radiograph after implant loading (restoration, Dr C. Jansen).

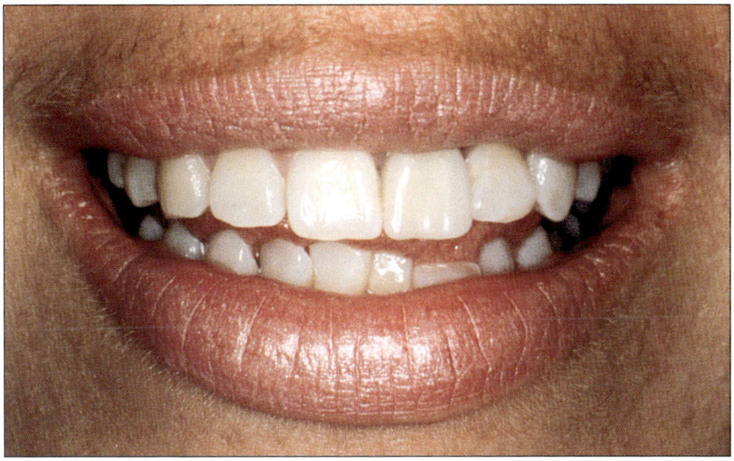

Fig 4-34 Patient's smile.

C. Intermediate components in implant-supported prosthodontics

1. *Definitions*

a. *Abutment*

The abutment is an intermediate component that is always titanium machined. It must not be modified, as it allows screwing of the implant-supported prosthesis. As a general rule, each abutment has a laboratory analogue.

—The abutment may be placed either by the surgeon at stage-two surgery or by the prosthodontist after soft tissue healing.
—The abutment screws are tightened using a 20-Ncm torque. Once positioned, the abutments are never removed until the end of the prosthetic phase.

b. *Inlay core*

The inlay core is an intermediate component machined in titanium, precious alloy, or porcelain. It may be modified at intraoral try-in or at the laboratory:

—the titanium inlay core may be prepared by precision milling
—the precious-alloy machined-base inlay core (UCLA) must be cast on in a compatible metal
—the porcelain inlay core may be prepared by precision milling

2. *Screw-retained prostheses*

Numerous types of abutments are marketed (Fig 4-35). The most frequently used are:

—the conical abutment
—the UCLA gold abutment
—the standard abutment
—the 25-degree angulated abutment.

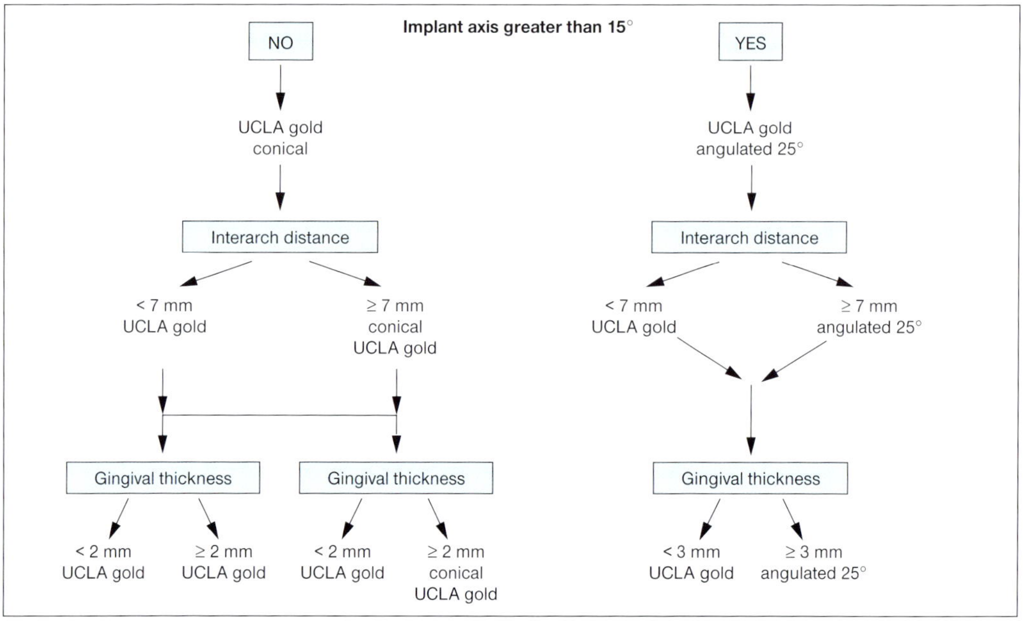

Fig 4-35 Intermediate components in screwed prosthodontics (3i system).

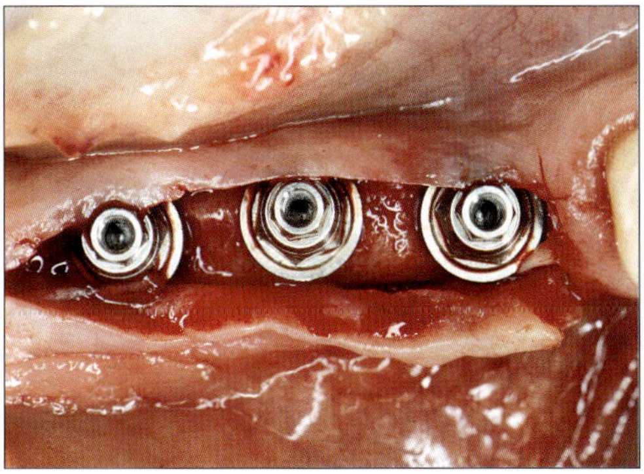

Fig 4-36 Occlusal view of three conical abutments placed at stage-two surgery.

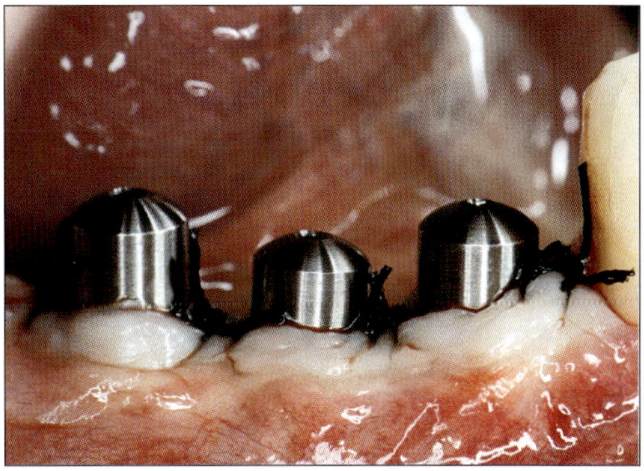

Fig 4-37 Buccal view of the titanium healing caps protecting the abutments.

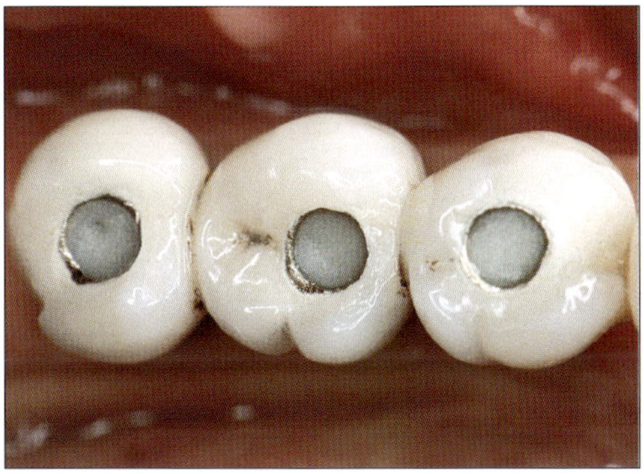

Fig 4-38 Occlusal view of the three splinted porcelain-fused-to-metal crowns (restoration, Dr P. Raygot).

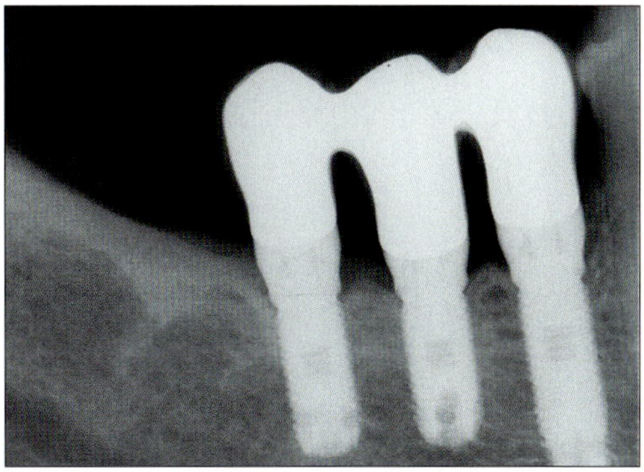

Fig 4-39 Radiographic control at 3 years.

In the presence of significant soft tissue thickness, the use of an intermediate component moves the working surface of the laboratory technician coronally. Abutment selection is most often performed at stage-two implant surgery. For a multiple prosthetic restoration, the abutments may be non-antirotating. For a single-unit restoration, the use of an antirotating abutment is essential.

a. Conical abutment (Figs 4-36 to 4-39)

Today, for esthetic and functional reasons, screw-retained fixed prostheses are most often fabricated on conical abutments. Indeed, these abutments allow improved stability and emergence profile compared to standard ones.

Indications:

—multiple restorations
—positioning the implants in a slightly convergent or divergent direction
—interarch distance of at least 7 mm
—soft tissue thickness of at least 2 mm

Some manufacturers do not market conical abutments presenting significant transmuco-

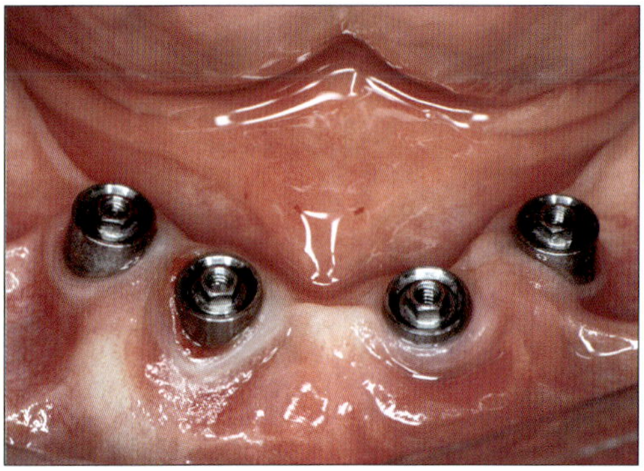

Fig 4-40 Buccal view of four standard abutments in a completely edentulous patient after 6 weeks of soft tissue healing.

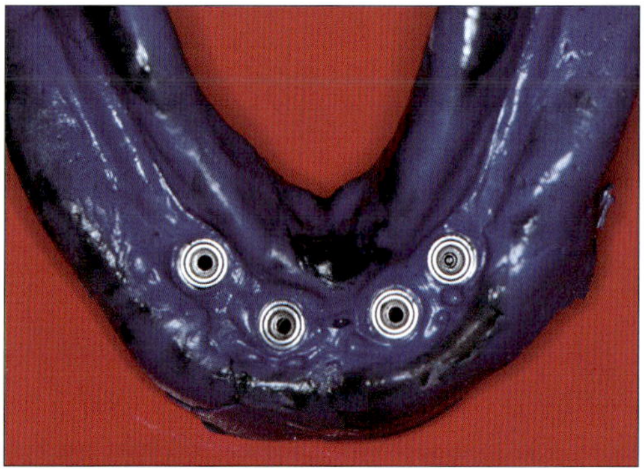

Fig 4-41 View of impression taking using pickup transfer copings.

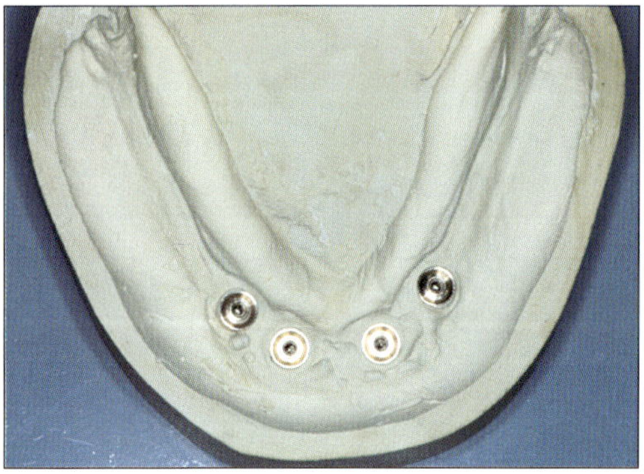

Fig 4-42 Working cast with the implant analogues.

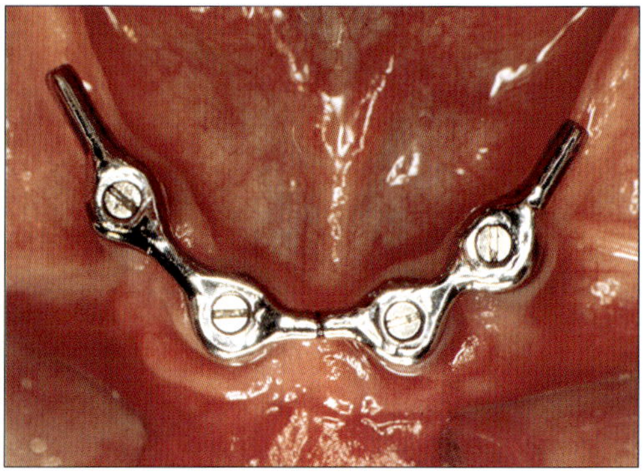

Fig 4-43 The screwed bar is placed on the abutments (restoration, Dr J. Moon).

sal height. The standard abutment is therefore preferable in the presence of thick soft tissues. Indeed, the use of a conical abutment that is too short for significant gingival height requires a very subgingival crown-abutment margin.

b. UCLA gold abutment

This abutment is often used as an inlay core for a cemented prosthesis. Nevertheless, it may sometimes be used to fabricate screw-retained prostheses.

Indications:

- single- or multiple-unit screw-retained restorations
- 30-degree maximum positioning of the implant axis
- interarch distance of at least 4.5 mm
- rehabilitation of esthetic segments with thin mucosa

c. Standard abutment (Figs 4-40 to 4-43)

These abutments are indicated to perform implant-supported fixed dentures and overdentures.

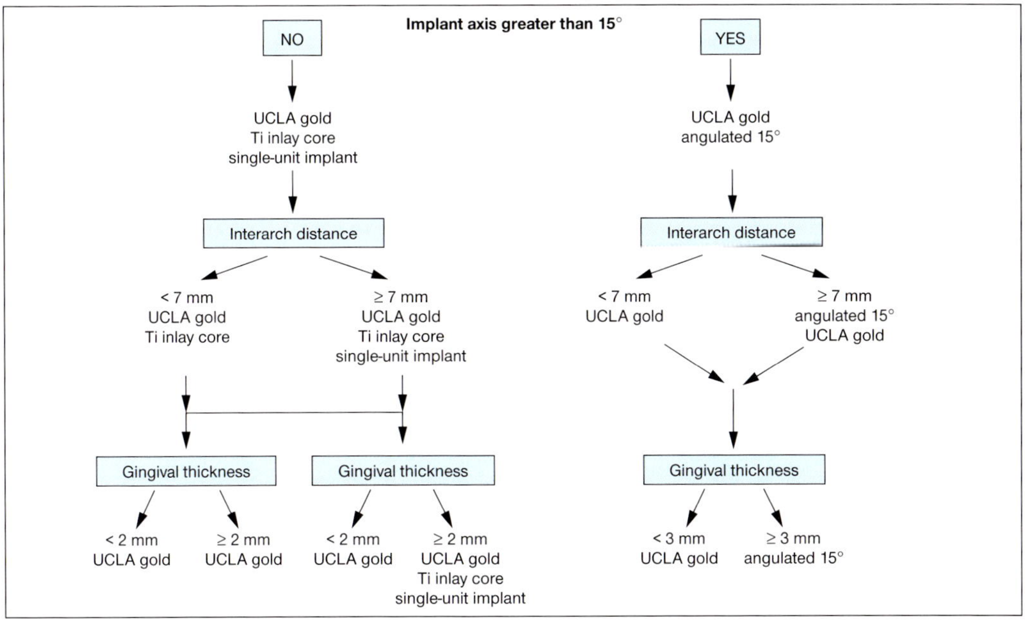

Fig 4-44 Intermediate components in screwed prosthodontics (3i system).

d. 25-degree angulated abutment

This abutment allows correction of angulation problems:

—screw access on the occlusal surfaces
—facilitated oral hygiene
—improved esthetics

Indications:

—multiple restorations
—implant axis correction
—interarch distance of at least 9.5 mm
—soft tissue thickness of at least 3 mm

—Angulated abutments are not advised for single-unit restorations. Prosthesis retention is often insufficient.
—This abutment also allows fabrication of cemented prostheses.

3. Cemented prostheses

Different intermediate components are used to fabricate the cemented prostheses (Fig 4-44):

—the UCLA gold abutment
—the titanium machined inlay core
—the abutment for a single-unit implant
—the gold conical abutment
—the 15-degree angulated abutment
—the porcelain inlay core (if necessary)

a. UCLA gold abutment (Figs 4-45 to 4-48)

Actually, this abutment consists of an inlay core. It offers all the esthetic and functional advantages when used as a screw-retained inlay core supporting a cemented restoration. It is composed of a gold base provided with a castable plastic tube. The latter is modified by

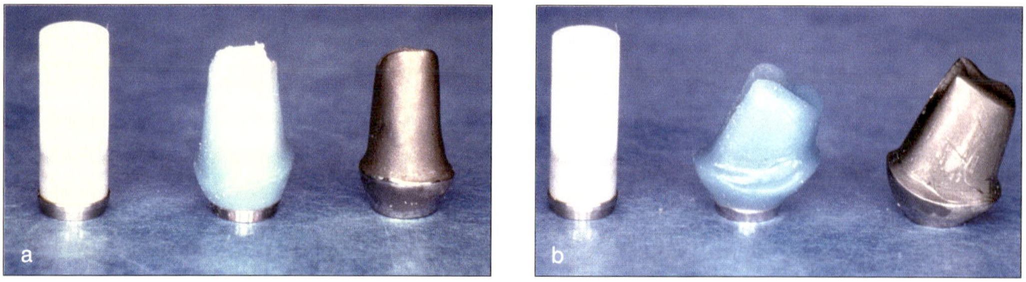

Figs 4-45a and 4-45b UCLA gold abutment allows an ideal emergence profile with various implant axes (angulation less than or greater than 15°).

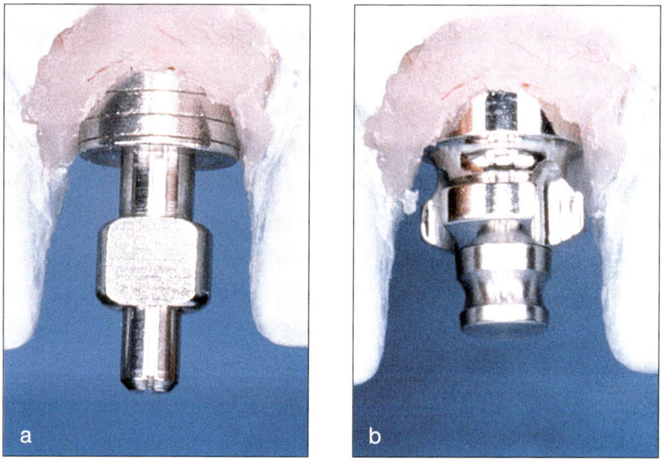

Figs 4-46a and 4-46b The impression may be taken using either a pickup or twist-lock transfer coping (3i).

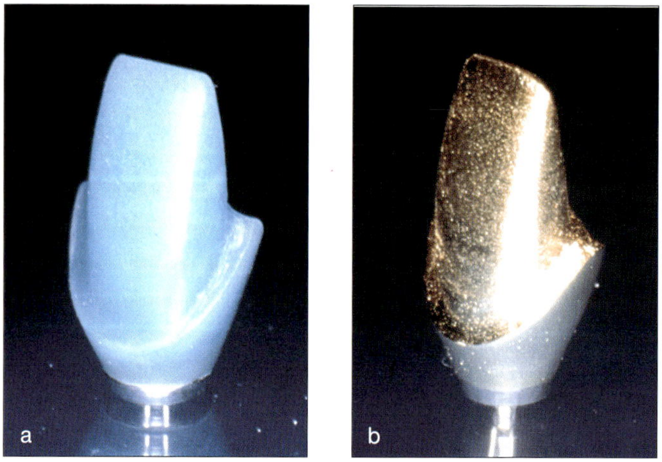

Figs 4-47a and 4-47b Fabrication of the wax pattern and the gold inlay core.

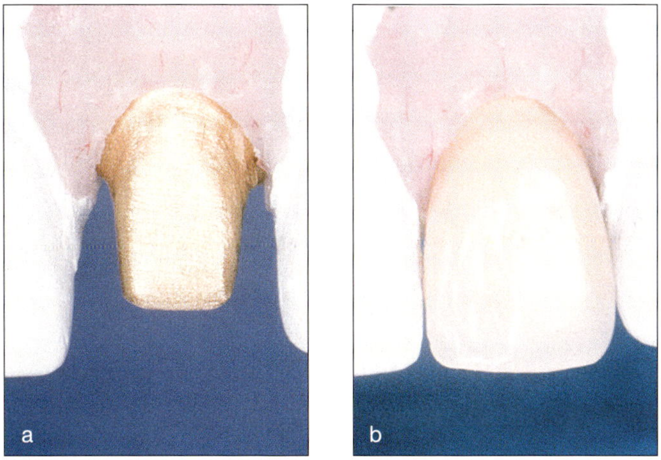

Figs 4-48a and 4-48b Buccal views of the metal coping and the ceramometal crown.

wax addition, then cast on using a precious metal compatible with the base.

Indications:

—single- or multiple-unit cemented restorations
—30-degree maximum positioning of the implant axis
—interarch distance of at least 7 mm
—rehabilitation of esthetic regions presenting a thin mucosa

—The different laboratory fabrication steps must not alter the gold base, which ensures fit accuracy.
—The castable UCLA abutment is strongly disadvised.
—The UCLA abutment with a machined gold base allows perfect fit over the implant.

b. Titanium machined inlay core (Prep-Tite) (Figs 4-49 to 4-52)

The titanium machined inlay core is modified by grinding in order to survey the implant axes. This type of abutment is screwed onto the implant. The limits of this system lie in the amount of titanium to be removed via a spark erosion process in order to compensate for the different implant axes without leading to fracture risk or significant retention loss. This abutment is secured using a gold screw torqued to 32 Ncm.

Indications:

—single- or multiple-unit cemented restorations
—10-degree maximum positioning of the implant axis
—interarch distance of at least 7 mm
—irregular soft tissue contour (modifiable abutment)

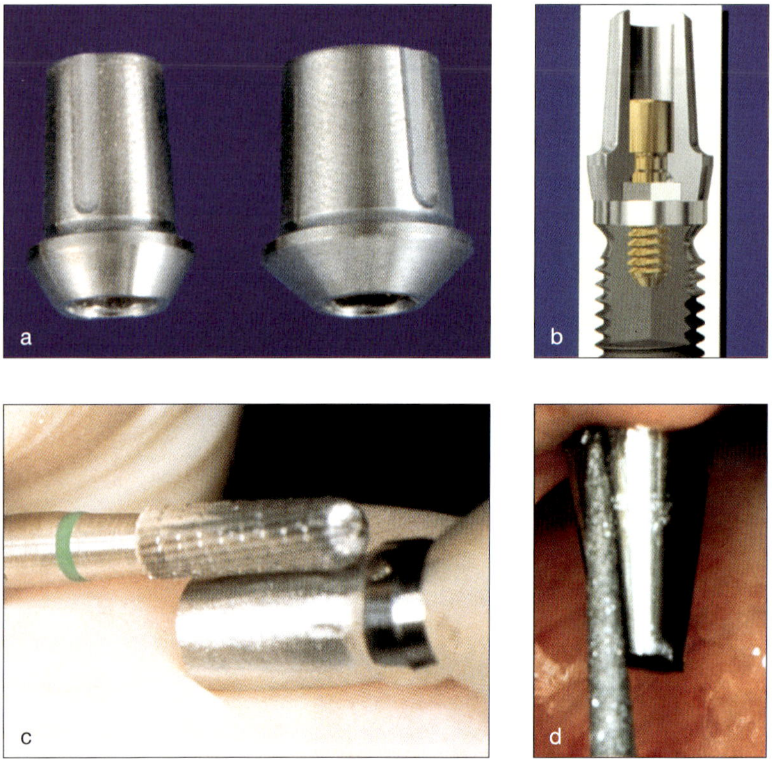

Figs 4-49a to 4-49d Titanium machined inlay core (Prep-Tite): a = view of the two different diameter titanium inlay cores; b = screwing the inlay core using a gold screw at 32 Ncm; c = preparation of the inlay core at the laboratory; d = checking the inlay core preparation for possible intraoral adjustment.

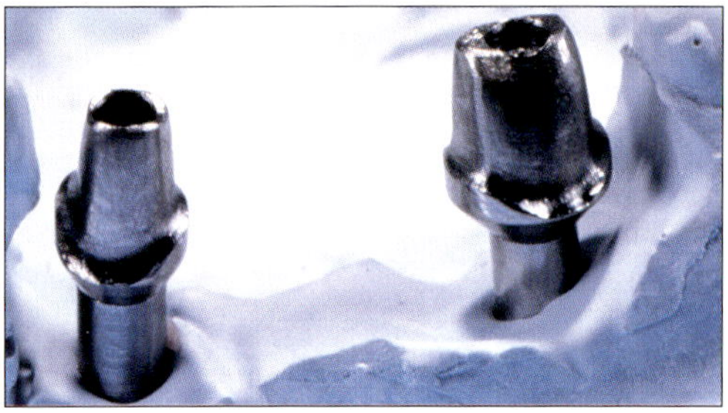

Fig 4-50 Laboratory preparation of the titanium machined inlay cores on the implant analogues.

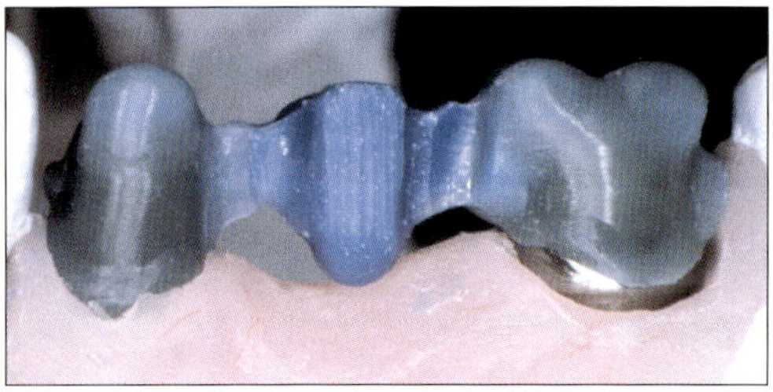

Fig 4-51 Buccal view of the wax pattern fabricated on the titanium inlay cores.

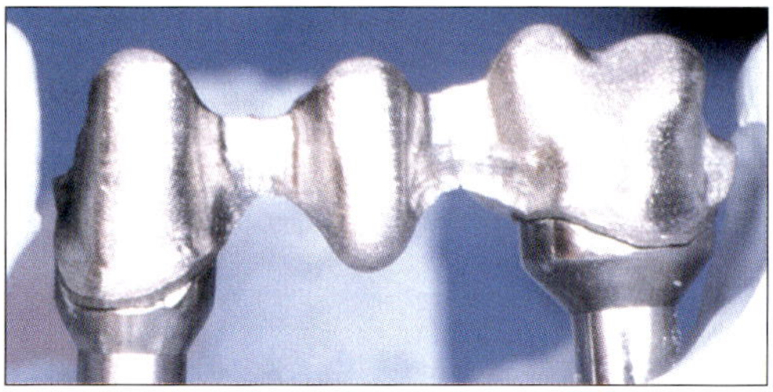

Fig 4-52 Buccal view of the metal framework.

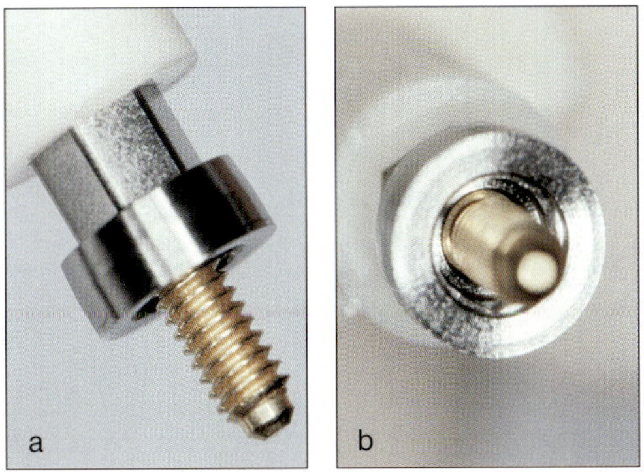

Figs 4-53a and 4-53b Abutment for a single-unit implant (STA) with a gold screw.

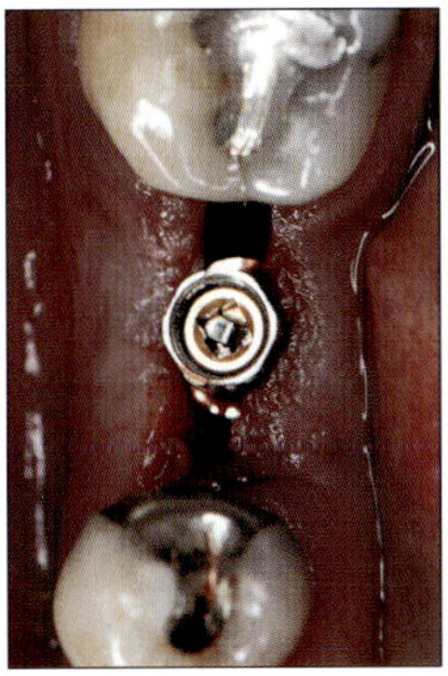

Fig 4-54 Placing the STA abutment at stage-two surgery.

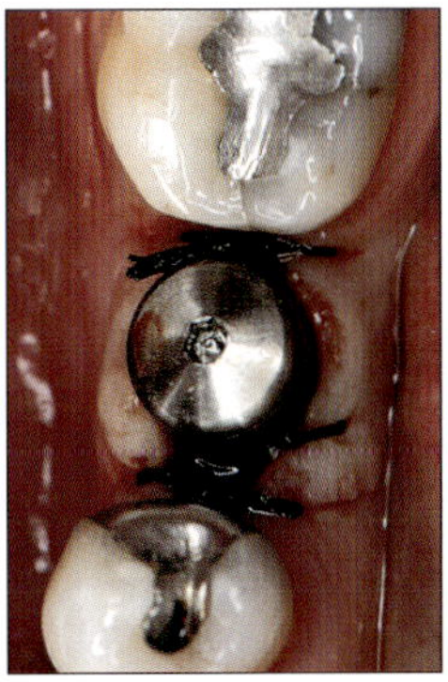

Fig 4-55 Placing the titanium healing cap.

Fig 4-56 Occlusal view of the final prosthetic work (restoration, Dr E. Cohen).

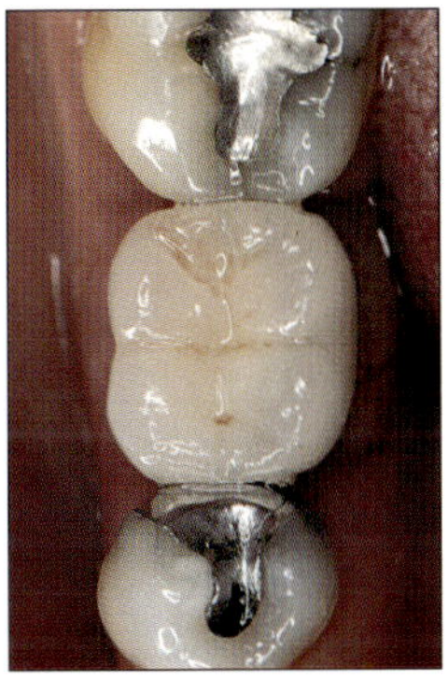

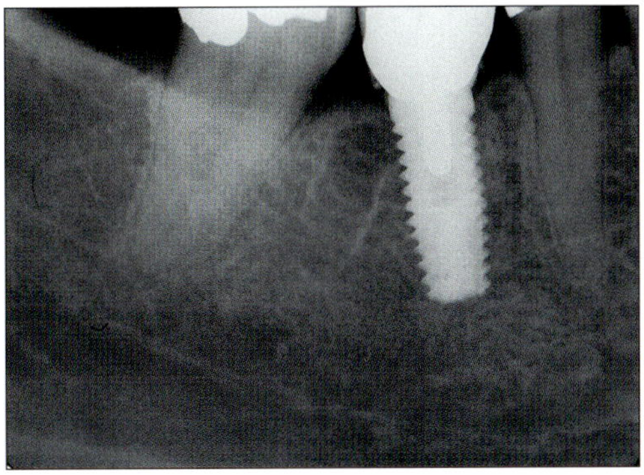

Fig 4-57 Radiographic control at 3 months.

c. *Single-unit implant abutment (STA) (Figs 4-53 to 4-57)*

The abutments for single-unit implants are not modifiable. Implant positioning must be ideal. The abutment may be placed by the surgeon at second-stage surgery. The abutment screw must be torqued using a torque wrench to 32 Ncm.

Indications:

—single-unit cemented restorations
—10-degree maximum positioning of the implant axis
—interarch distance of at least 7 mm
—soft tissue thickness of at least 2 mm, with even contours

The aim of the titanium machined inlay core and the single-unit implant abutment is to simplify the laboratory fabrication. These two abutments do not require a cast-on technique. The use of the titanium machined inlay core gives the clinician freedom to choose the metal for the framework fabrication.

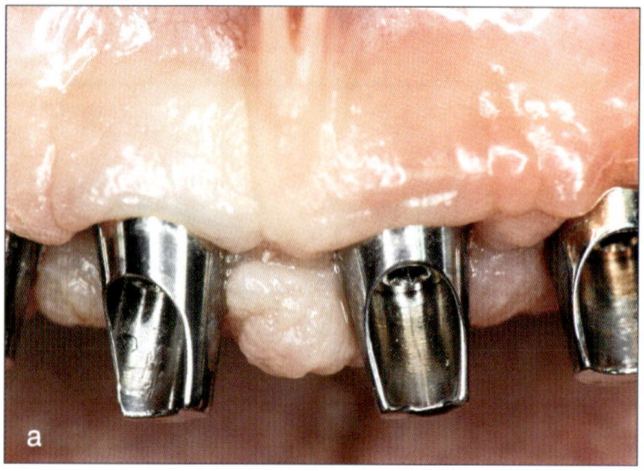

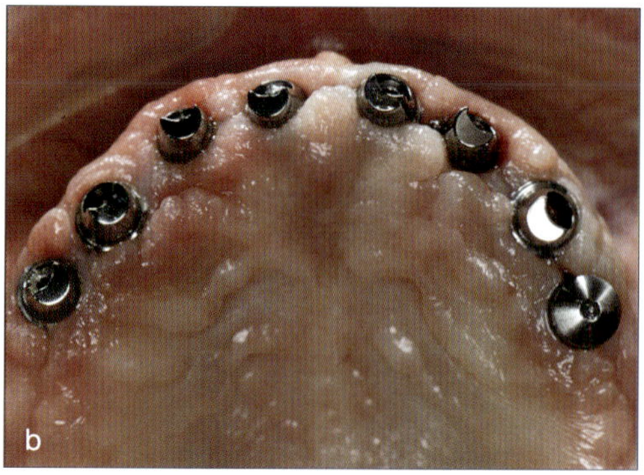

Figs 4-58a and 4-58b Buccal and occlusal views of 15-degree angulated abutments for the treatment of a completely edentulous patient. Note the correction of the implant axes.

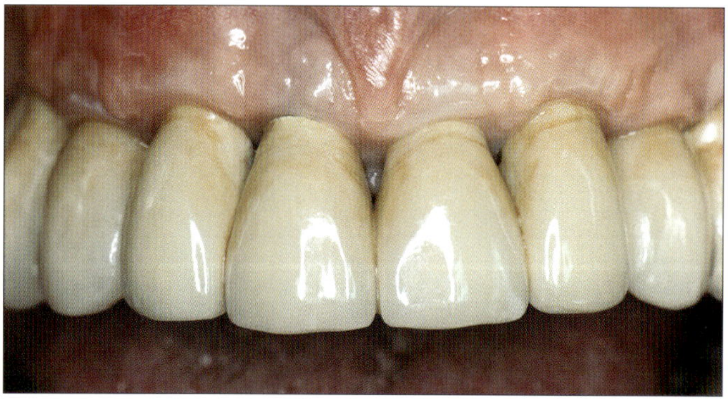

Fig 4-59 Buccal view of the final implant-supported fixed partial denture (restoration, Dr E. Cohen).

d. 15-degree angulated abutment (Gold Post) (Figs 4-58 and 4-59)

This abutment allows correction of the implant axis.

Indications:

—multiple prosthetic restorations
—interarch distance of at least 7.4 mm
—soft tissue thickness of at least 3 mm

D. Prosthesis fabrication

1. Screw-retained prostheses on a conical abutment

a. Impression taking

Two types of impression transfer copings are available:

—Standard transfer copings are screwed into the implants during impression taking. They are repositioned inside the impression prior to pouring. Impression taking is difficult, indeed impossible, if the implant axes are too divergent or convergent.

–Pickup transfer copings remain inside the impression. Their use requires a custom impression tray in order to provide screw access. The splinting of the transfer copings to each other may be achieved using floss and cold-curing acrylic resin. Radiographic control is essential in order to check the fit of the transfer copings over the implants.

b. Casting (impression pouring)

The abutment analogues must be placed on the impression transfer copings prior to plaster pouring. It is essential to fabricate the soft tissue analogue in order to check the fit and allow achievement of an anatomic emergence profile.

c. Removal from the impression

- For the pickup technique, unscrew the transfer screws.
- Carefully separate the plaster cast from the impression.

d. Mounting of casts to the articulator (using a facebow)

e. Fabrication of the framework and provisional restoration at the laboratory

- Use the gold cylinders with the cast-on process for the framework.
- Use titanium or plastic posts for the provisional restoration.

f. Intraoral framework try-in

- It is sometimes necessary to cut the framework and splint it intraorally using cold-curing acrylic resin.
- Perform soldering at the laboratory in order to obtain passive fit.

Method to determine fit quality:
–screwing of the framework at one end and checking the fit on the opposite end
–tactile check using a probe; the average precision is about 100 μm
–radiographic (periapical) control; the average precision is about 200 μm
–checking with direct visual control

g. Biscuit try-in

- Check passivity and fit.
- Adjust occlusion.
- Check function, speech, and esthetics.

h. Placing the final restoration

- Control tightening of the abutment screws at 20 Ncm.
- Tighten the gold screws at 10 Ncm.
- Perform temporary obturation of the screw access holes (cotton pellet covered with temporary cement).
- Control tightening of the gold screws (10 Ncm) at 7 and 15 days.

i. Obturation of the screw access holes

The screw access holes are obturated using composite after having interposed a cotton pellet. The use of impression transfer copings recording the hex position of the antirotating abutment is essential for a single-unit restoration and optional for a multiple-unit restoration. The UCLA gold abutment may be used for a screw-retained restoration.

2. *Cemented prostheses*

The prosthetic fabrication using the different abutments will be described.

a. *UCLA gold abutment*

I. Impression taking

The impression transfer copings (pickup or standard) are positioned: the diameter of the transfer coping used must correspond with that of the implant and the healing abutment. It is essential to check the fit of the transfer copings over the implants on a radiograph.

II. Casting (impression pouring)

The implant analogues are placed on the impression transfer copings prior to plaster pouring. The use of a soft tissue analogue is essential in order to check the fit and allow an anatomic emergence profile.

III. Removal from the impression

- For the pickup technique, unscrew the transfer screws.
- Carefully separate the plaster cast from the impression.

IV. Mounting the casts to an articulator (using a facebow)

V. Fabrication of the screwed inlay cores

The waxup technique facilitates the achievement of an anatomic morphology.

VI. Fabrication of the framework and the provisional denture

It is advised to place a notch at the cervical limit in the waxup on the lingual aspect in order to allow insertion of a crown remover in case retrieval is necessary.

VII. Framework try-in

- The screwed inlay cores are placed.
- A periapical radiograph is obtained for fit control.
- Tighten screw at 32 Ncm.
- Place the framework.
- If the fit is perfect, occlusion is recorded using a polyvinyl siloxane material or a type of recording wax.
- If the fit is inadequate, the framework is cut and splinted.
- Take a full impression of the positioning (silicone).

VIII. Placing the provisional restoration

- Tighten the abutment screws at 32 Ncm.
- Splint the components intraorally.
- Cement using temporary cement.

IX. Biscuit try-in

- Attain visual control (on the lingual aspect) and radiographic control of the fit.
- Make occlusal adjustment.
- Check function, speech, and esthetics.

X. Placing the final restoration

- Cement using a temporary cement.
- Remove excess cement using a probe.

b. *Titanium machined inlay cores (Prep-Tite)*

I. Impression taking

The impression transfer copings (pickup or standard) are positioned: the diameter of the transfer coping used must correspond with that of the implant and the healing abutment. It is essential to check the fit of the transfer copings over the implants on a radiograph.

II. Casting (impression pouring)

The implant analogues are placed on the impression transfer copings prior to plaster pouring.

III. Removal from the impression

- For the pickup technique, unscrew the transfer screws.
- Carefully separate the plaster cast from the impression.

IV. Mounting the casts to an articulator (using a facebow)

V. Survey and coronal adjustment of the laboratory abutments

- Select the abutment that best corresponds to the clinical situation.
- Prepare the abutments by grinding with a bur.

VI. Fabrication of the framework and the provisional denture

It is advised to place a notch at the cervical limit in the waxup on the lingual aspect.

VII. Framework try-in

- The screwed inlay cores are placed.
- A periapical radiograph is obtained for fit control.
- Place the framework.
- If the fit is perfect, occlusion is recorded using a polyvinyl siloxane material.
- If the fit is inadequate, the framework is cut and splinted.

VIII. Placing the provisional restoration

- Tighten the abutment screws at 32 Ncm.
- Splint the components intraorally.
- Cement using temporary cement.

IX. Biscuit try-in

- Achieve visual control (on the lingual aspect) and radiographic control of the fit.
- Make occlusal adjustment.
- Check function, speech, and esthetics.

X. Placing the final restoration

- Cement using a temporary cement.
- Eliminate excess cement using a probe.

c. *Single-unit implant abutment (STA)*

The abutment may be placed by the surgeon at second-stage surgery and covered with a healing abutment. Selection of abutment height for the single-unit implant may be performed more accurately after complete healing of the soft tissues surrounding a healing abutment.

I. Impression taking

The impression is taken using a specific friction-secured transfer coping on the abutment. The transfer remains inside the impression.

II. Casting (impression pouring)

The implant analogues are placed on the impression transfer copings prior to plaster pouring.

III. Removal from the impression

Carefully separate the plaster cast from the impression.

IV. Mounting the casts to an articulator (using a facebow)

V. Fabrication of the framework and building the porcelain and provisional restoration

Fabricate a metal coping. It is possible to use an aluminum coping instead of the metal coping and to build the porcelain crown onto it. The esthetic outcome is improved by this technique. However, some authors emphasize the fragility of this aluminum coping.

VI. Biscuit try-in

- Achieve control of contact points, occlusion, and esthetics.
- Achieve control of the marginal fit.

VII. Placing the provisional restoration

- Cement using a temporary cement.
- Perform fit control.

VIII. Placing the final restoration

- Cement using a temporary cement.
- Perform fit control.

The final restoration success depends on good diagnosis, prosthetic design, and good cooperation between the surgeon, the prosthodontist, and the laboratory technician.

References

1. Henry PJ, Tan AE, Uzawa S. Fit discrimination of implant-supported fixed partial dentures fabricated from implant level impressions made at stage I surgery. J Prosthet Dent 1997;77:265–270.
2. Hochwald DA. Surgical template impression during stage I surgery for fabrication of a provisional restoration to be placed at stage II surgery. J Prosthet Dent 1991;66:796–798.
3. Prestipino V, Ingber A. Implant fixture position registration at the time of fixture placement surgery. Pract Periodontics Aesthet Dent 1994;6:73–82.
4. Brånemark P-I, Zarb GA, Albrektsson T. Tissue-Integrated Prostheses. Chicago: Quintessence, 1985.
5. Fenton AH, Jamshaid A, Davis D. Osseointegrated fixture mobility [abstract 62]. J Dent Res 1987;66:144.
6. Spector MR, Donovan TE, Nicholls JI. An evaluation of impression techniques for osseointegrated implants. J Prosthet Dent 1990;63:444–447.
7. Adell RM, Lekholm U, Rockler B, Brånemark P-I. A 15-year study of osseointegrated implants in the treatment of the edentulous jaw. Int J Oral Surg 1981;10:387–416.
8. Albrektsson T, Jansson T, Lekholm U. Osseointegrated dental implants. Dent Clin North Am 1986;30:151–174.
9. Worthington P, Bolender CL, Taylor TD. The Swedish system of osseointegrated implants: Problems and complications encountered during a 4 year trial period. Int J Oral Maxillofac Implants 1987;2:77–84.
10. Sydiskis RJ, Gerhardt DE. Cytotoxicity of impression materials. J Prosthet Dent 1993;69:431–435.
11. Guez G, Hary F. Les empreintes en prothèse implantaire. Implant 1998;4:165–169.
12. Jendresen MD, Allen EP, Bayne SC, et al. Annual review of selected dental literature: Report of the American Academy of Restorative Dentistry. J Prosthet Dent 1994;72:68.
13. Carr AB. A comparison of impression techniques for a five-implant mandibular model. Int J Oral Maxillofac Implants 1991;6:445–455.
14. Mojon P, Oberholzer J, Meyer JM, Belser UC. Polymerization shrinkage of index and pattern acrylic resins. J Prosthet Dent 1990;64:684–688.
15. Assif D, Fenton A, Zarb G, Schmitt A. Comparative accuracy of implant impression procedures. Int J Periodontics Restorative Dent 1992;12:113–121.
16. Hsu CC, Millstein PL, Stein RS. A comparative analysis of the accuracy of implant transfer techniques. J Prosthet Dent 1993;69:588–593.
17. Humphries RM, Yaman P, Bloem TJ. The accuracy of implant master casts constructed from transfer impressions. Int J Oral Maxillofac Implants 1990;5:331–336.
18. Agar JR, Cameron SM, Hughbanks JC. Cement removal from restorations luted to titanium abutments with simulated subgingival margins. J Prosthet Dent 1997;78:43–47.
19. Jornéus L, Jemt T, Carlsson L. Loads and designs of screw joints for single crowns supported by osseointegrated implants. Int J Oral Maxillofac Implants 1992;7:353–359.
20. Kenneth SH, Reena CG. Cement-retained versus screw-retained implant restorations: Achieving optimal occlusion and esthetics in implant dentistry. J Prosthet Dent 1997;77:28–35.
21. Misch CE. Screw-retained versus cement-retained implant supported prostheses. Pract Periodontics Aesthet Dent 1995;7:15–18.
22. Misch CE. Principles for cement retained fixed implant prosthodontics. In: Contemporary Implant Dentistry. St Louis: Mosby, 1999:549–573.
23. Singer A, Serfaty V. Cement retained implant supported fixed partial dentures. Int J Oral Maxillofac Implants 1996;11:645–649.

CHAPTER 5

Treatment Considerations for Complete Edentulism

M. Davarpanah/E. Cohen/O. Fromentin/H. Martínez/J.-L. Sauvan

For a completely edentulous patient, the treatment choice depends on several parameters:

–prosthetic and esthetic patient demands
–edentulism etiology
–duration of the edentulous situation
–patient's psychologic profile
–esthetic and functional quality of the existing prostheses

Indications for implants are:

–absence of stability of the removable prostheses
–discomfort caused by the removable prostheses
–realistic prosthetic patient demands
–psychologic problems related to the wear of removable prostheses

Some contraindications are absolute:

–unrealistic prosthetic and/or esthetic patient demands
–psychologic disorders
–uncontrolled systemic disease
–alcohol, drug, or tobacco dependence

Some contraindications are relative:

–insufficient bone volume
–poor bone quality
–insufficient hygiene

I. Diagnosis

Different clinical and radiographic means allow establishment of the diagnosis for the completely edentulous patient:

–The panoramic roentgenogram and the study casts mounted on an articulator in centric relation, with an appropriately determined vertical dimension of occlusion, provide the first data required for choosing a prosthesis type.
–Skeletal jaw relationships and available prosthetic space must be assessed.[1]
–The existing complete denture or the temporary diagnostic prosthesis confirms the vertical dimension of occlusion and available prosthetic space for the different implants and prosthetic components. It gives a previsualization of the esthetic and functional outcome.
–The computed tomogram (CT scan) using a radiographic template evaluates the residual bone quality and volume at the implant sites.
–An appointment (between the surgeon and clinician) is required to decide on implant number, type, and position, and to confirm the prosthetic design.

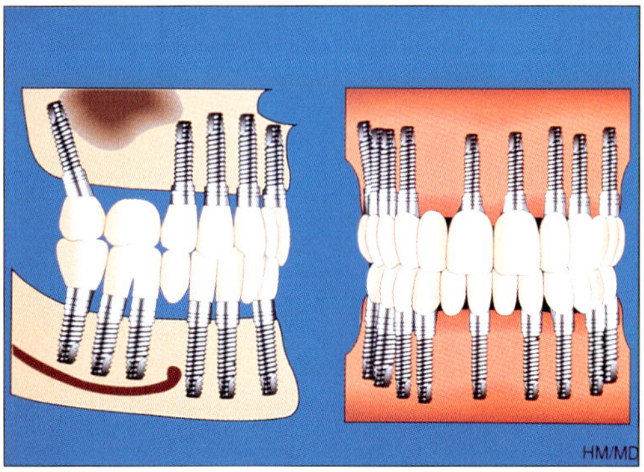

Fig 5-1 Implant-supported fixed bridge indicated in the presence of a slightly resorbed ridge.

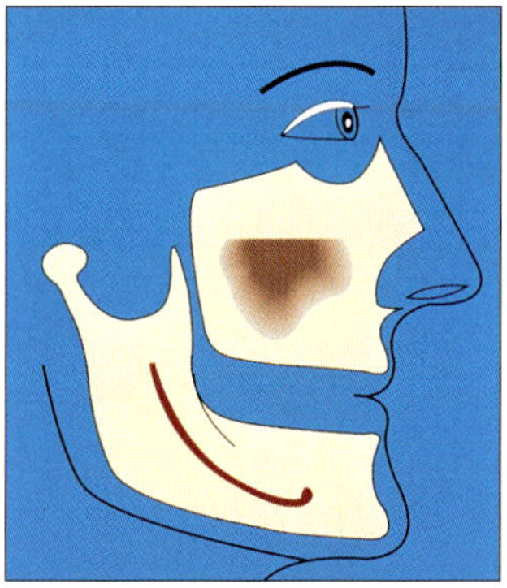

Fig 5-2 Slightly resorbed ridges with an adequate interarch ratio.

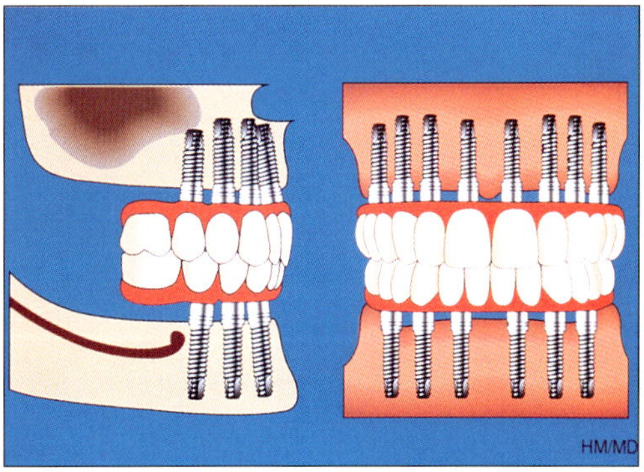

Fig 5-3 Implant-supported fixed prosthesis indicated in the presence of a slightly or moderately resorbed alveolar ridge.

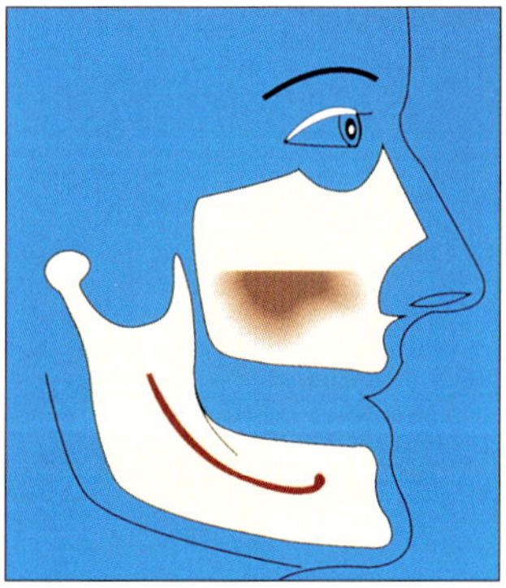

Fig 5-4 Moderately resorbed ridges.

II. Treatment options

They are determined by:

—extent of alveolar bone resorption
—interarch ratio
—patient demands
—conclusions from the esthetic and functional analysis[2]

The options include:

- Implant-supported fixed bridge (Figs 5-1 and 5-2)
  —Slightly resorbed bone ridge associated with an adequate interarch ratio.
- Implant-supported fixed prosthesis (Figs 5-3 and 5-4)
  —Slightly resorbed bone ridge associated with an adequate interarch ratio.
  —Moderate resorption of bone ridge associated with a good interarch ratio or with a slight maxillomandibular discrepancy.
- Implant-supported overdenture (Figs 5-5 and 5-6)
  —Advanced bone resorption associated with a significant interarch discrepancy and/or insufficient lip support.
- Contraindication for implants (Fig 5-7)
  —Extensive bone resorption. Bone augmentation may then be considered.

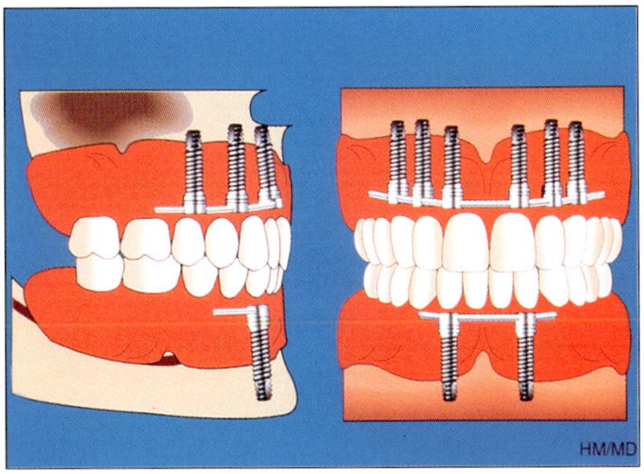

Fig 5-5 Implant-supported overdenture: the implants are used to stabilize the prosthesis.

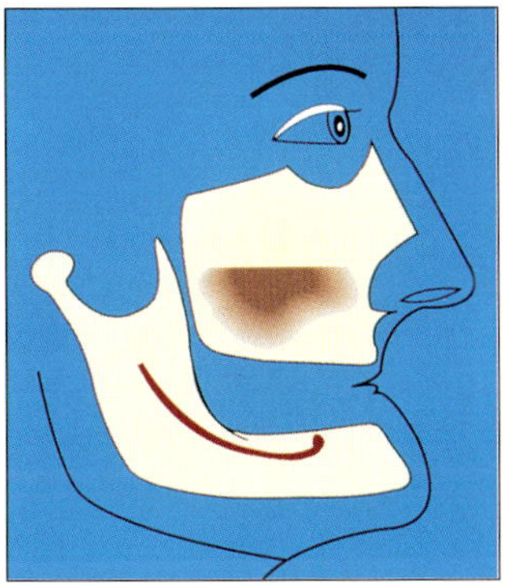

Fig 5-6 Alveolar ridges with advanced resorption.

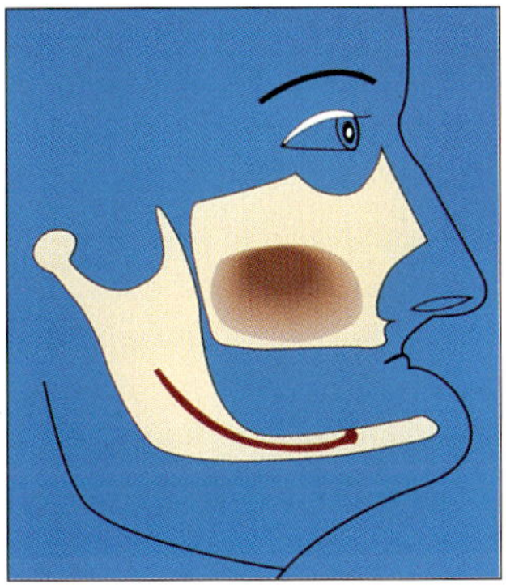

Fig 5-7 Alveolar ridges with extensive resorption.

III. Treatment

A. Prosthetic assessment

If the existing prosthesis shows esthetic or functional design defects, it must be remade. This the mandatory first stage of the treatment, whatever prosthetic solution is considered.

B. Stage-one surgery: Implant placement

A prosthetic replica may judiciously be used as a surgical template; implant positioning problems (localization, emergence, orientation) may thus be avoided.

C. Postoperative follow-up

Removable denture wearing must be avoided as much as possible during the 10 to 15 days following surgery. During the initial tissue healing period, any compression on the soft tissue may compromise the osseointegration process. Ten to 15 days following surgery, sutures are removed, and denture relief and relining are performed in relation to the implant site. An elastic material is used for relining.

D. Stage-two surgery

During abutment connection, the cover screws are replaced by the transmucosal healing abutments or by the final abutments. The denture interface area surrounding the healing abutments must be hollowed and relined using an elastic material (resin or silicone). The prosthetic stability is thus preserved, and functional implant overloads are controlled. Any alteration of the denture interface must be followed by a relining procedure.

E. Impression taking

After 4 to 8 weeks of soft tissue healing, the healing abutments are removed, and impression taking may be performed. The impression allows judgment of the accurate position of implants as well as their cervical emergence. For tissue-supported prostheses, the impression must record the maximum prosthetic-supporting surface as well as the marginal contours during function.

The impressions are made using transfer copings, which are available in two forms, standard screwed transfers or pickup screwed transfers:

- —standard transfer copings, used with a stock impression tray, are recommended in the posterior regions, where screwing of the pickups is difficult
- —pickup transfer copings are used with an impression tray hollowed out for screw access

Screwing of the pickup transfer copings after impression material has set avoids the repositioning required with the standard transfer copings. For some, screwed transfer copings may lead to inaccuracies.

F. Prosthetic phase

The study casts are mounted on an articulator using the occlusal patterns adjusted in the anterior (vertical dimension) and sagittal planes (centric occlusion). It is essential to conceive of a rational and judicious occlusion and disclusion design according to the number of implants, their localization, the type of prosthesis, and the opposing arch.

The occlusal design may be:

- —a lingually tipped occlusion bilaterally balanced in the eccentric movements
- —a so-called mutually protected occlusion, the different parameters of which (canine guidance, vertical overbite) must be perfectly under control
- —a group function type of occlusion and disclusion

The following prosthetic steps depend on the type of prosthesis that is fabricated. Nevertheless, the protocols are similar in two points:

- —the esthetic and functional validations must be performed at each intraoral try-in (pattern framework, biscuit, porcelain)
- —clinical and radiographic control for fit accuracy of the implant connection components is essential; passive insertion and tension-free screwing must be sought

G. Maintenance phase

Following the final prosthetic fabrication, a custom maintenance program is recommended to the patient.

IV. Skeletal relationships and treatment choice

The nature of the opposing arch, extent of residual ridge resorption, as well as the skeletal jaw relationship are essential parameters for treatment choice. These parameters influence the number and position of the implants, as well as the type of prosthesis.[2]

It is essential to determine the skeletal class, especially in the presence of a severe resorption that does not allow implant placement in the whole arch. Long-span posterior cantilevers increase the risk for complications and implant failures.

A. Class I

In the presence of a Class I relationship (ideal interarch relationships), the treatment option is determined by the residual bone volume.

B. Class II

A Class II relationship presents a mesial position of the maxilla in relation to the mandible. The patient's smile and esthetic demands must be seriously assessed.

A lingual angulation of the anterior maxillary implants and buccal angulation of the mandibular implants is very difficult to achieve. It may lead to lip support alteration and/or significant esthetic facial change, which is hardly acceptable for the patient. A prosthetic compensation of the skeletal discrepancy must be considered.

1. In the maxilla

- A complete implant-supported fixed bridge leads to anterior open bite.
- An implant-supported fixed prosthesis will undergo occlusal overload on the posterior implants. A greater number of posterior implants will allow compensation for the occlusal forces. The distal cantilever must not exceed 10 mm. A preview of the esthetic and phonetic outcome must be performed.
- An implant-supported overdenture is the optimal treatment choice in the presence of a significant discrepancy.

2. In the mandible

- In the presence of a significant discrepancy, a complete implant-supported fixed bridge will lead to an anterior open bite. In the presence of a moderate discrepancy, a more anterior angulation of the symphysis implants may compensate for this space.
- A complete implant-supported fixed prosthesis (implants placed between the mental foramina) requires a less distal cantilever in relation to a Class I relationship in order to obtain molar occlusion. The esthetic and functional results must be previewed if a mesial cantilever is to be used to compensate for the open bite.
- An implant-supported overdenture is again the optimal treatment choice in the presence of a significant discrepancy of the osseous bases.

C. Class III

A Class III relationship presents a distal position of the maxilla in relation to the mandible. The esthetic and functional imperatives must be determined.

1. In the maxilla

- In the presence of adequate bone volume, a more buccal angulation of the implants and an appropriate prosthetic design allow reduction, indeed correction, of the skeletal discrepancy.
- In the presence of a reduced bone volume, only the prosthetic design may compensate for this discrepancy. The implant-supported overdenture is the best treatment choice in the presence of a significant discrepancy.

2. In the mandible

- In the presence of adequate bone volume, a more lingual angulation of the implants and

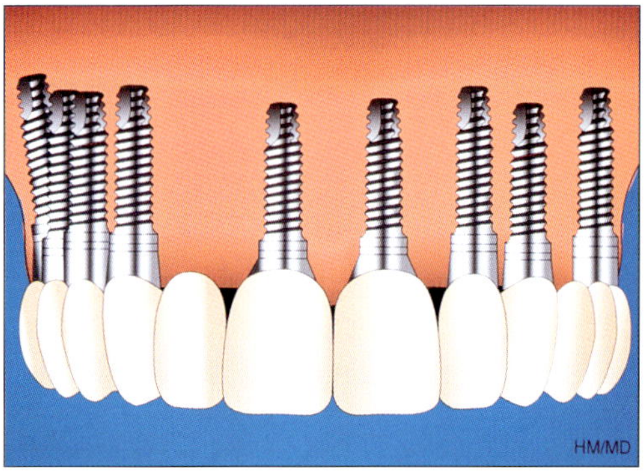

Fig 5-8 Implant-supported fixed bridge in the maxilla.

an appropriate prosthetic design may reduce, indeed correct, the skeletal discrepancy.

- In the presence of reduced bone volume, only the prosthetic design may compensate for this discrepancy. The removable implant-supported overdenture becomes, here again, the best treatment choice in the presence of a significant discrepancy.

In skeletal Classes II and III, an excessive discrepancy of the osseous bases indicates a need for corrective orthognathic surgery.

V. Prosthetic designs

A. Implant-supported fixed bridge

The prosthetic structure may be either screwed or cemented on the abutments (Fig 5-8). This type of prosthesis may be retrieved by the surgeon.

The advantages are those of fixed prosthodontics:

—esthetics often satisfactory
—a prosthesis that is retrievable by the surgeon
—excellent comfort for the patient
—personal maintenance similar to that of natural teeth

The disadvantages are as follows:

—adequate lip support may be difficult to obtain
—an esthetic and phonetic result may be difficult to obtain
—management of the interarch discrepancy is impossible

1. Surgical considerations

a. Number of implants

The number of implants depends on the extent of bone resorption. In some cases, each edentulous site may be provided with an implant. A greater bone anchorage surface will thus be developed (Figs 5-9 to 5-16). An adequate interimplant distance, prosthetic requirements, and an appropriate emergence profile are essential.

b. Implant diameter

The choice of the implant diameter depends on the edentulous site and the residual bone morphology. In the presence of an adequate ridge width, the selected diameter must correspond to the cervical diameter of the tooth to be replaced (Tables 5-1 and 5-2). An ideal emergence profile allows a better esthetic result. In the posterior regions, the anatomic limits (maxillary sinus and inferior dental canal) often limit the length of the implants. In the presence of a large ridge, the use of large-diameter implants allows increased anchoring surface.

c. Implant positioning

The available bone volume must be evaluated in the three dimensions of space in order to

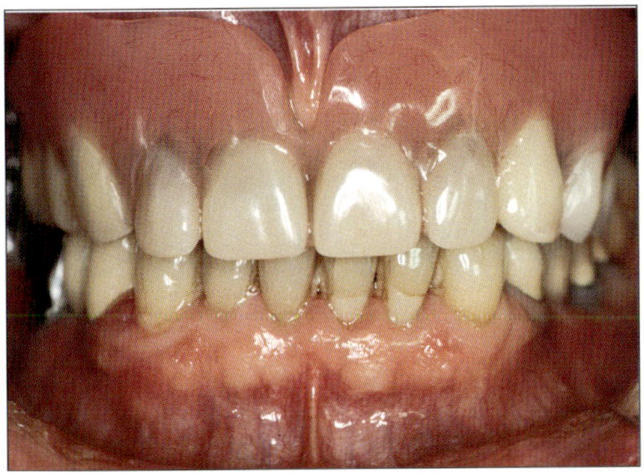

Fig 5-9 Patient presenting a complete removable prosthesis in the maxilla with discomfort because of the buccal anterior flange.

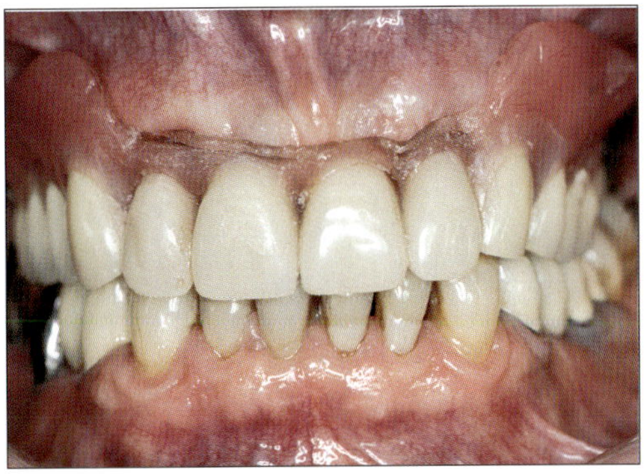

Fig 5-10 Clinical view after eliminating the acrylic resin buccal flange.

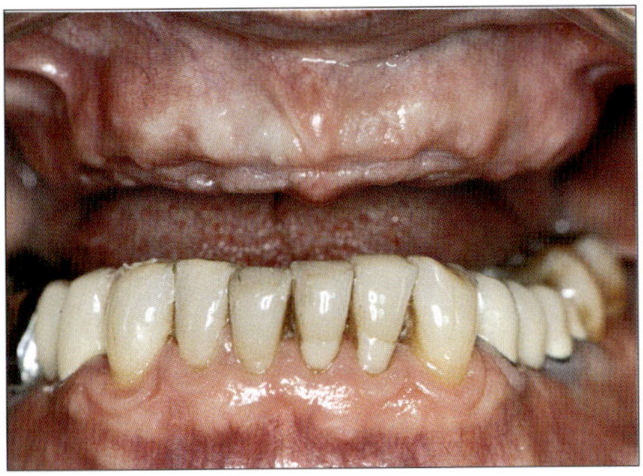

Fig 5-11 Alveolar ridge showing slight resorption.

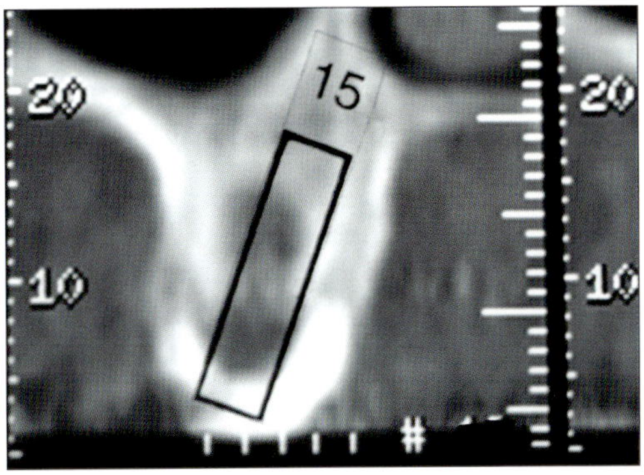

Fig 5-12 Oblique CT scan shows very good bone volume.

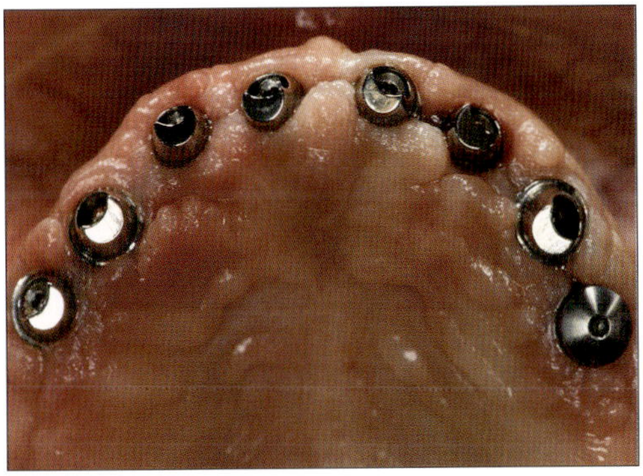

Fig 5-13 Occlusal view of the angulated abutments (15 degrees, 3i) 15 days following stage-two surgery.

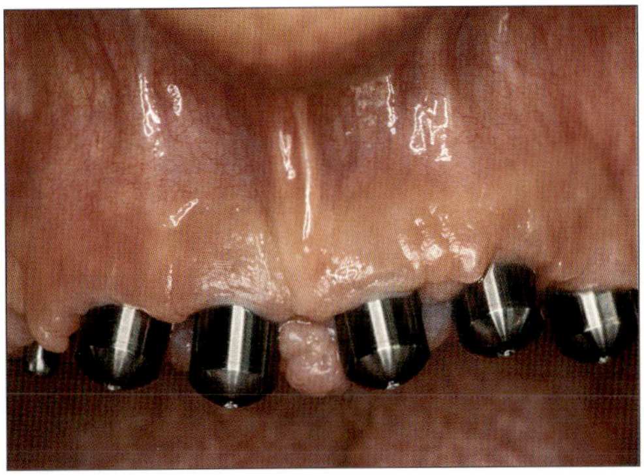

Fig 5-14 Healing is guided by the titanium healing caps.

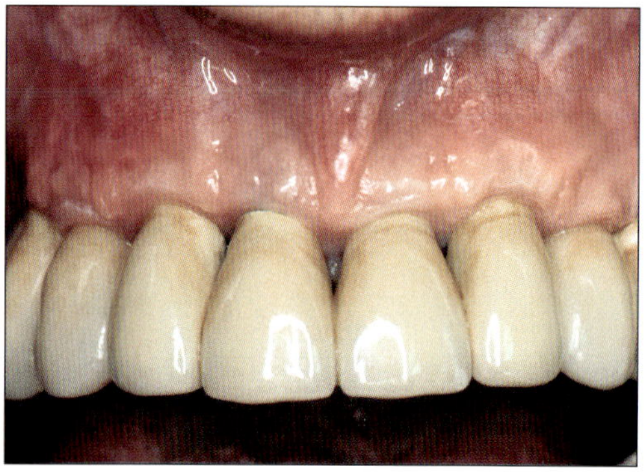

Fig 5-15a View of the implant-supported complete fixed bridge following 6 months of loading (restoration, Dr E. Cohen).

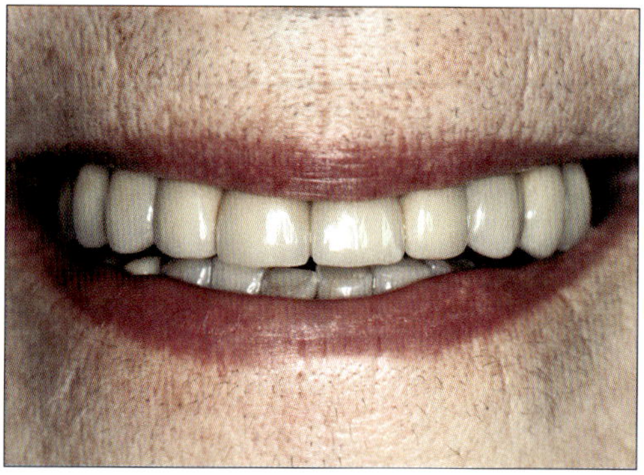

Fig 5-15b Patient's smile. Note the good esthetic result.

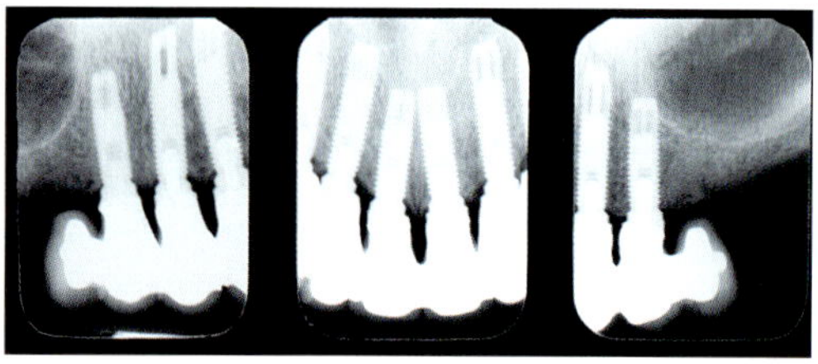

Fig 5-16 Periapical radiograph after 1 year of loading.

make a decision for the implant diameter and length.

- Mesiodistal plane. In the presence of an adequate bone width (at least 6 mm), the number of implants (standard) is calculated according to the available mesiodistal space. The use of small-diameter implants inevitably changes this calculation. A minimum distance of 3 mm must be observed between the implants.
- Buccolingual plane. The implants must be surrounded with at least 1 mm of bone on the buccal and lingual aspects:

—for a standard implant, a ridge width of at least 6 mm is required
—for a large-diameter implant (5 mm), a ridge width of at least 7 mm is essential
—for a small-diameter implant (3.25 mm), a ridge width of at least 5 mm is required

Ideally, the implants must be placed in the center of the future prosthetic crowns. The fabrication of study casts mounted on an articulator and a diagnostic waxup allow definition of the ideal prosthetic axis in relation to the residual ridge. The radiographic template allows transfer of this axis on the reconstructed CT scans. The oblique CT scan sections allow visualization of the possibility of positioning the implant according to the ideal prosthetic axis.

The posterior mandibular morphology often presents a highly increased lingual concavity. In this situation, two solutions may be considered:

—shorter large-diameter implants (if possible)
—changing the implant axis

- Apicocoronal plane. An appropriate implant length allows use of a maximum portion of

Table 5-1 Mean measurements for the maxillary teeth and recommended implant diameter

Tooth	Mesiodistal cervical diameter (mm)	Buccolingual cervical diameter (mm)	Implant diameter
Central incisor	7.0	6.0	Standard or large
Lateral incisor	5.0	5.0	Standard or small
Canine	5.5	7.0	Standard or large
First premolar	5.0	8.0	Standard
Second premolar	5.0	8.0	Standard
First molar	8.0	10.0	Large
Second molar	8.0	9.0	Large

Table 5-2 Mean measurements for the mandibular teeth and recommended implant diameter

Tooth	Mesiodistal cervical diameter (mm)	Buccolingual cervical diameter (mm)	Implant diameter
Central incisor	3.5	5.5	Small
Lateral incisor	4.0	5.5	Small
Canine	5.0	6.5	Standard
First premolar	5.0	7.0	Standard
Second premolar	5.0	8.0	Standard
First molar	8.5	9.0	Large
Second molar	8.0	9.0	Large

the residual ridge. A bicortical anchorage increases the primary stability of the implants. In the presence of a reduced bone height, the number and, if possible, the diameter of the implants must be increased in order to obtain an adequate anchoring surface.

–In the posterior regions, 8 to 10 mm of residual bone height associated with a thin ridge indicates the use of short standard implants.
–Increased failure rates have been reported with short standard implants.
–An adequate implant submerging avoids excessive force transmission by the removable prosthesis during the osseointegration period.

2. *Prosthetic considerations*

a. *Prosthetic space*

The vertical dimension determines the available prosthetic space (Figs 5-17 to 5-22). An adequate crown:implant ratio is essential for a good prognosis of the reconstruction. The longer an implant, the better its prognosis. Analysis of residual bone and available prosthetic space determines implant selection and prosthetic design.

b. *Implant angulation*

Ideally, the implants must be positioned according to the prosthetic axis. The implant axis may possibly be corrected using angulated abutments. If an implant presents a significant angulation or a difficult prosthetic positioning, its integration in the prosthetic reconstruction must be reconsidered.

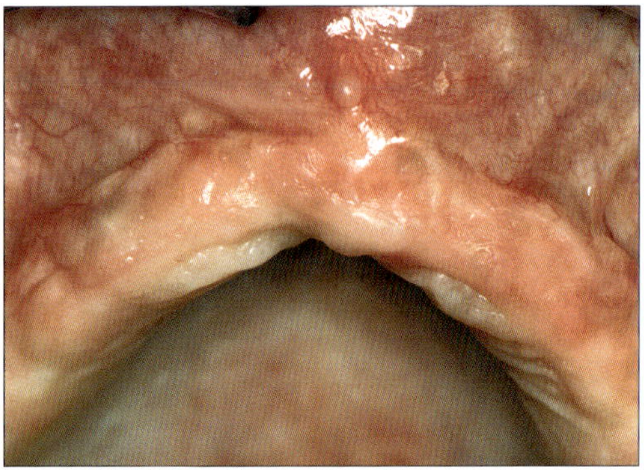

Fig 5-17 Occlusal view of a maxillary ridge showing advanced resorption. The patient's esthetic demands are high.

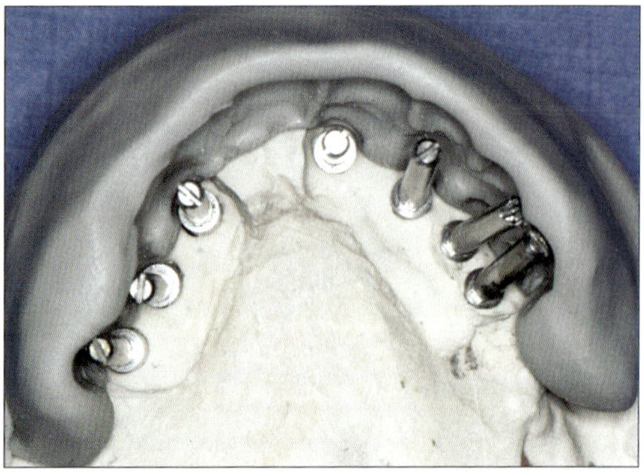

Fig 5-18 The impression was taken directly on the implant heads. View of the master cast with the buccal index.

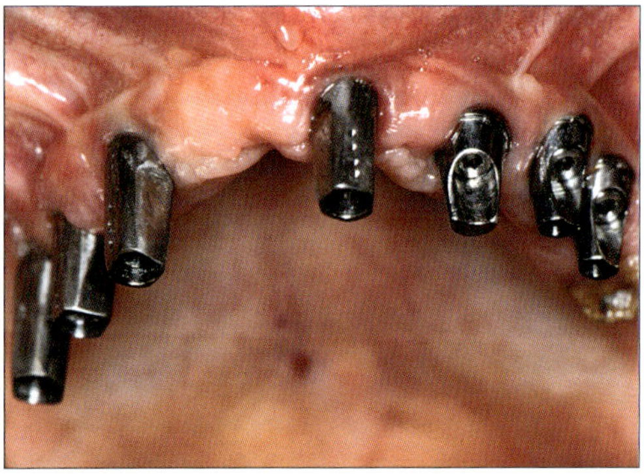

Fig 5-19 Abutment selection: inlay cores on the right and angulated abutments (15 and 25 degrees) on the left to correct the axes of the implants.

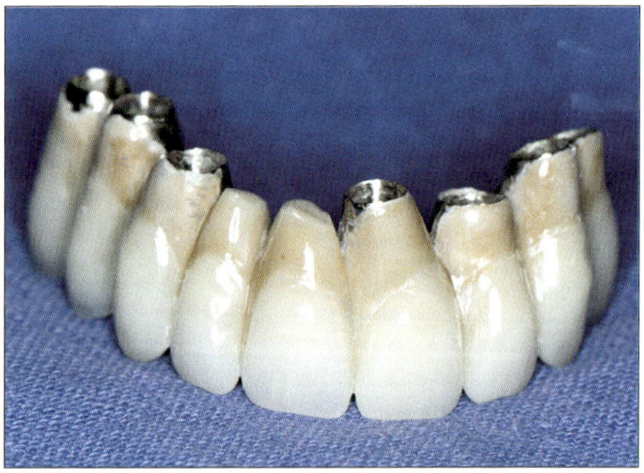

Fig 5-20 View of the final bridge at the laboratory.

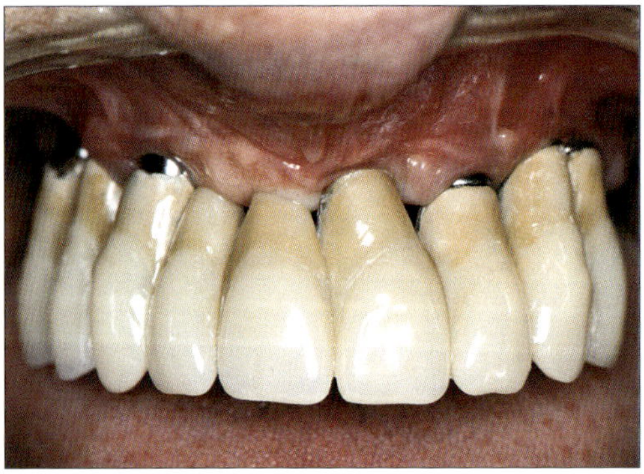

Fig 5-21 Clinical view of the implant-supported complete fixed bridge. This case is a borderline indication for an implant-supported complete fixed bridge.

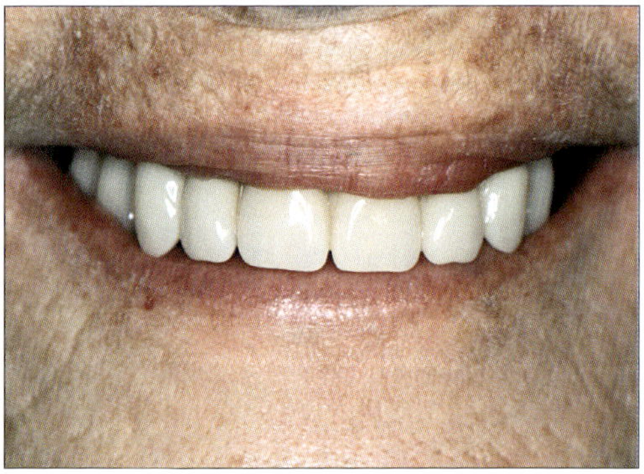

Fig 5-22 Patient's smile (restoration, Dr E. Cohen).

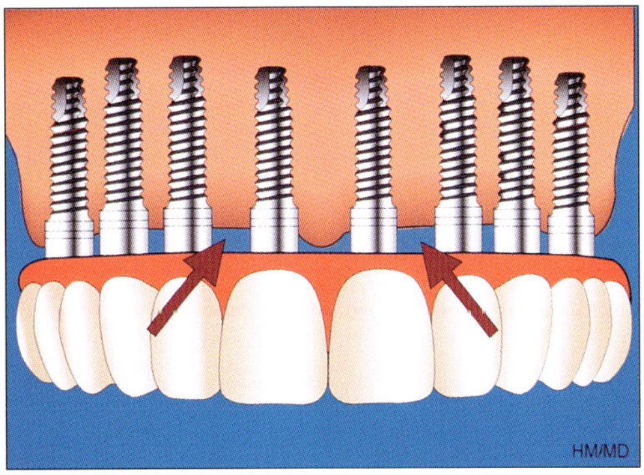

Fig 5-23 Implant-supported maxillary fixed prosthesis.

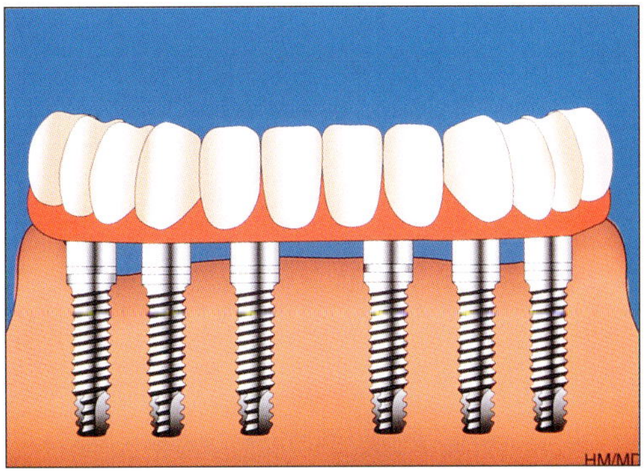

Fig 5-24 Implant-supported mandibular fixed prosthesis.

c. *Implant emergence site*

An implant emerging through an embrasure leads to a disastrous esthetic result and difficulty ensuring good oral hygiene and maintenance. In this situation, the use of this implant must be reconsidered.

d. *Progressive loading*

Progressive loading of the posterior implants is recommended in the presence of insufficient bone quality and/or volume. The use of provisional acrylic resin restorations during at least 1 year allows reduction of the occlusal stresses at the bone-implant interface and thus reinforces osseointegration.

e. *Type of prosthesis: Screw-retained or cemented*

Actually, the prosthetic choice of either screw-retained or cemented restorations is often philosophical. It must of course be based on implant positioning, angulation, and esthetic imperatives. Whatever choice is made, we recommend a prosthetic design that facilitates restoration retrievability.

B. Implant-supported complete fixed prosthesis

The implant-supported complete fixed prosthesis is screwed on the abutments (Figs 5-23 and 5-24). It is specifically indicated in the presence of moderate ridge resorption, when an implant-supported bridge cannot be acceptably placed.

The advantages of this prosthesis are:

- fixed prosthesis
- uncovered palate
- prosthesis that is retrievable by the dentist
- acceptable comfort for the patient

Its possible disadvantages are:

- maintenance sometimes difficult
- speech problems (maxillary)
- esthetic problems in the presence of a high smile line (visibility of the metal components)[3]
- inadequate lip support

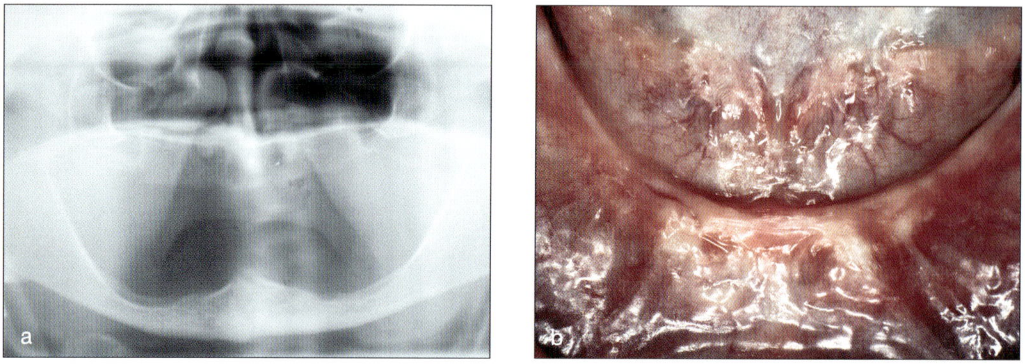

Figs 5-25a and 5-25b Clinical and radiographic views of an edentulous alveolar ridge with advanced posterior resorption.

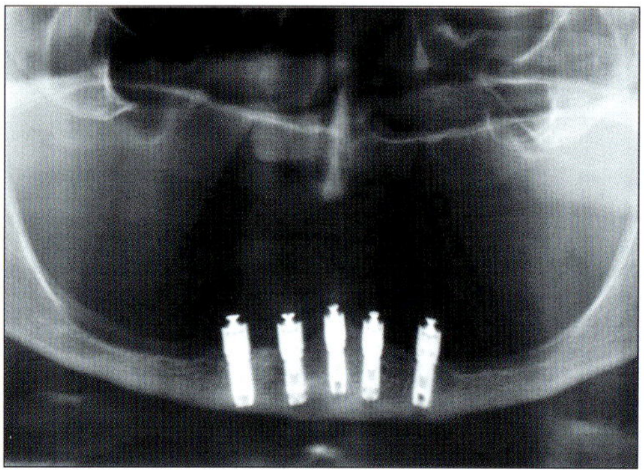

Fig 5-26 Control panoramic roentgenogram following abutment placement.

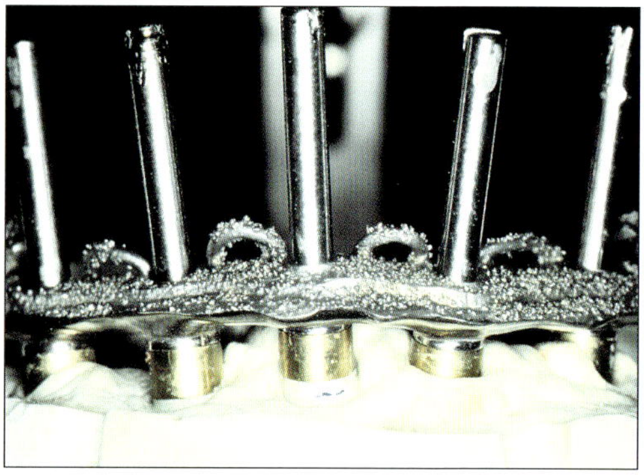

Fig 5-27 View of the metal framework with the guide pins at the laboratory.

1. Surgical considerations

a. Number of implants

The number of implants depends on arch form and residual bone volume. In the mandible (Figs 5-25 to 5-30), ideally, six implants placed mesial to the mental foramina allow excellent results.[4] However, in some cases, the use of four or five implants may be considered (Figs 5-31 and 5-32). In the maxilla (Figs 5-33 to 5-38), a minimum of six implants (length greater than 10 mm) is recommended. Ideally, eight implants are recommended.[5]

b. Implant positioning

The available bone volume must be evaluated in the three dimensions of space in order to select implant number, diameter, and length. Adequate bone width (at least 6 mm) is needed to place standard diameter implants. The number of implants is often calculated according to the mesiodistal distance available mesial to the maxillary sinuses or between the mental foramina (Table 5-3).

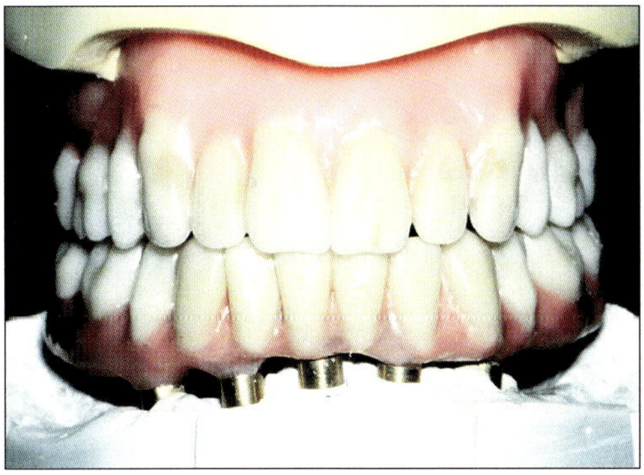

Fig 5-28 View of the wax patterns mounted on an articulator.

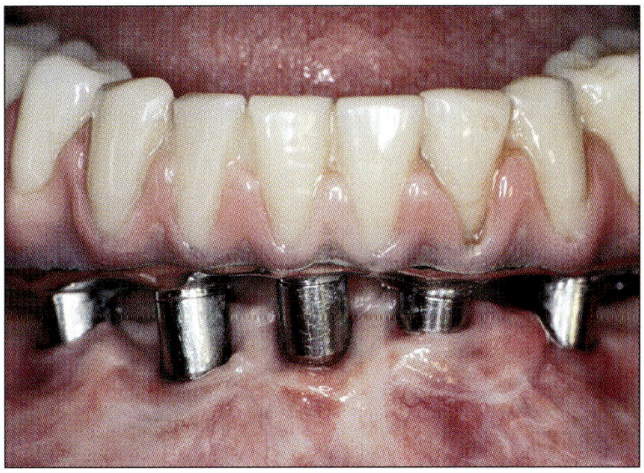

Fig 5-29 Clinical view of the fixed complete prosthesis (restoration, Dr F. Vidjak).

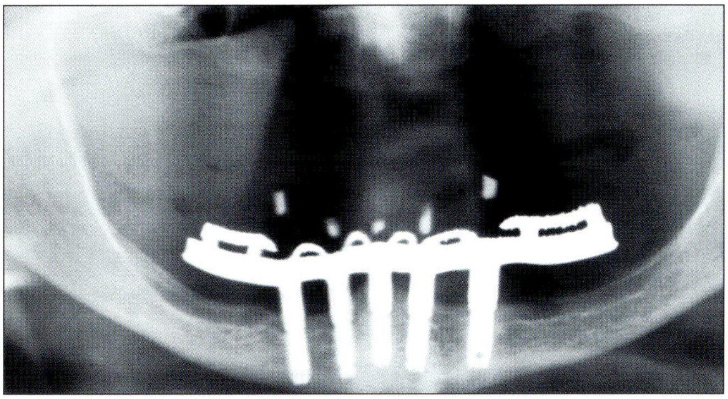

Fig 5-30 Control panoramic radiograph following 1 year of loading.

c. Residual ridge anatomy and implant angulation

A long-term edentulous situation leads to a more extensive vertical and/or horizontal bone resorption. This bone loss clinically appears as a ridge contour alteration. An interarch discrepancy is often present due to the reversed resorption pattern of the maxilla (centripetal for the maxilla, and centrifugal for the mandible). The clinically observed discrepancy is confirmed by mounting to the articulator. The implant position must be modified in order to compensate for a slight shift.

In presence of a significant interarch shift, two solutions may be considered:

—a removable implant-supported overdenture
—a surgical reconstruction of bone volume

Table 5-3 Available mesiodistal space and recommended number of implants

Available mesiodistal bone distance (mm)	No. of implants (standard) recommended
29	4
36	5
43	6
50	7
57	8

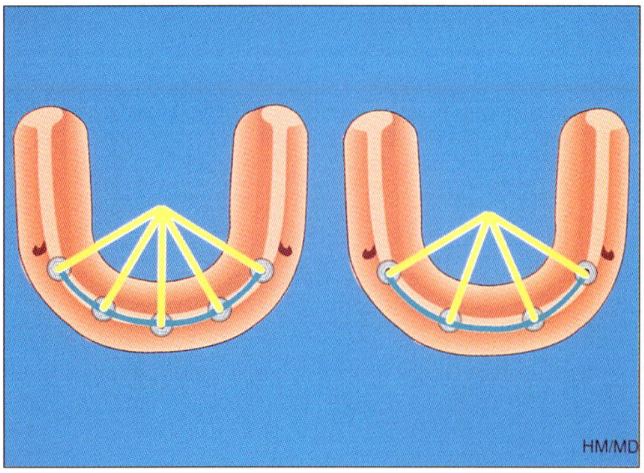

Fig 5-31 In the mandible, the number of implants depends on the available distance between the mental foramina.

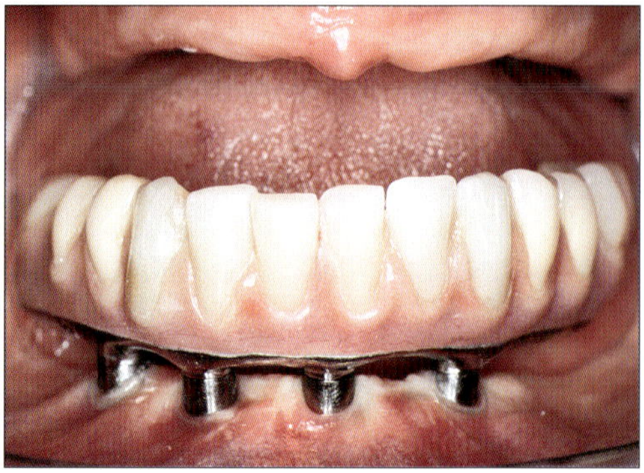

Fig 5-32 Clinical view of a mandibular fixed complete prosthesis built on four 18-mm-long implants (restoration, Dr F. Vidjak).

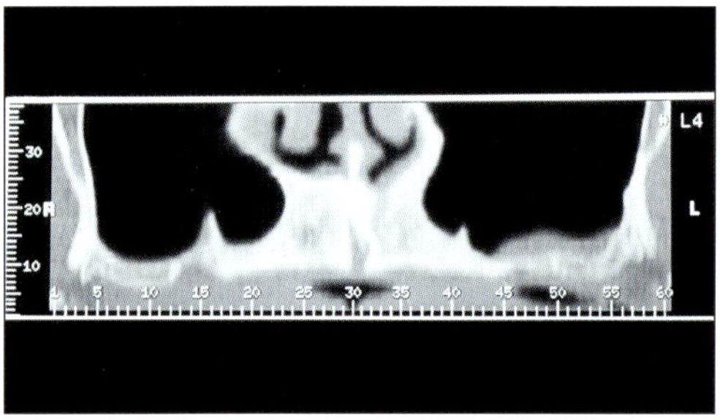

Fig 5-33 Panoramic CT scan showing advanced bone resorption.

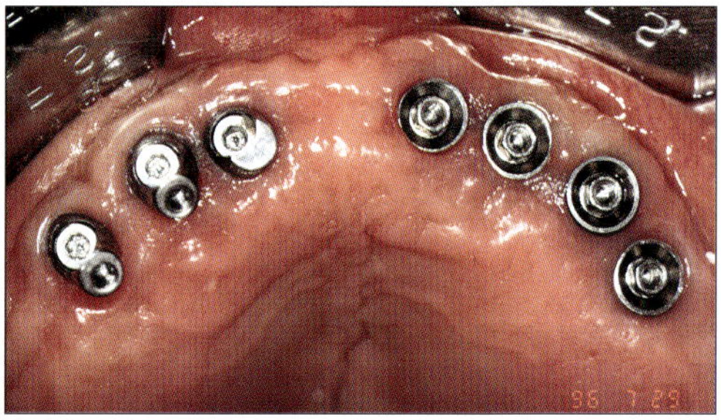

Fig 5-34 Occlusal view of seven 3i standard implants following stage-two surgery. On the left, placement of four conventional abutments. On the right, placement of mesial 15-degree angulated abutment and a distal 25-degree angulated abutment.

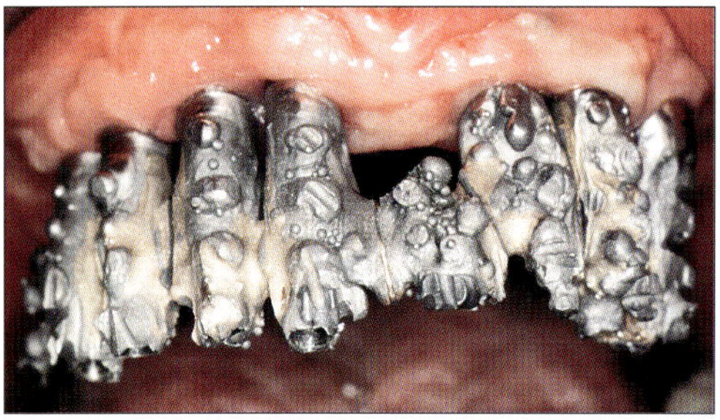

Fig 5-35a Framework try-in before splinting. The aim is to obtain a passive adaptation of the framework.

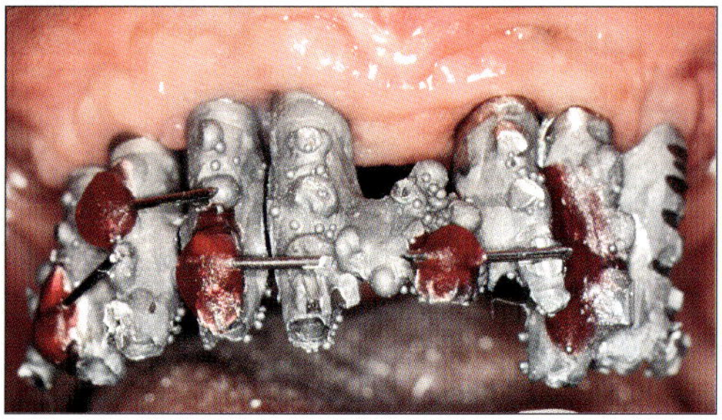

Fig 5-35b Splinting of the framework in the mouth.

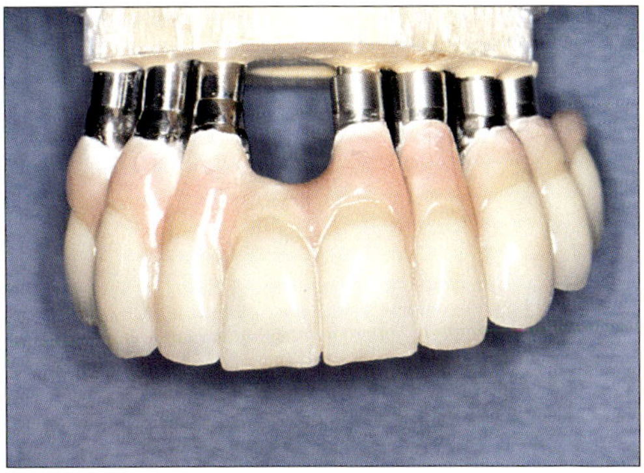

Fig 5-36 View of the maxillary denture at the laboratory. Note the amount of pink acrylic required to compensate for the alveolar bone loss.

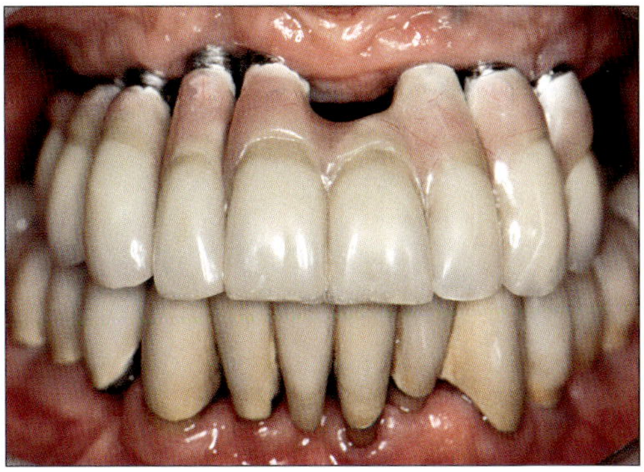

Fig 5-37 Clinical view of the final prosthetic work (restoration, Dr P. Raygot).

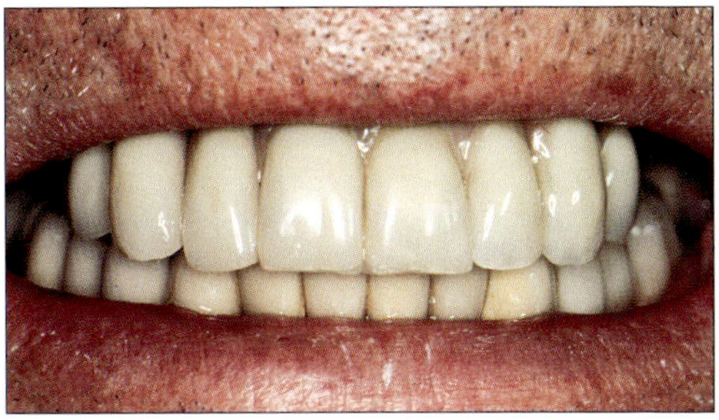

Fig 5-38 Patient's smile.

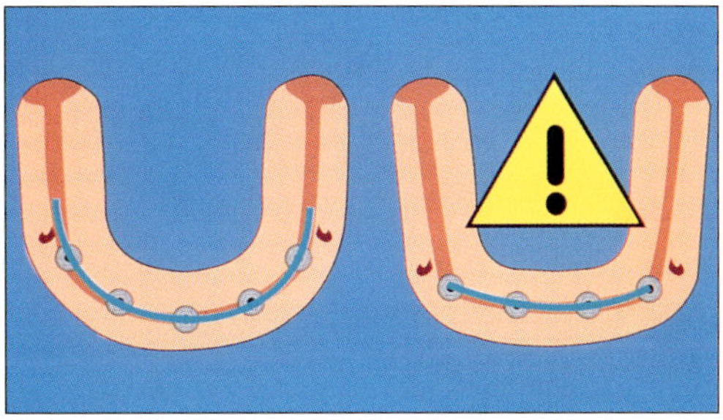

Fig 5-39 On the left, view of an ovoid arch allowing implant placement in a circular distribution, a very favorable distribution from a mechanical point of view. On the right, rectangular arch imposing a linear implant distribution. This distribution is much less favorable from a mechanical point of view.

2. *Prosthetic considerations*

a. *Arch form and prosthetic design (Fig 5-39)*

- An ovoid arch allows placement of the implants in a circular distribution. From a biomechanical aspect, this implant distribution is very favorable and allows consideration of longer distal cantilevers. The length of the latter is calculated according to the distance between the most distal implants.
- A rectangular arch associated with mesial inferior dental nerve emergence requires a linear implant distribution. This implant distribution contraindicates extended cantilevers.

b. *Prosthetic space*

The residual vertical dimension determines the available prosthetic space. The prosthetic structure requires a minimum height of 7 mm (framework and cosmetic material mechanical

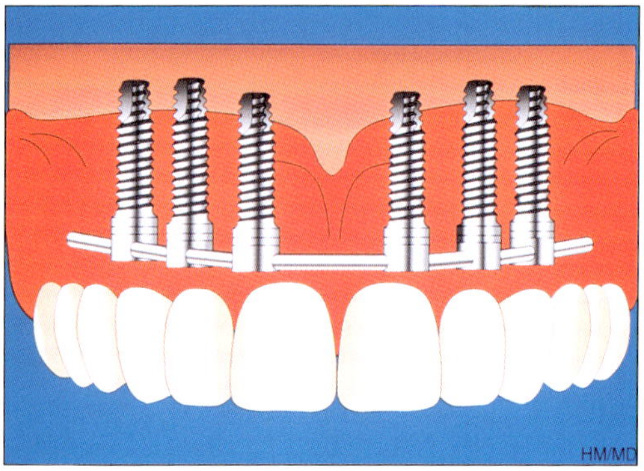

Fig 5-40 Implant-supported overdenture in the maxilla.

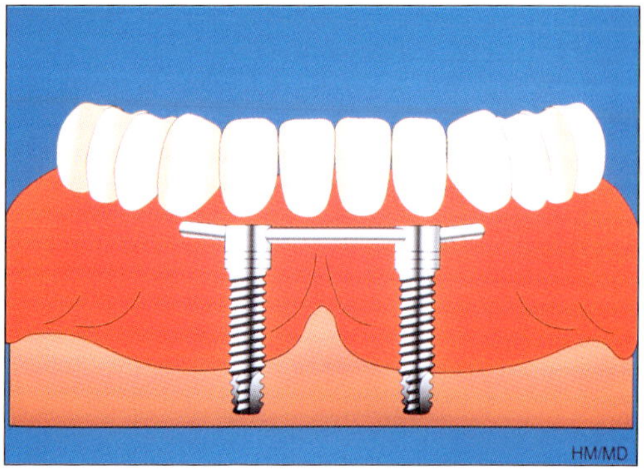

Fig 5-41 Implant-supported overdenture in the mandible.

resistance). A good implant:prosthesis anchorage ratio is essential for a good prognosis. The implant number, length, and diameter must be analyzed according to the available prosthetic space.

Chewing forces in the long-term completely edentulous patient dramatically increase after implant loading (85% after 2 months). This increase of forces may lead to prosthetic fractures.

c. Implant angulation and esthetics

An appropriate implant angulation in the buccolingual plane is essential to obtain a good prosthetic and esthetic result. An implant emerging on the buccal aspect leads to an unesthetic result. This type of disadvantage may sometimes be corrected using angulated abutments. In the maxilla, apparent prosthetic limits and inadequate lip support are synonymous with prosthetic failure for the patient.

d. Prosthetic alternative

In the maxilla, inadequate lip support associated with an interarch discrepancy may indicate a very specific type of fixed-removable, implant-supported prosthesis (double-bar prosthesis). Retention, stabilization, and support are ensured by the implant system. The connection is ensured by a precision-milled bar system screwed on a variable number of implants. A metal counterpart of this bar is fabricated within the removable prosthesis. The splinting of these two parts is ensured by a lateral lock or axial precision attachments.

C. Implant-supported overdenture

This is a removable osseous tissue–supported prosthesis (Figs 5-40 and 5-41). Stability and retention are shared between the prosthesis and the implants. Support is ensured by the osseous tissue surface. The prosthesis is connected to the implants using mechanical, magnet, or conjunction bar axial connections, available in various forms.[6,7] This type of prosthesis must be removed and cleaned by the patient.

The advantages are:

- stability of the removable prosthesis
- facilitated personal maintenance
- achievement of a good esthetic result in the presence of a "gummy" smile (high smile line)

—easier control of lip profile and support
—interarch discrepancy easier to manage

1. Surgical considerations

a. Number of implants

In the maxilla, in the past, four implants placed in the anterior region were recommended. Recent longitudinal studies recommend a number of implants similar to that of an implant-supported denture. A minimum of six implants at least 10 mm in length is strongly advised. For the implant-supported overdenture, a significant implant failure rate in the maxilla (25%) has been reported, especially if the number of implants is insufficient (less than or equal to four).[3,8–10]

In the mandible, two to four symphysis implants (length of at least 10 mm) allow an excellent result.[11] Parallelism between the implant axes facilitates the prosthetic fabrication.

b. Treatment evolution

Implant positioning to stabilize a complete removable prosthesis must consider a possible evolution of the case toward a fixed implant-supported prosthesis. Indeed, implants placed in the maxillary and mandibular anterior regions must allow the positioning of other implants in a second-stage surgery. Treatment planning modification may be justified by psychologic, functional, or esthetic reasons.

2. Prosthetic considerations

a. Prosthetic space

The residual vertical dimension determines the available prosthetic space. The intermediate prosthetic structure requires a minimum height of 7 mm in order to ensure the solidity of the stabilization system. In the presence of a reduced prosthetic space, connections that are directly screwed onto the implants will allow a better management of the prosthetic imperatives.

b. Implant angulation

Implant parallelism facilitates fabrication of the implant-supported stabilization system. Absence of parallelism of the implant axes under an axial ball attachment system may lead to premature wear of the different connection components. An angulation-compensating system is often required.

c. Prosthetic connections means

- The conjunction bar (Figs 5-42 to 5-46). Fabricated at the laboratory, it is screwed onto the intermediate components. These intermediate components are directly screwed on the implants. A retention clip allows stabilization of the prosthesis on the bar.[12]

  One or several clips or a retention splint allows stabilization of the prosthesis on the bar according to the bar morphology (Hadder, Dolder, or Ackermann) and length and the number and localization of the clips; we try to find a balance between the prosthetic retention:stability ratio and the functional load release.[10] If the prosthetic space is limited, this bar may be directly screwed onto the implants without using any intermediate components.

- The axial magnet connection. The lack of direct mechanical connection between the prosthesis and the implants is a major characteristic of axial magnet connections. Direct transmission of functional loads to the implant is limited.

  Numerous disadvantages have been reported with magnet connections:

  —corrosion and wear of the magnet components

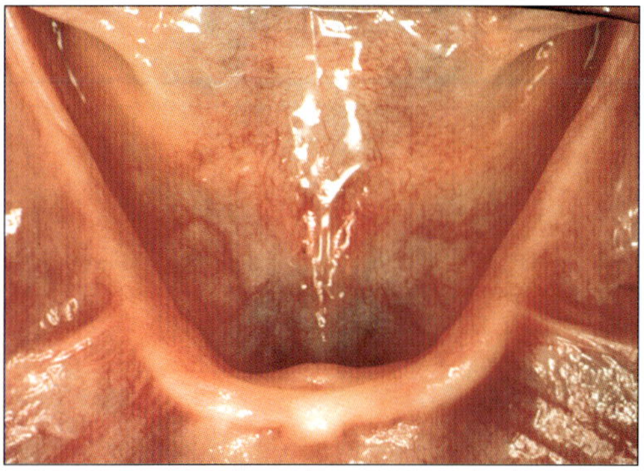

Fig 5-42 Occlusal view of a mandibular edentulous ridge.

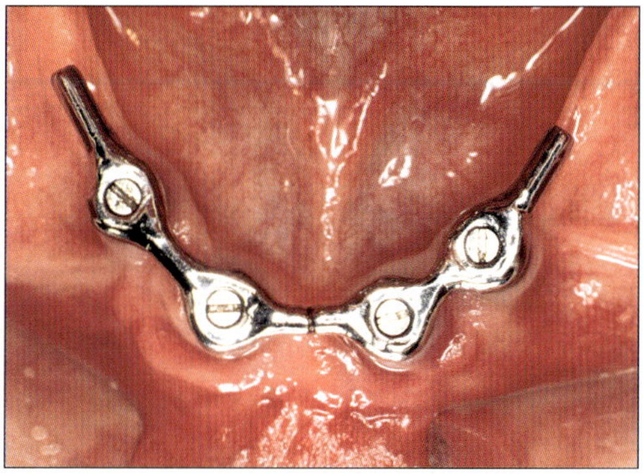

Fig 5-43 Clinical view following placement of the bar on four implants.

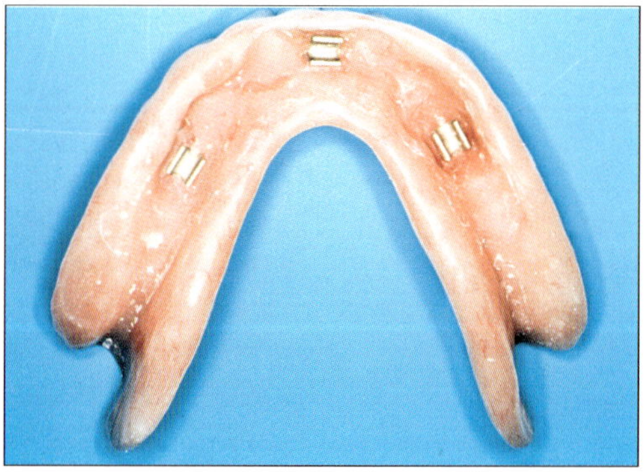

Fig 5-44 View of the prosthetic interface with three clips allowing stabilization of the prosthesis on the bar (restoration, Dr J. Moon).

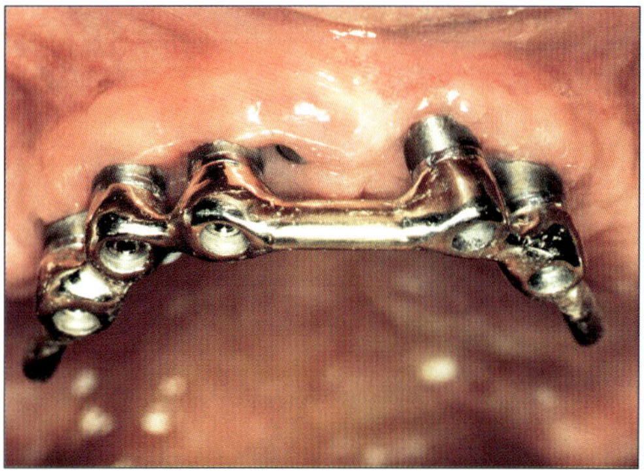

Fig 5-45 Clinical view of a maxillary bar screwed on five implants with lengths of at least 13 mm.

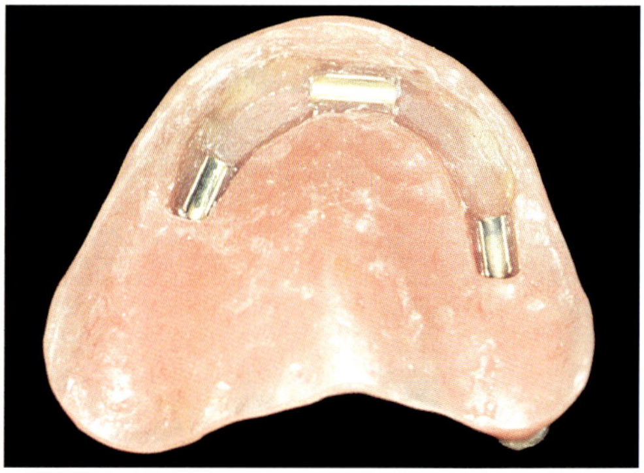

Fig 5-46 View of the three clips stabilizing the removable prosthesis (restoration, Dr E. Cohen).

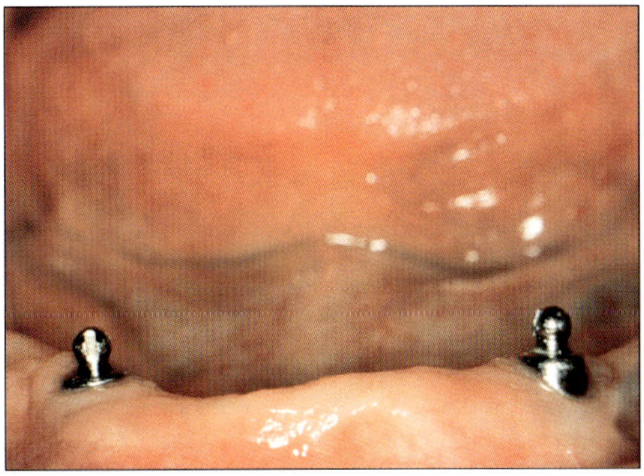

Fig 5-47 Clinical view of two axial ball connections in the mandible.

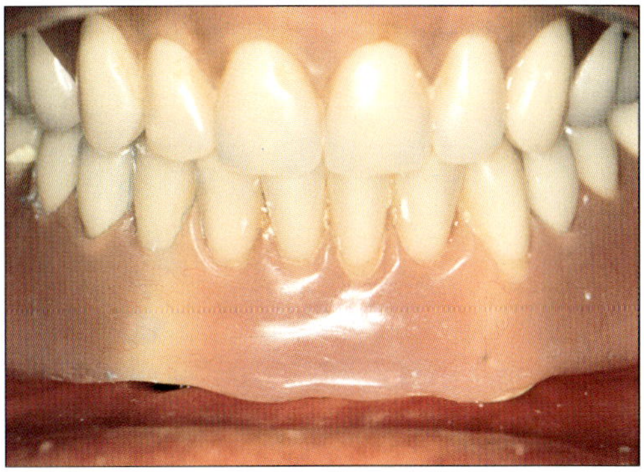

Fig 5-48 View of the prostheses: removable complete denture in the maxilla and implant-supported overdenture in the mandible (restoration, Dr O. Fromentin).

—inability to assess resiliency within the device
—permanent sliding of the prostheses on the magnets; this sliding leads to connection wear and may be related to prosthesis-induced stomatitis or gingival hyperplasia
—less efficiency in relation to the mechanical connections

- The axial ball connector (Figs 5-47 and 5-48). This is a male-female type of attachment system. The male part is generally screwed onto the implant; the female part is adapted to the interface of the prosthesis. While positioning the prosthesis, the male part adapts to the female part, which usually presents the retention device (metal wings, elastic silicone rubber ring, nylon or Teflon caps).[10]
- The mechanical axial connectors are devices that use metal (precious or nonprecious), elastic, or viscoelastic (nylon, Teflon, silicone rubber) retention components.

Variations:

—Reduced height axial connections or "reversed" designs (male part integrated in the prosthesis) facilitate treatment of cases with a reduced prosthetic space (vertical dimension and reduced inter-ridge heights, macroglossia).
—Axial connections allowing angulation correction compensate for divergent implants axes a single insertion axis; this avoids premature wear of the retention device.
—Axial connections allowing a release of functional loads may be rigid or stress breaking.

The more play allowed by the device (vertical ranging from 4 to 8 or 10 mm as well as rotation), the more it is meant to relieve the implants from the loads transmitted during function. The prosthetic support is then only ensured by the mucosa. The implant axial connection will only participate in lateral stabilization and resistance to prosthesis dislodging. The implant success rate in the mandible is excellent, inverse to that of the maxilla.[10]

References

1. Engelman MJ. Clinical Decision Making and Treatment Planning in Osseointegration. Chicago: Quintessence, 1996.
2. Desjardins RP. Prosthesis design for osseointegrated implants in the edentulous maxilla. Int J Oral Maxillofac Implants 1992;7:311–320.
3. Hemmings KW, Schmitt A, Zarb GA. Complications and maintenance requirements for fixed prostheses and overdentures in the edentulous mandible: A 5-year report. Int J Oral Maxillofac Implants 1994;9:191–196.
4. Quirynen M, Naert I, van Steenberghe D. A study of 589 consecutive implants supporting complete fixed prostheses. Part I: Periodontal aspects. J Prosthet Dent 1992;68:655–663.
5. Jemt T. Fixed implant-supported prostheses in the edentulous maxilla: A five-year follow-up report. Clin Oral Implants Res 1994;5:142–147.
6. Cune MS, De Putter C. A comparative evaluation of some outcome measures of implant systems and suprastructure types in mandibular implant overdenture treatment. Int J Oral Maxillofac Implants 1994;9:548–555.
7. Quirynen M, Naert I, van Steenberghe D, Teerlinck J, Dekeyser C, Theuniers G. Periodontal aspects of osseointegrated fixtures supporting an overdenture: A 4-year retrospective study. J Clin Periodontol 1991;18:719–728.
8. Engquist B, Bergendal T, Kallus T, Linden U. A retrospective multicenter evaluation of osseointegrated implants supporting overdentures. Int J Oral Maxillofac Implants 1988;3:129–134.
9. Johns RB, Jemt T, Heath MR. A multicenter study of overdentures supported by Brånemark implants. Int J Oral Maxillofac Implants 1992;7:513–522.
10. Slonim C, Fromentin O, Tarounine M. Les prothèses adjointes supra-implantaires. J Parodontol Implantol Orale 1995;14:295–306.
11. Naert I, Quirynen M, Hooghe M. A comparative prospective study of splinted and unsplinted Brånemark implants in mandibular overdenture therapy. A preliminary report. Int J Prosthodont 1994;7:486–492.
12. Kramer A, Weber H, Benzing U. Implant and prosthetic treatment of the edentulous maxilla using a bar-supported prosthesis. Int J Oral Maxillofac Implants 1992;7:251–255.

CHAPTER 6

Treatment Considerations for Partial Edentulism

H. Martínez/M. Davarpanah/F. Lamond/G. Audi/J.-F. Tecucianu

For the partially edentulous patient, whether the edentulous space is tooth-bound or distal, treatment decisions will depend on:

—the prosthetic value of the residual teeth
—the extent of edentulism
—the edentulous situation
—patient age
—etiology of tooth loss
—the available prosthetic space
—prosthetic and esthetic patient demands[1]

Implant indications are:

—absence of or poor tooth abutments
—edentulousness associated with sound adjacent teeth (Fig 6-1)
—realistic patient prosthetic demands
—discomfort caused by the removable prostheses
—patient's psychologic profile

I. Treatment planning

The treatment planning includes the following steps:

—possible treatment of an emergency
—motivation for oral hygiene
—initial periodontal preparation
—extraction of hopeless teeth
—dental care (conservative dentistry and endodontics)
—provisional restorations

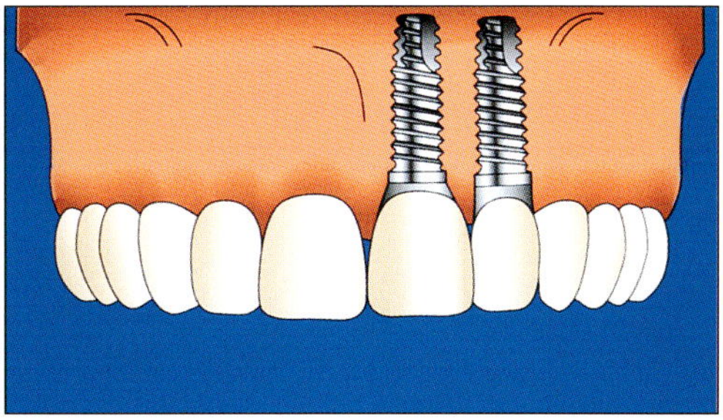

Fig 6-1 Partial anterior edentulism: implant-supported prosthesis.

—periodontal reassessment
—first-stage surgery (implant placement)
—second-stage surgery (abutment connection)
—temporary restorations
—final restorations
—maintenance phase

II. Partial edentulism in the anterior regions

A. Surgical considerations

In the anterior regions, patient esthetic demands are often considerable.[2]

1. Smile analysis

Concerning the smile, the position and thickness of the upper lip are defined by:

—the degree of contraction of the mimic muscles
—bone and overlying soft tissue anatomy

The level of the inferior edge of the upper lip determines the degree of visibility of the maxillary anterior teeth. Treatment choice must consider the type of smile:

—a low lip line slightly reveals the teeth
—a moderate lip smile reveals the teeth and the interdental papillae
—a high smile line, or "gummy" smile, reveals teeth and gingiva (10% of patients)

The extent of gingival visibility is of major importance to the final esthetic outcome. Soft tissue management is often a long and delicate process. The esthetic result is not always predictable. Implant treatment in an anterior partially edentulous maxilla may be contraindicated.

2. *Anatomic limits*

The position and morphology of the nasopalatal canal are determined by the radiographic analysis (CT scan). A large canal imposes malpositioning of the implants and inevitably leads to a poor esthetic result.[3] The midline must also be considered. Mesiodistal and apicocoronal harmony in both anterior regions allows a balanced, harmonious smile.

3. *Implant positioning*

The available bone volume (width and length) must be assessed in the three dimensions of space in order to select implant number, diameter, and length[4] (Figs 6-2 to 6-5).

a. Edentulous extent (mesiodistal space)

Starting from the midline, each edentulous segment must be measured separately. In the presence of an adequate bone ridge width (at least 6 mm), the number of implants (standard) is calculated in relation to the unilateral mesiodistal distance of the edentulous space (Table 6-1).

For mesiodistal spaces smaller than the standard values, it is preferable to place fewer implants. Implant proximity leads to difficulties regarding prosthetic fabrication and oral hygiene. An implant placed too near a tooth may lead to the loss of the papilla and/or subsequent gingival recession.

The different implant diameters allow an optimal management of the available space. In the presence of a significant mesiodistal distance associated with a large ridge, large-diameter implants may be considered for the central incisors, and possibly for the canines. Inversely, if the available distance is borderline for the placement of three standard implants, the use of small-diameter implants may be considered for the mandibular incisors or the maxillary lateral incisors.

b. Buccolingual plane

The implant must ideally be surrounded with at least 1 mm of bone on its overall surface. For a standard-diameter implant (3.75 mm), a minimum of 5.75 mm of ridge width is required. For a small-diameter implant (3.25 mm), a minimum of 5.25 mm of ridge width is required. For a large-diameter implant (5 mm), a ridge width greater than 7 mm is essential. The coronal emergence point determines the type of implant prosthesis: cemented or screw retained.

- For screw-retained restorations, the access hole of the abutment screw must be located on the lingual or palatal aspect, ideally between the incisor edge and the cingulum of the future crown.
- For cemented restorations, the abutment screw may also emerge on the buccal aspect.

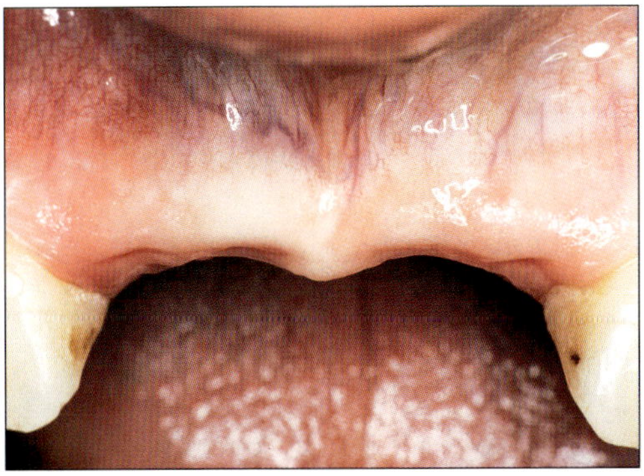

Fig 6-2 Partial anterior tooth-bound edentulous space in the maxilla.

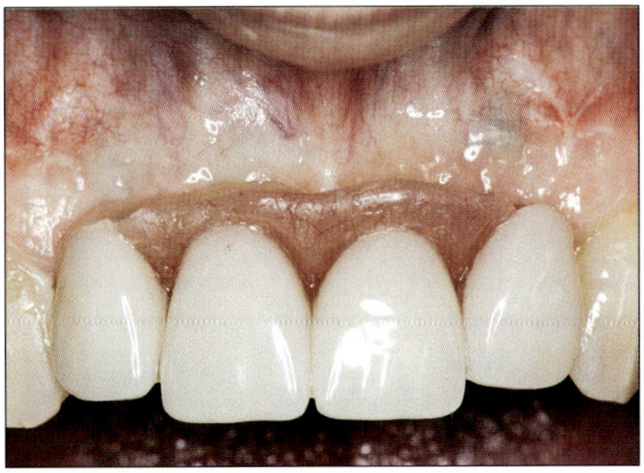

Fig 6-3 Clinical view of the provisional removable prosthesis 6 months after implant placement.

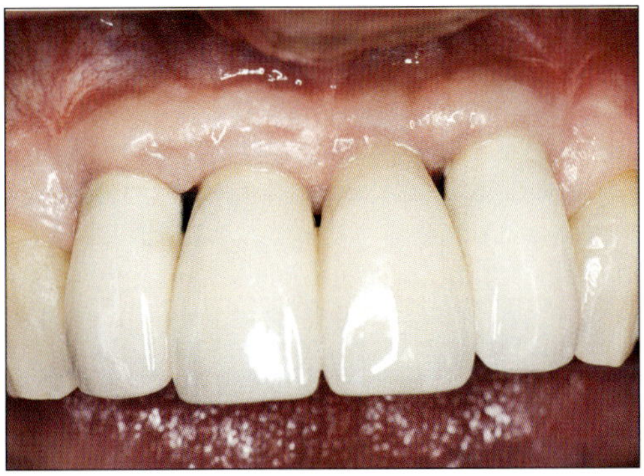

Fig 6-4 View of the final denture supported by three implants at the positions of the maxillary lateral incisors and the right central incisor (restoration, Dr E. Cohen).

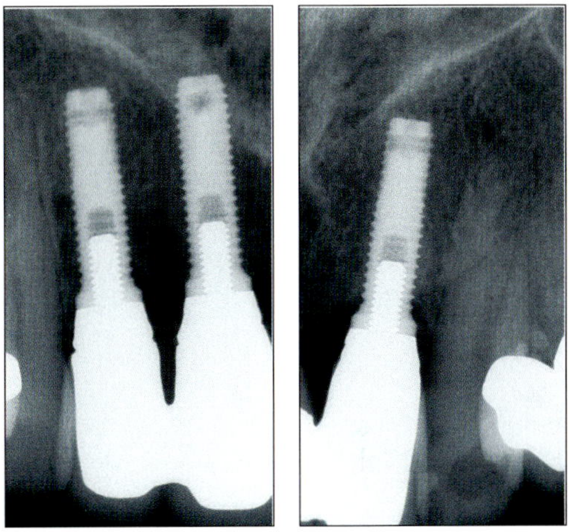

Fig 6-5 Radiographic control after 1 year of loading.

- Excessive buccal angulation leads to an unesthetic emergence profile associated with a subsequent gingival recession risk. The metal framework often becomes visible.
- Excessive lingual tipping must be compensated for by a buccal prosthetic ridge lap with difficult, indeed impossible, access for oral hygiene and maintenance.

Table 6-1 Number of implants in relation to the available mesiodistal space

Mesiodistal prosthetic space (mm)	Recommended number of standard implants
7	1
15	2
22	3
29	4
36	5

c. Apicocoronal plane

It is preferable to use implant lengths of at least 10 mm. In the mandibular symphysis region, the placement of long implants (at least 13 mm) is often possible. The implant neck is submerged apical to the cemento-enamel junction of the adjacent teeth. The submerging is limited by the alveolar cortical bone thickness. In the presence of a thin cortical alveolar crest, excessive submerging may compromise implant stability.

3. Residual ridge contour

Tooth loss leads to more or less mid- and long-term bone resorption (vertical and/or horizontal). This bone loss appears clinically as an alteration of the buccal, crestal, or lingual contour. Contour alteration is often unilateral. In the anterior regions, an extensive bone defect may lead to a change in the patient's profile and compromise the number and positioning of the implants. In cases of extensive tissue loss, the clinical crown:implant ratio would be reversed.

These ridge contour alterations may lead to prosthetic failure or a number of complications:

—poor implant angulations
—poor esthetic result
—phonetic problems
—insufficient lip support
—difficult oral hygiene and maintenance

4. Residual ridge contour and treatment choice

The different diagnostic means and the patient's esthetic demands will guide the treatment choice, depending on the residual ridge contour.

a. Normal or slightly resorbed residual ridge contour

The ridge circumference is intact. Implants of appropriate diameter and length may be placed in an ideal prosthetic axis. The ridge contour as well as the prosthetic space are respected.

b. Moderately resorbed residual ridge contour

The treatment choice will depend on:

—the residual bone volume
—edentulous situation (maxilla or mandible)
—patient demands
—type of smile

An edentulous anterior maxilla with a partially resorbed ridge associated with a gummy smile and major esthetic demands requires implant placement according to an ideal prosthetic axis. This positioning may create peri-implant bone defects (dehiscence or fenestration). Guided tissue regeneration and/or bone grafting before or during implant placement are sometimes indicated.

c. Severely resorbed residual ridge contour

The ridge circumference is totally altered and often associated with horizontal bone loss. The mesiodistal space is thus limited by the curved alveolar arch decrease. Bone augmentation (onlay bone grafting) is the treatment of choice in the maxilla. In the mandible, esthetic demands in the anterior region are less important. Bone ridge height may be reduced by several millimeters. The implants are placed in a more apical position.

B. Prosthetic considerations

1. Available vertical prosthetic space

A minimum vertical space of 5 mm (from the implant neck to the opposite tooth) is necessary for the prosthetic rehabilitation. The abutment is chosen according to this space.

In the presence of a reduced prosthetic space, several options must be considered:

- —coronoplasty of the opposing teeth
- —prosthetic rehabilitation of the opposing teeth in order to increase the prosthetic space, combined with a possible preprosthetic periodontal surgery
- —orthodontic treatment
- —orthodontic surgery (for borderline cases)

2. *Implant emergence point*

The mesiodistal aspect of the implant emergence point is essential for the prosthetic work (Figs 6-6 to 6-11). An implant emerging in the interproximal space leads to an unesthetic result and makes it impossible to ensure adequate oral hygiene and maintenance. In the anterior maxillary regions, an esthetic analysis is essential in order to avoid prosthetic failures. The use of a surgical template allows ideal implant positioning.

3. *Emergence profile*

In the anterior regions, anatomy of the contralateral tooth must be precisely assessed in order to obtain a more natural emergence profile. The mesiodistal prosthetic space available for the mandibular incisors, and sometimes for the maxillary lateral incisors, is less than 4.5 mm. Using a standard implant (neck diameter 4.1 mm), it is often impossible to achieve a good esthetic outcome. The narrow-neck implants (3.4 mm) allow a more natural emergence profile. For the maxillary central incisors, a more adapted emergence profile is obtained using wide-neck implants. The parallel between the implant and prosthetic margins allows a more natural crown anatomy.

4. *Occlusion*

The analysis of occlusion must be performed before considering the implant option (mounting the models to a simulator and diagnostic waxup). The static interarch relationships (centric relation, maximum intercuspation) and the dynamic ones (lateral movements, protrusion) are thus analyzed. Simultaneous contacts on the implant prosthesis and on the posterior teeth must be sought. It is preferable that the occlusal stresses apply to the implant's long axis.[5]

5. *Type of prosthesis: Screw-retained or cemented*

The prosthesis must be cemented if the implant axes emerge on the buccal aspect or at the incisor edge level. The prosthesis can be screw retained if the screw access holes of the abutments are located on the palatal or lingual aspect of the clinical crown. Angulated abutments allow correction of the implant axis.

III. Partial edentulism in the posterior regions

This type of edentulous situation may be combined with the presence or absence of the posterior teeth (tooth bound or distal).

For a tooth-bound edentulous space, the parameters governing the prosthetic choice are:

- —patient demand
- —state of the adjacent teeth in relation to the edentulous space
- —the prosthetic value of the adjacent teeth as abutments for a fixed partial denture
- —the available bone
- —the available prosthetic space

For a distal edentulous region, the prosthetic options will depend on:

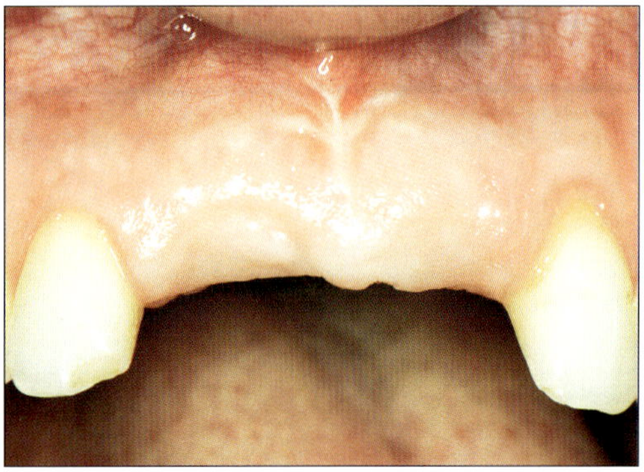

Fig 6-6 Tooth-bound edentulous space in a patient presenting diastemas.

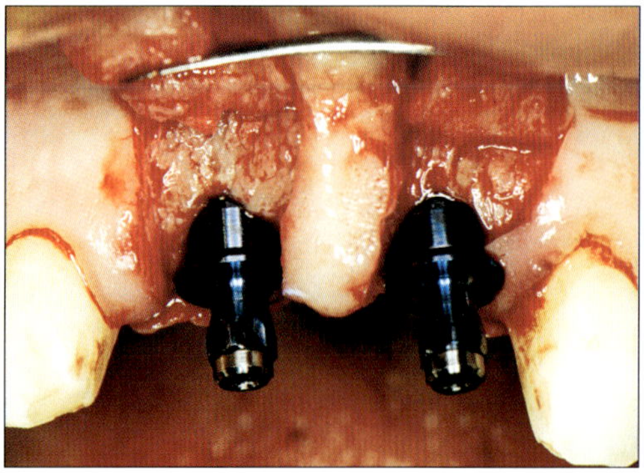

Fig 6-7 Placement of two 3i implants: double flap technique preserving the interdental papilla (surgery, Dr D. Etienne).

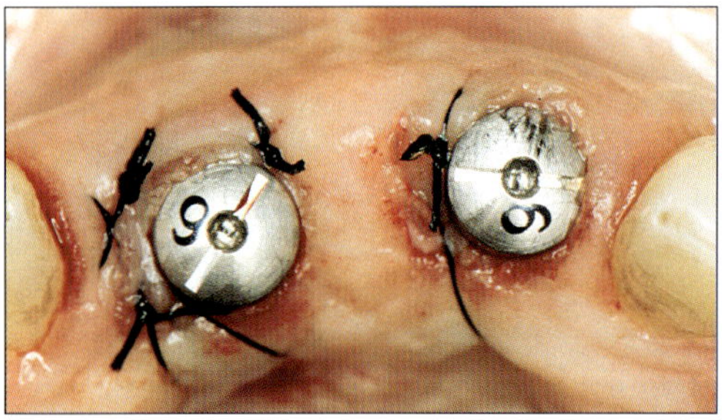

Fig 6-8 Occlusal view of stage-two surgery. Placing the 3i healing abutments (5-mm diameter and 6-mm height).

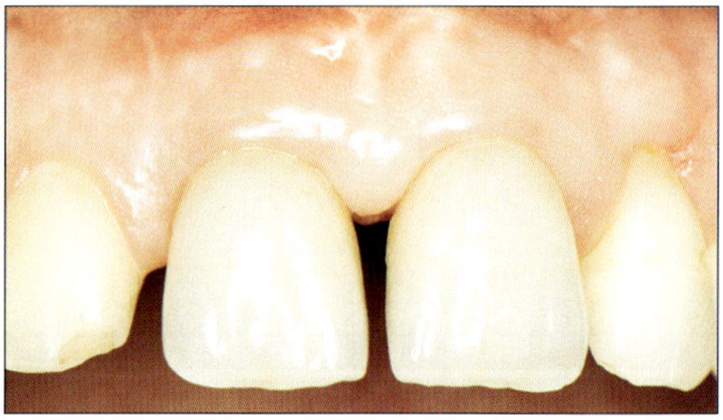

Fig 6-9 Clinical view of two final single-unit crowns replacing the maxillary central incisors (restoration, Dr P.-L. Menger).

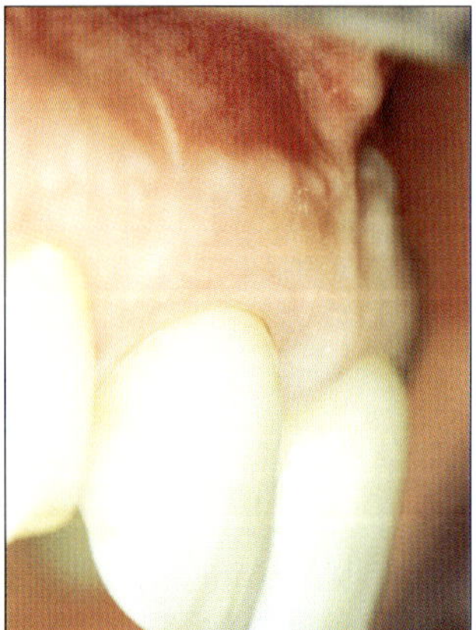

Fig 6-10 Note the very good emergence profile.

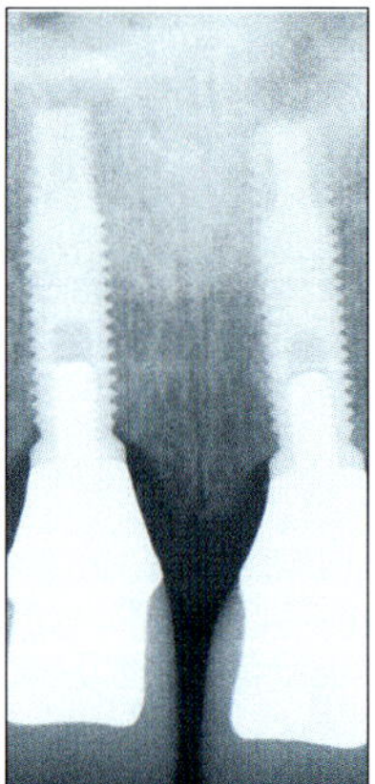

Fig 6-11 Radiographic control after 1 year of loading.

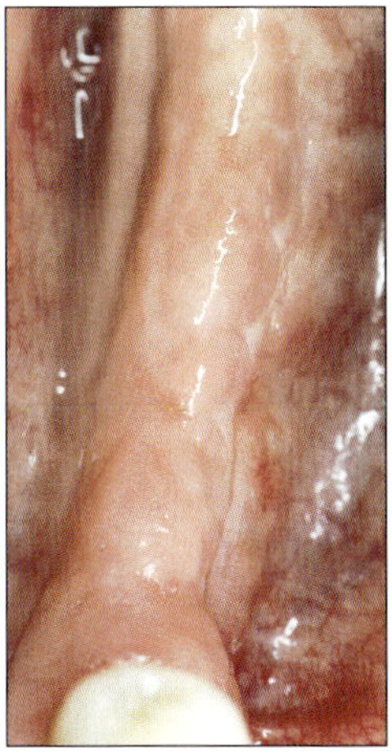

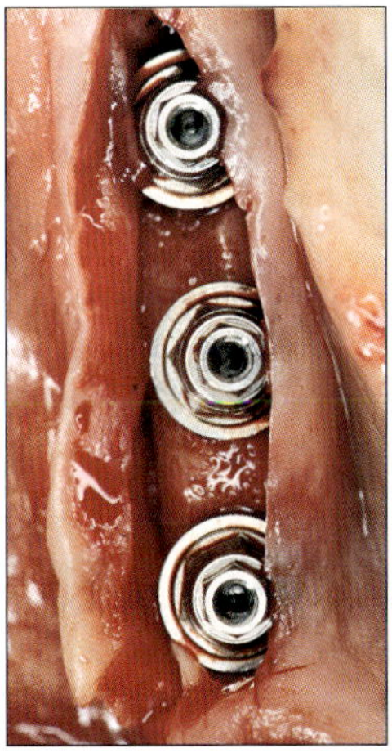

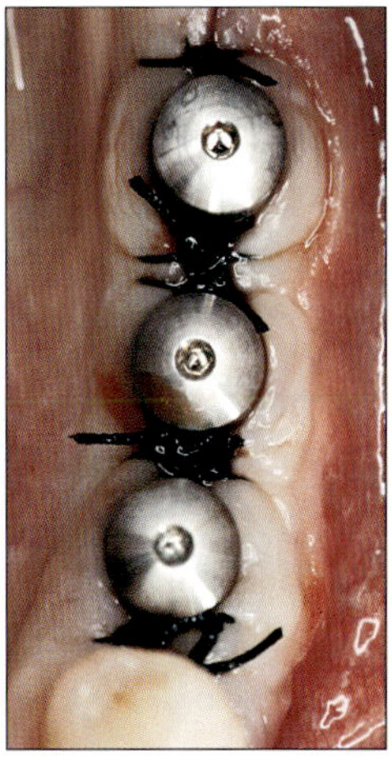

Fig 6-12 *(left)* Posterior edentulous space in the left mandibular region.

Fig 6-13 *(center)* Clinical view of stage-two surgery. Placement of three conical abutments (3i).

Fig 6-14 *(right)* Occlusal view after placing the titanium healing caps protecting the conical abutments.

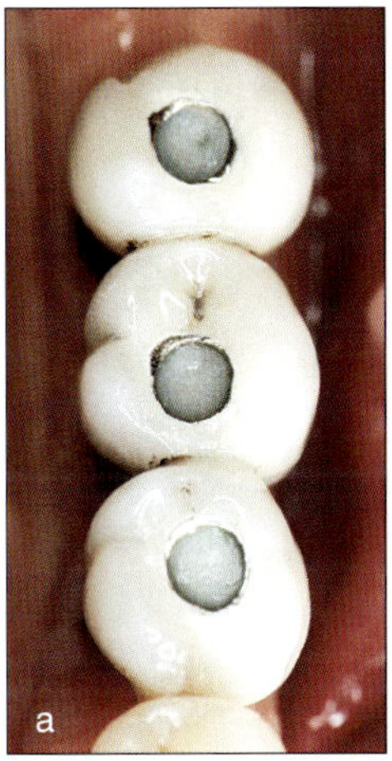

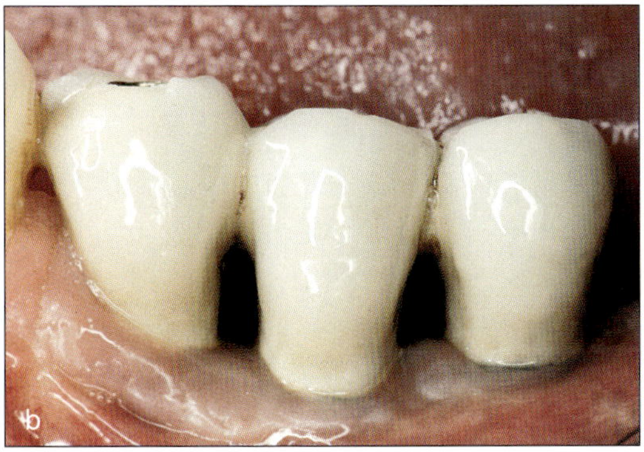

Fig 6-15a Occlusal view of the three splinted and screwed crowns (restoration, Dr P. Raygot).

Fig 6-15b Buccal view of the final prosthesis.

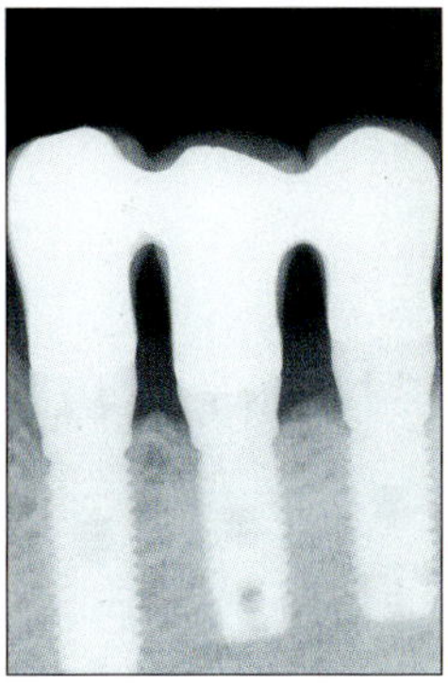

Fig 6-16 Radiographic view after 3 years of loading. Note the perfect osseointegration of the implants.

—patient demand
—the available bone
—the available prosthetic space[6]

A. Surgical considerations

1. Implant positioning

The available bone volume (width and height) must be assessed in the three dimensions of space in order to select the number, diameter, and length of the implants.

a. Mesiodistal plane

In presence of an adequate bone width, the number of implants (standard) is calculated in relation to the unilateral mesiodistal distance of the edentulous space. The aim is to place one implant per tooth (Figs 6-12 to 6-16; see Table 6-1).

Alternatively, in the posterior regions, large-diameter implants may be placed in the presence of large bone ridges. The different implant diameters allow adaptation of the

Table 6-2 Mean cervical measurements of the posterior maxillary teeth and recommended implant diameter

Tooth	Mesiodistal cervical diameter (mm)	Buccolingual cervical diameter (mm)	Implant diameter
Canine	5.5	7.0	Standard or large
First premolar	5.0	8.0	Standard
Second premolar	5.0	8.0	Standard
First molar	8.0	10.0	Large
Second premolar	8.0	9.0	Large

Table 6-3 Mean cervical measurements of the posterior mandibular teeth and recommended implant diameter

Tooth	Mesiodistal cervical diameter (mm)	Buccolingual cervical diameter (mm)	Implant diameter
Canine	5.0	6.5	Standard
First premolar	5.0	7.0	Standard
Second premolar	5.0	8.0	Standard
First molar	8.5	9.0	Large
Second premolar	8.0	9.0	Large

prosthetic emergence profile to the replaced natural tooth (Tables 6-2 and 6-3). If the available ridge width limits the placement of large-diameter implants, a greater number of standard implants must then be considered. In the presence of an adequate mesiodistal space, some clinicians recommend two standard implants to replace one molar.

b. Buccolingual plane

The implants must ideally be surrounded by at least 1 mm of bone on all sides. For a standard implant, a ridge width of at least 6 mm is necessary. For a large-diameter implant, a ridge width of at least 7 mm is essential.

Ideally, the implants must be placed in the center of the future prosthetic crowns; however, the respective bone resorption (centripetal for the maxilla and centrifugal for the mandible) prevents ideal positioning. The study casts mounted to a simulator and the diagnostic wax pattern allow consideration of the ideal prosthetic axis according to the residual ridge. This axis is transferred to the scan reconstructions using the radiographic template. The oblique scans confirm the possible positioning of the implant in the anticipated prosthetic axis.

The posterior mandibular bone morphology often presents a highly increased lingual concavity. In this situation, two solutions may be considered:

—the use of shorter implants
—modification of the implant axis

c. Apicocoronal plane

When a residual 8 to 10 mm of bone height is available, the use of short standard implants may be considered for the prosthetic restoration in the posterior region. Higher failure rates

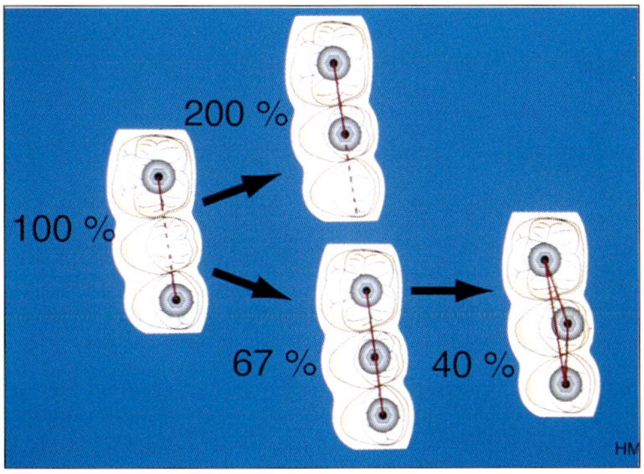

Fig 6-17 Distribution of the occlusal forces in relation to implant number and position (according to Rangert et al[8]).

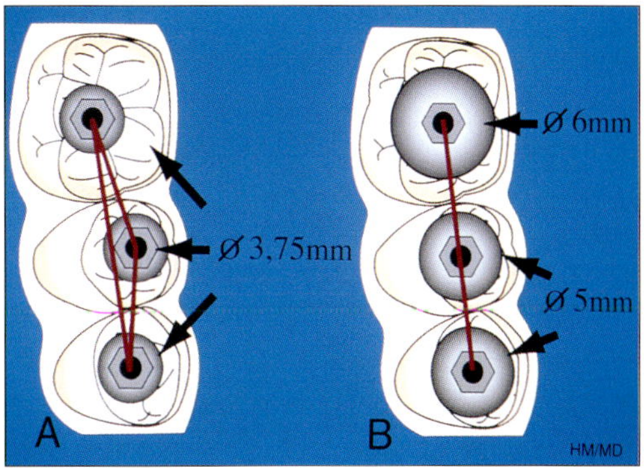

Fig 6-18 (A) Positioning of the standard implants in a tripod arrangement; (B) in the presence of a large ridge, large-diameter implants may be placed in a linear arrangement.

have been reported with the short standard implants.

2. *Inadequate implant angulations*

Frequently, the residual bone volume does not allow implant placement according to ideal axes.[7] A slightly modified axis will be corrected during the prosthetic fabrication. A significant cantilever increases the risk for fracture of the prosthetic and/or implant components. A significant implant angulation may be corrected using angulated abutments. It is preferable to splint significantly angled implants in order to reduce mechanical stress.

3. *Implant diameter*

In the posterior regions, the use of an implant diameter that is adapted to the cervical diameter of the replaced tooth allows a good esthetic result and an adequate emergence profile. At the cervical level, the mesiodistal diameter of the implant must be slightly smaller than that of the future prosthetic tooth. In the presence of a large ridge (greater than 7 mm), the use of large-diameter implants is recommended for molar replacement. However, this recommendation must take other factors into account (anatomic structures, residual bone quality and quantity, available prosthetic space), which will allow selection of the appropriate implant diameter.

B. Prosthetic considerations

1. *The tripod concept*

In the posterior regions, it is preferable to place the implants (standard) according to a tripod arrangement (Fig 6-17). This type of positioning for three implants is more favorable from a biomechanical point of view. The tripod arrangement allows an axial distribution of the occlusal forces, increases the stability of the restoration, and reduces the stress on the implants.[8,9]

In the presence of a wide ridge, large-diameter implants may be placed in a linear arrangement. This allows a good distribution of the occlusal forces and an optimal esthetic result (Fig 6-18).

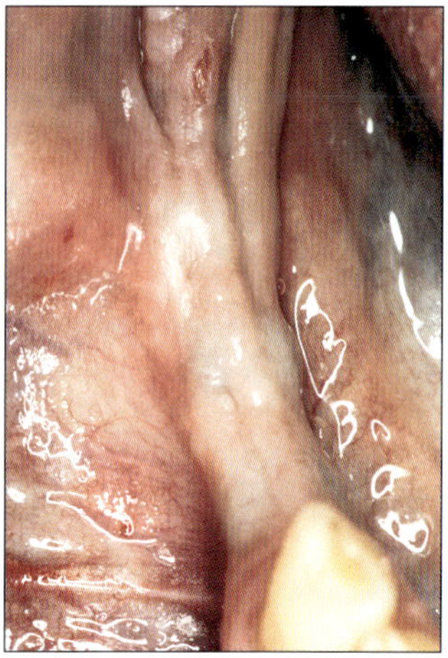

Fig 6-19 Distal edentulous space in the right mandibular region.

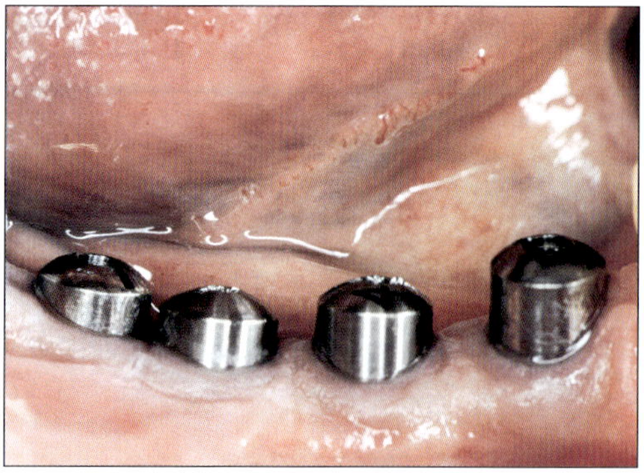

Fig 6-20 Buccal view of the healing abutments 6 weeks after loading.

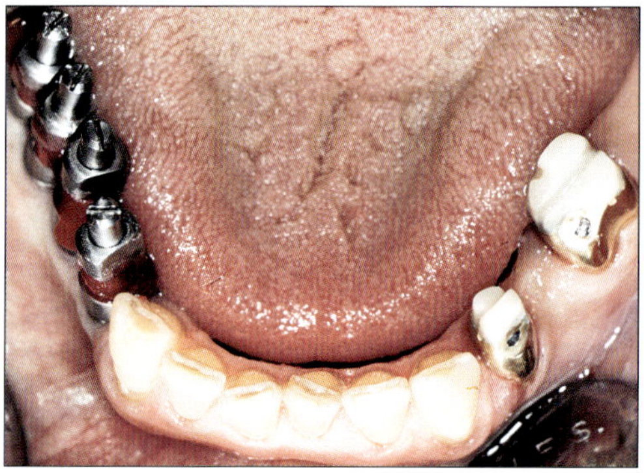

Fig 6-21 Occlusal view of the five transfer copings placed directly on the implant heads. The transfer copings are splinted using Duralay.

2. *Progressive loading*

Progressive loading has often been recommended for posterior implants. Indeed, insufficient bone quality and quantity in the posterior regions, combined with significant occlusal forces, may lead to implant complications. The use of an acrylic resin provisional restoration for 6 to 12 months may reduce the stress at the implant-bone interface.

During the loading, it is imperative to fabricate a metal framework supporting the acrylic resin. In the absence of a metal framework, the lack of rigidity offered by the resin may generate adverse forces on the implants.

3. *Occlusion*

During the prosthetic fabrication, simultaneous contacts on the implant-supported prosthesis and maximum intercuspation of the residual teeth must be sought.[10] The occlusal stress must ideally be applied along the implant axes.[11]

4. *Type of prosthesis: Screw-retained or cemented*

The implant-supported prosthesis must be cemented if the implant screws emerge on the buccal aspect. The prosthesis can be screw

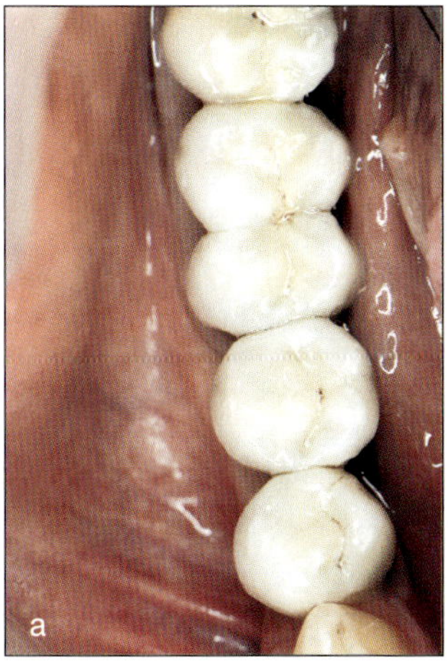

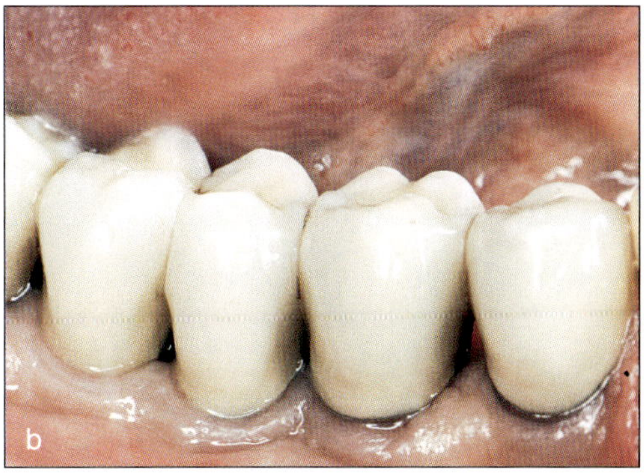

Figs 6-22a and 6-22b Final prosthetic restoration: buccal and occlusal views of the denture cemented to the implants (restoration, Dr P. Raygot).

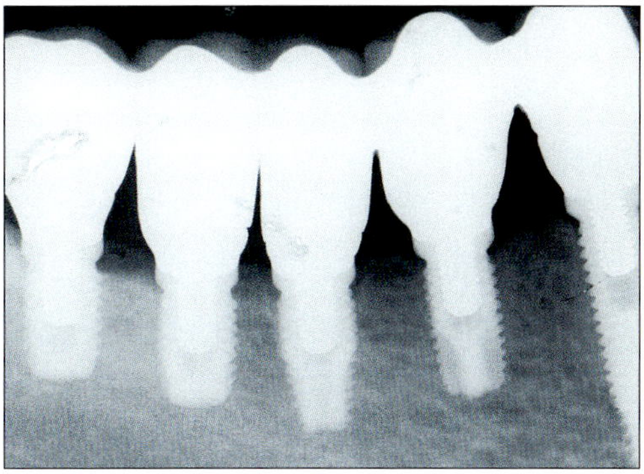

Fig 6-23 Radiographic view after 1 year of loading.

retained if the screw access holes of the abutments are located occlusally (Figs 6-19 to 6-23). Angulated abutments allow correction of the implant axis.

5. *Available vertical prosthetic space*

The available vertical prosthetic space is an essential factor in treatment planning. The absence of maxillary or mandibular molars may lead to overeruption of the opposing teeth. This overeruption limits the interarch distance for the future prosthetic fabrication. Management of the interarch space must therefore be performed before considering implant treatment. A vertical prosthetic space of at least 5 mm (from the implant neck to the opposing tooth) is required for the prosthetic restoration. The abutment selection is made according to that distance.

6. *Implant-tooth prosthetic connection*

Splinting natural teeth and endosseous implants still incites much controversy. The physiologic tooth mobility contrasts with the implant ankylosis. This relationship theoretically leads to biomechanical complications because of the difference of axial mobility between the tooth and the implant.[10] During masticatory function, the forces will concentrate on the implant. These stresses may compromise the bone-implant interface.

Indications include:

—insufficient sound natural abutments
—limited residual bone volume combined with a significant edentulous space
—presence of anatomic limitations

7. Tooth-implant resilience

Several theories and appliances have been developed in order to compensate for and justify the different tooth-implant resilience:

—the use of acrylic resin as a cosmetic material (instead of porcelain and metal); acrylic resin reduces the transmitted occlusal forces compared to the other materials
—interposition of resilient components between the implant and the prosthesis
—elastic property of the implant-abutment system (Brånemark system)
—use of nonrigid attachments

However, the results of the different options mentioned above vary considerably and are contradictory. They naturally depend on the mobility of each tooth. For some, the presence of natural teeth may compensate for the absence of periodontal membrane receptors at the implant level even if other receptors (mucoperiosteal, muscular, capsular) may play an important role.

Rigid prosthetic restorations splinting teeth and implants have reported good short-term results.[12] The number and follow-up of the published studies are still lacking, and further investigations are required. It is preferable not to splint natural abutments and implants, except if specifically required for some borderline situations.

References

1. Bernard JP, Belser UC, Marchand D, Gebran G. Implants in partially edentulous patients: Surgical and prosthetic considerations. Cah Prothet 1996;96: 85–95.
2. Engelman MJ. Clinical Decision Making and Treatment Planning in Osseointegration. Chicago: Quintessence, 1996.
3. Henry PJ, Tolman DE, Bolender G. The applicability of osseointegrated implants in the treatment of partially edentulous patients: Three-year results of a prospective multicenter study. Quintessence Int 1993;24: 123–129.
4. Lazzara R. Effect of implant position on implant restoration design. J Esthet Dent 1993;5:265–269.
5. Zarb GA, Schmitt A. The longitudinal effectiveness of osseointegrated implants in anterior partially edentulous patients. Int J Prosthodont 1993;6:180–188.
6. Parein AM, Eckert SE, Wollan PC, Keller EE. Implant reconstruction in the posterior mandible: A long-term retrospective study. J Prosthet Dent 1997;78:34–42.
7. Naert I, Quirynen M, van Steenberghe D, Darius P. Six-year prosthodontic study of 509 consecutively inserted implants for the treatment of partial edentulism. J Prosthet Dent 1992;67:236–245.
8. Rangert B, Sullivan RM, Jemt TM. Load factor control for implants in the posterior partially edentulous segment. Int J Oral Maxillofac Implants 1997;12:360–370.
9. Rangert B, Krogh O, Langer B. Bending overload and implant fracture: A retrospective clinical analysis. Int J Oral Maxillofac Implants 1995;10:326–334.
10. Rangert B. Biomechanical considerations for partial prostheses. Nobelpharma News 1992;6:2.
11. Zarb GA, Schmitt A. The longitudinal effectiveness of osseointegrated implants in posterior partially edentulous patients. Int J Prosthodont 1993;6:189–196.
12. van Steenberghe D, Lekholm U, Bolender C. The applicability of osseointegrated oral implants in the rehabilitation of partial edentulism: A prospective multicenter study on 588 fixtures. Int J Oral Maxillofac Implants 1990;5:272–281.

CHAPTER 7

Treatment Considerations for the Single Missing Tooth

M. Davarpanah/M. Kebir/H. Martínez/J.-P. Bressand/D. Etienne

Treatment of single missing teeth is demanding and delicate. Success depends on the indications and respect of the surgical and prosthetic imperatives (Figs 7-1 to 7-4).[1-6]

Indications include:

- tooth agenesis
- edentulous situation combined with sound adjacent teeth
- edentulous situation combined with diastemas

- During single-unit implant placement, respect of the periodontal tissues surrounding the adjacent teeth is essential. At the cervical level, a minimum distance of 1 mm between the implant and the adjacent teeth allows papilla preservation or new formation (Fig 7-8).
- New implant diameters allow adaptation of the prosthetic emergence profile to the replaced tooth and to the available mesiodistal space.

I. Surgical considerations

A. Bone volume and implant position

The minimum bone volume required for the placement of a standard implant (3.75- or 4-mm diameter) must be assessed in the three dimensions of space.[3,7,8]

1. Mesiodistal plane

A distance greater than or equal to 6 mm in relation to the adjacent roots is essential. The implant axis must be placed in the center of the available mesiodistal width. The incisions must respect the papillae. In the presence of converging adjacent roots, management of the inter-root space using an orthodontic treatment is indicated (Figs 7-5 to 7-7).

2. Buccolingual plane

The implant must ideally be surrounded on its overall perimeter by at least 1 mm of bone. For a standard implant, a ridge width greater than or equal to 6 mm is necessary.

- The implant emergence point has an major influence on the type of prosthesis (cemented or screw retained).[9] For screw-retained restorations, the abutment screw access must be located on the lingual, palatal, or occlusal aspect. For cemented restorations, the abutment screw may be located on the buccal aspect.
- An excessively buccal axis leads to an unesthetic prosthetic emergence profile that is likely to induce subsequent gingival recession (Fig 7-9). An excessively lingual

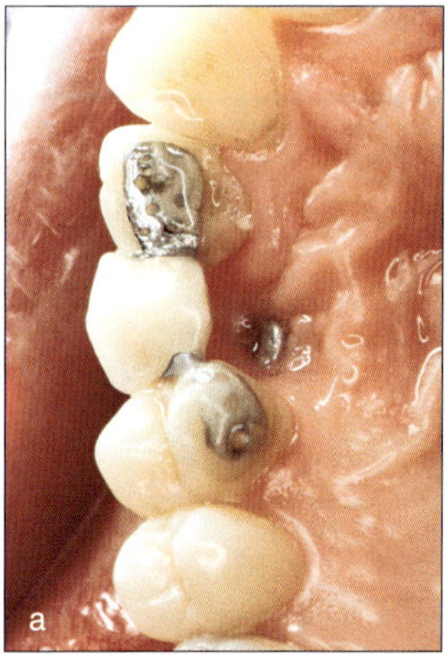

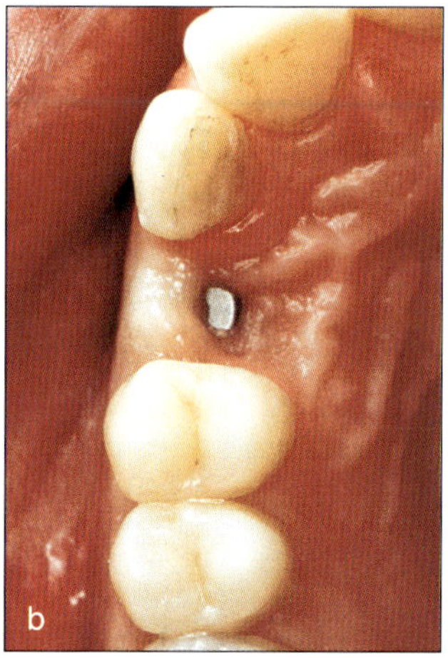

Fig 7-1a Single missing canine situation prior to retrieving the bonded fixed partial denture. Note the implant cover screw exposure.

Fig 7-1b Occlusal view following removal of the bonded partial denture.

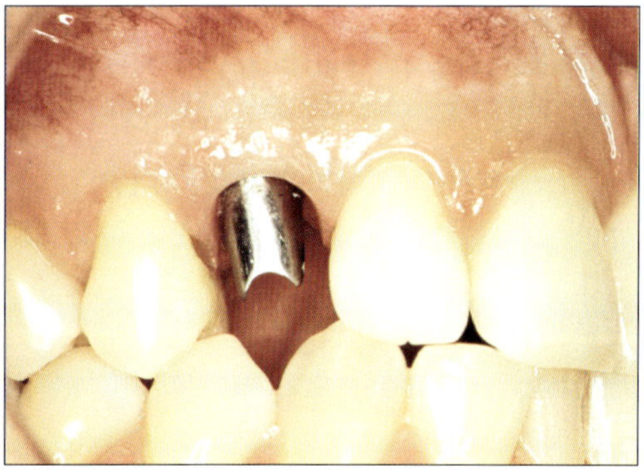

Fig 7-2 View of the gold UCLA abutment following removal of the provisional restoration at 3 months.

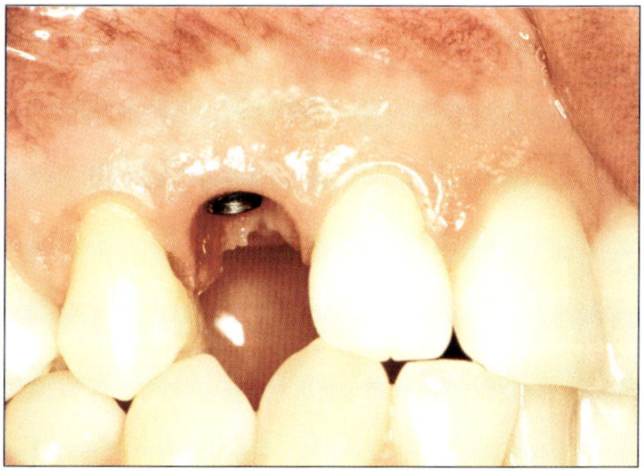

Fig 7-3 View of the tissue environment following removal of the gold UCLA abutment.

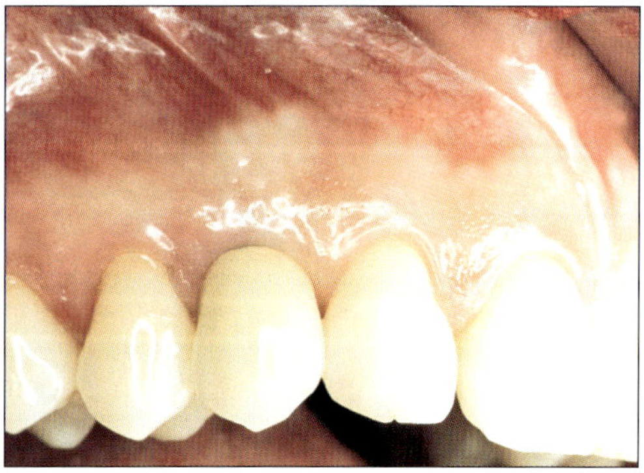

Fig 7-4a Clinical view of the final restoration (restoration, Dr J.-P. Bressand).

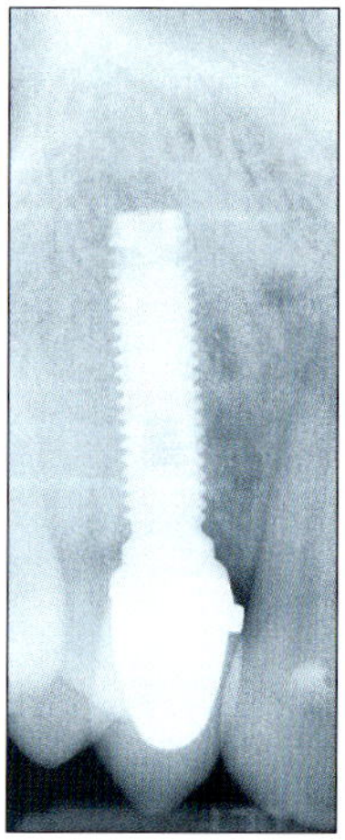

Fig 7-4b Radiographic control after 3 months of loading.

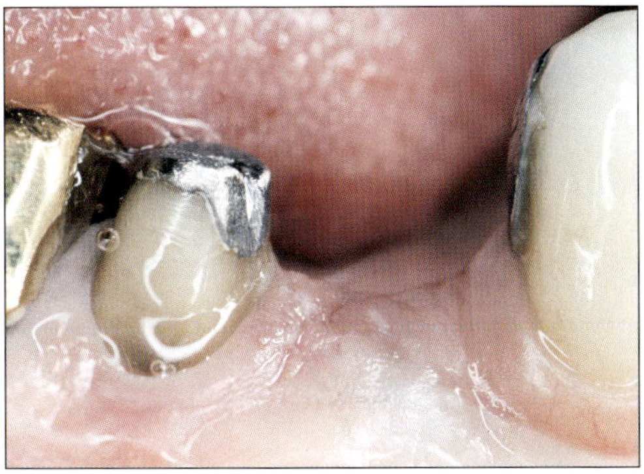

Fig 7-5a Missing mandibular right first premolar.

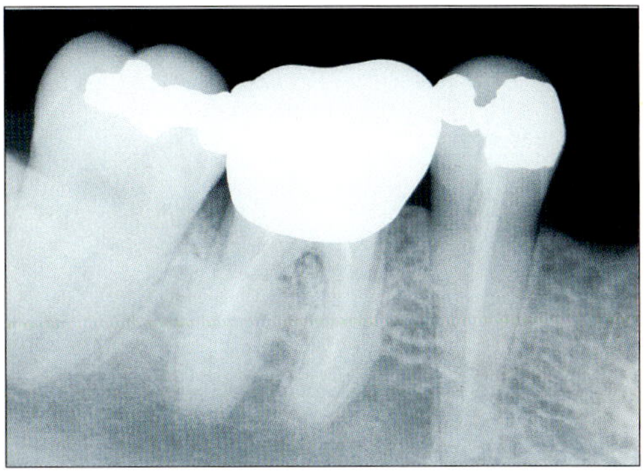

Fig 7-5b Radiographic view.

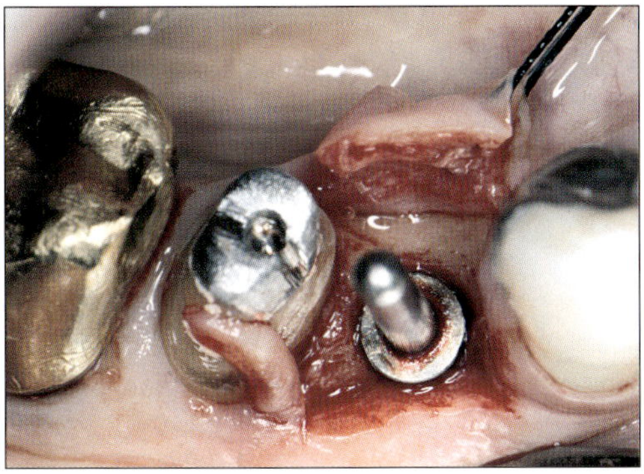

Fig 7-6 Occlusal view at stage-one surgery with the positioned direction indicator.

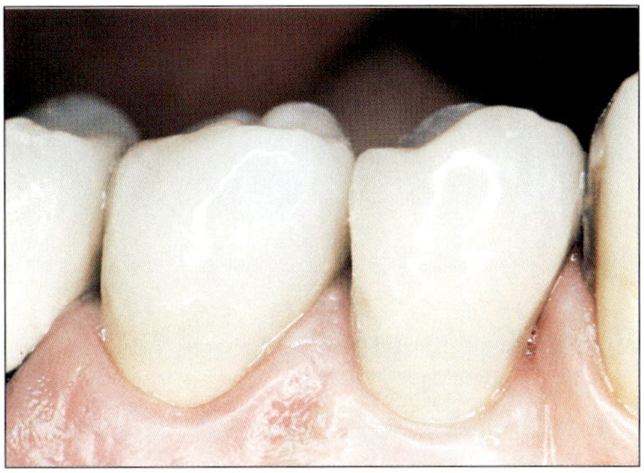

Fig 7-7 Clinical view after 2 years of loading (restoration, Dr P. Raygot).

axis must be compensated for with a buccal prosthetic overcontour, thus rendering oral hygiene and maintenance difficult.

3. *Apicocoronal plane*

It is recommended to use an implant with a length of at least 10 mm. A residual bone height of 12 mm is then necessary to prepare an implant site in the posterior mandibular regions. In the absence of gingival recession on the adjacent teeth, the coronal part of the implant is submerged 2 to 4 mm apical to the gingival margin of the adjacent teeth.

- A standard single-unit implant with a length of at least 10 mm has an uncertain prognosis that will depend on the bone quality (type I or II) of the implant site.
- In the mandible, a 2-mm space above the inferior dental canal must be strictly respected.
- In the presence of a thin cortical alveolar crest, implant stability may be compromised by excessive submerging.

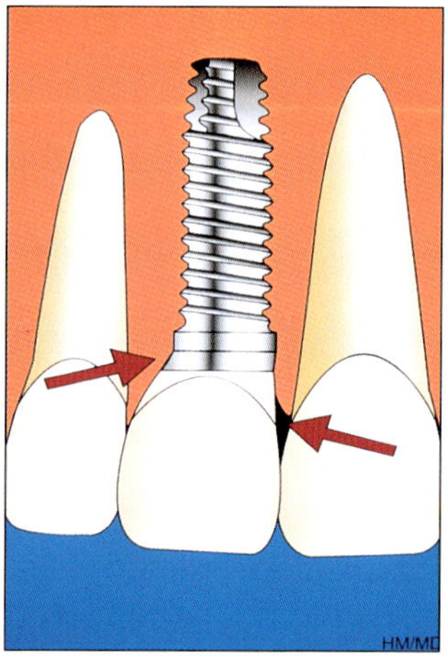

Fig 7-8 Positioning an implant too close to the adjacent tooth prevents papilla neoformation and leads to an adverse esthetic result.

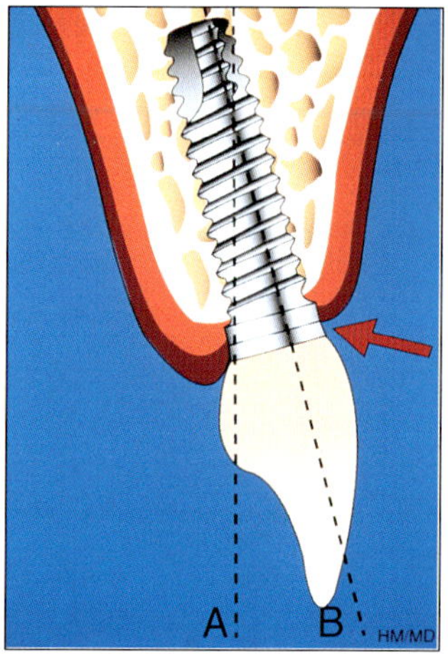

Fig 7-9 Diagram illustrating (A) implant axis in the center of the alveolar ridge and (B) excessively buccal implant axis. The emergence point leads to an inadequate esthetic result.

B. Anatomic limitations

The position and morphology of the nasopalatine canal, the maxillary sinus, and the mandibular canal must be determined by radiographic analysis. An large canal may dictate inadequate implant positioning and lead to an unesthetic outcome.

C. Implant diameter

The use of an implant diameter adapted to the cervical diameter of the replaced tooth allows a good esthetic result and an appropriate emergence profile. At the cervical level, the mesiodistal diameter of the implant must be slightly smaller than that of the future prosthetic tooth. In the apicocoronal aspect, and in the absence of gingival recession, the implant must be submerged 2 to 4 mm apical to the cementoenamel junction of the adjacent teeth. At that level, the root diameter is inevitably smaller than that of the cementoenamel junction.

II. Prosthetic considerations

A. Available prosthetic space

A vertical interarch height greater than 5 mm (from the implant neck to the opposing tooth) is required for the prosthetic restoration. Abutment selection depends on this distance.

A long-lasting edentulous situation is frequently combined with overeruption of the opposing teeth. The residual space is assessed clinically and on the study casts. The mean soft tissue thickness is 1 mm in the mandible and 2 mm in the maxilla. A precise evaluation may be performed under local anesthesia.

In the presence of insufficient prosthetic height, several options may be considered:

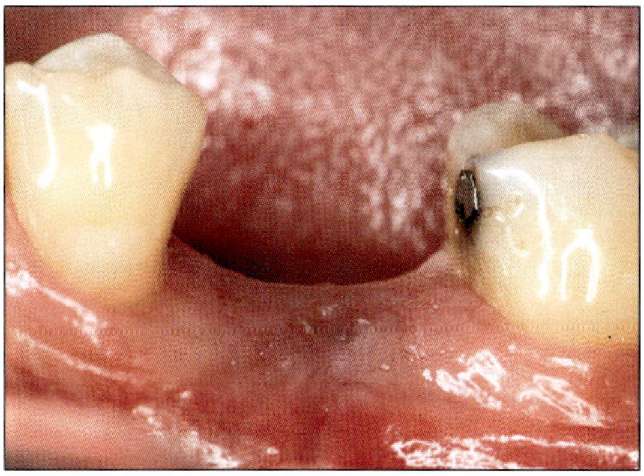

Fig 7-10 Single missing molar.

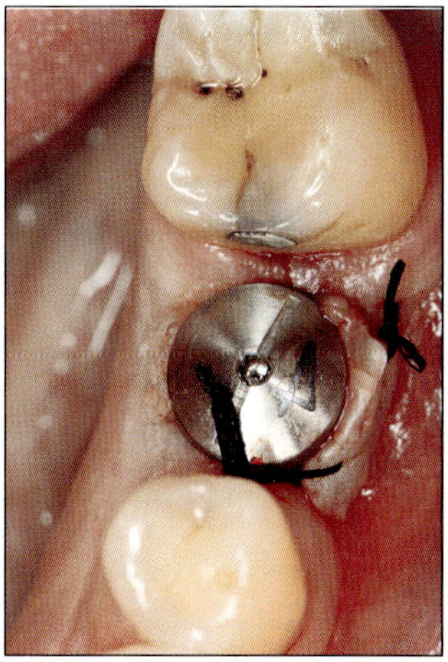

Fig 7-11 Occlusal view at stage-two surgery with the placement of a 3i abutment (7.5-mm diameter on 4 mm of height).

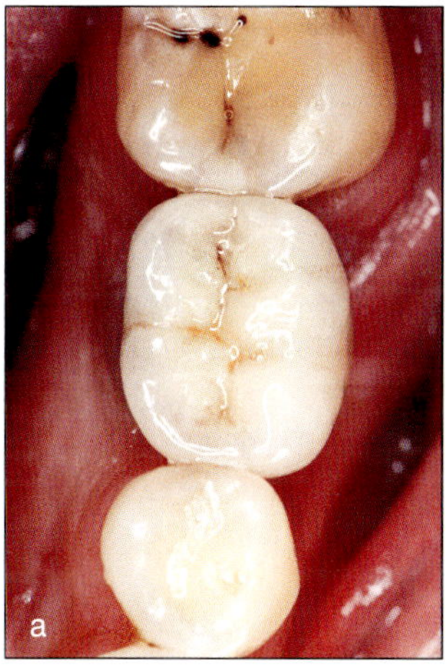

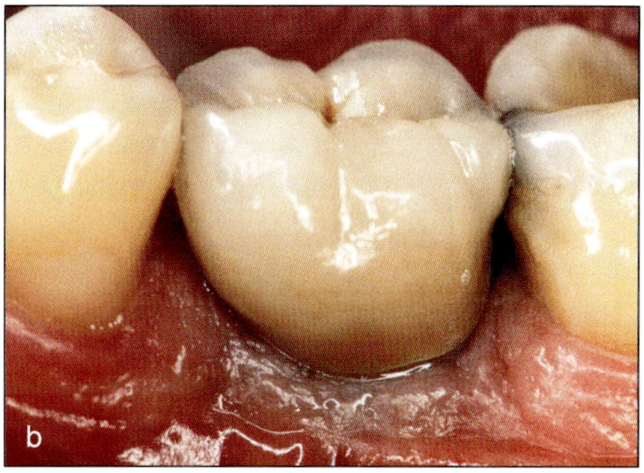

Figs 7-12a and 7-12b Occlusal and buccal views of the final restoration after 1 year of loading (restoration, Dr J.-P. Bressand).

—coronoplasty of the opposing tooth
—prosthetic restoration of the opposing tooth in order to reduce its clinical crown height, possibly preceded by preprosthetic surgery
—orthodontic ingression

B. Emergence profile

In the anterior regions, the anatomy of the contralateral tooth must be precisely assessed in order to obtain a more natural emergence profile. The available mesiodistal prosthetic space for the mandibular incisors, and sometimes for the maxillary lateral incisors, is less than

4.5 mm. A successful esthetic result is often impossible to obtain using a standard implant (neck diameter 4.1 mm).[3]

For the posterior teeth or the maxillary central incisors, a more adapted emergence profile is obtained using wide-neck implants (Figs 7-10 to 7-12). The parallel between the implant and prosthetic perimeters allows a more natural crown anatomy.

C. Clinical implant:crown ratio

Ideally, the clinical implant:crown ratio must be 1:2. A 1:1 ratio with poor bone density and/or heavy occlusal forces may compromise implant prognosis.

D. Occlusion

The occlusal analysis is performed before considering implant treatment. Some clinicians consider overbites and parafunctions contraindications to single-unit implant placement (especially for molars). Indeed, excessive occlusal forces may lead to screw loosening of the prosthetic components, fracture of the prosthetic parts, or even implant fracture and/or excessive bone resorption.[3] On a single-unit, implant-supported prosthesis, the occlusal contacts are adapted to the type of occlusion and to the patient's masticatory forces. Ideally, lateral contacts must be avoided or limited. In centric relation, contacts are harmoniously distributed simultaneously on the implant prosthesis as well as on the natural teeth. It is preferable that the resulting occlusal stress be applied along the implant axis. The best method to determine the occlusal pattern remains cast mounting to a simulator and fabrication of a diagnostic waxup.

E. Type of prosthesis: screwed or cemented

For the anterior teeth, the prosthesis may be screw retained if the abutment screw access is located on the palatal or lingual aspect of the clinical crown. For the posterior teeth, this access must be located on the occlusal aspect. The prosthesis must be cemented if the screw emerges on the buccal aspect.[3]

Esthetic demands vary from one patient to another. The esthetic outcome depends on the form, contours, cervical limits, emergence profile, and peri-implant soft tissue quality and quantity. A very successful esthetic result is often difficult to acheive.[3]

References

1. Balshi TJ. Candidates and requirements for single tooth implant prostheses. Int J Periodontics Restorative Dent 1994;14:317–331.
2. Boudrias P. The implant-supported single-tooth restoration. Preoperative evaluation and clinical procedure. Dent Clin North Am 1993;37:497–511.
3. Davarpanah M, Kebir M, Tecucianu JF, Etienne D, Martínez H. Implants unitaires: Impératifs chirurgicaux et prothétiques. J Parodontol Implantol Orale 1995;14:423–434.
4. Ekfeldt A, Carlsson GE, Borjesson G. Clinical evaluation of single-tooth restorations supported by osseointegrated implants: A retrospective study. Int J Oral Maxillofac Implants 1994;9:179–183.
5. Lekholm U, Jemt T. Principles for single tooth replacement. In: Albrektsson T, Zarb GA (eds). The Brånemark Osseointegrated Implant. Chicago: Quintessence, 1989:117–126.
6. Saadoun AP, Sullivan DY, Krischek M, Le Gall M. Single tooth implant management for success. Pract Periodontics Aesthet Dent 1994;6:73–82.
7. Lazzara R. Effect of implant position on implant restoration design. J Esthet Dent 1993;5:265–269.
8. Engquist B, Nilson H, Astrand P. Single-tooth replacement by osseointegrated Brånemark implants. Clin Oral Implants Res 1995;6:238–245.
9. Katona TR, Goodacre CJ, Brown DT, Roberts WE. Force-moment systems on single maxillary anterior implants: Effects of incisal guidance, fixture orientation and loss of bone support. Int J Oral Maxillofac Implants 1993;8:512–522.

CHAPTER 8

Implant Treatment for the Posterior Regions: Classification

H. Martínez/M. Davarpanah/P. Missika

In the posterior regions, the available bone volume may be insufficient due to bone resorption and/or anatomic limitations.

I. Type of bone loss

A. Maxillary bone loss

In the maxilla, bone loss in the region located beneath the sinus is:

—centripetal and related to postextraction bone resorption[1]
—centrifugal and related to a physiologic pneumatization of the maxillary sinus[2]

B. Mandibular bone loss

In the mandible, the bone loss is centrifugal.[3] This resorption leads to a residual ridge circumference that is larger than in the maxilla. A coronal position of the inferior dental canal may contraindicate implant placement. Long-lasting untreated posterior edentulism leads to overeruption of the opposing teeth. Adjustment of the interarch distance must be considered before the final prosthetic treatment. The position and state of the residual teeth must be assessed. The possible extractions will be performed according to the treatment planning. Some hopeless teeth are preserved during the osseointegration period as abutments for provisional restorations. An adequate clinical crown:implant ratio is essential for a good prognosis. The assessment of the available interarch distance and residual bone volume determines the surgical and prosthetic options.[1]

II. Classification and treatment options

A. Prosthetic space and maxillary bone volume (Table 8-1)

1. Limited bone volume and reduced prosthetic space (Fig 8-1)

a. In the maxilla

Placing implants in the subsinus region is possible when 8 to 10 mm of residual bone height is available. A sinus lift procedure may also be considered with an immediate implant placement.[4]

b. In the mandible

It is necessary to adjust the prosthetic space in order to obtain an adequate occlusal curve and an interarch distance greater than 5 mm. Depending on the overeruption degree of the opposing teeth, several options may be considered:

—coronoplasty of the mandibular teeth if the overeruption is slight
—crown lengthening combined with endodon-

Table 8-1 Prosthetic and surgical treatment according to the maxillary bone volume and available prosthetic space

Prosthetic space	Limited bone volume	Insufficient bone volume
Reduced	Prosthetic treatment in the mandible: —Coronoplasty in presence of a slight tooth overeruption —Crown lengthening and fixed prosthesis if overeruption is extensive	Prosthetic treatment in the mandible: —Coronoplasty in presence of a slight tooth overeruption —Crown lengthening and fixed prosthesis if overeruption is extensive
	Surgical treatment: —Implants penetrating the sinus —Large-diameter implants	Surgical treatment: —Tuberosity implants —Osteotomy and grafting —Sinus elevation and grafting
Adequate	Prosthetic treatment in the mandible: —Preservation of the prosthetic space	Prosthetic treatment in the mandible: —Preservation of the prosthetic space
	Surgical treatment: —Implants penetrating the sinus —Large-diameter implants	Surgical treatment: —Tuberosity implants —Osteotomy procedure —Sinus elevation and grafting
Increased	Prosthetic treatment in the mandible: —Preservation of the prosthetic space if the curve of Spee is normal —Fixed prosthesis if the curve of Spee is altered	Prosthetic treatment in the mandible: —Preservation of the prosthetic space if the curve of Spee is normal —Fixed prosthesis if the curve of Spee is altered
	Surgical treatment: —Implants penetrating the sinus —Large-diameter implants	Surgical treatment: —Osteotomy procedure —Sinus elevation and grafting —Onlay graft if the bone loss is extensive with a small-sized sinus

tic and prosthetic treatment if the overeruption is significant

2. *Insufficient bone volume and adequate prosthetic space (Fig 8-2)*

Pneumatization of the sinus is associated with this situation. Different treatment options may be offered in the maxilla according to:

—location of the residual teeth
—edentulous extent
—available bone volume mesial and distal to the sinus

a. *In the maxilla*

Different options may be considered:

—placing a tuberosity implant combined with one or two implants in the premolar region if the bone volume is sufficient[5]
—osteotomy procedure in the presence of a subsinus bone height between 5 and 7 mm[6]
—sinus grafting procedure (if the residual height is less than 6 mm) combined with implant placement[7]

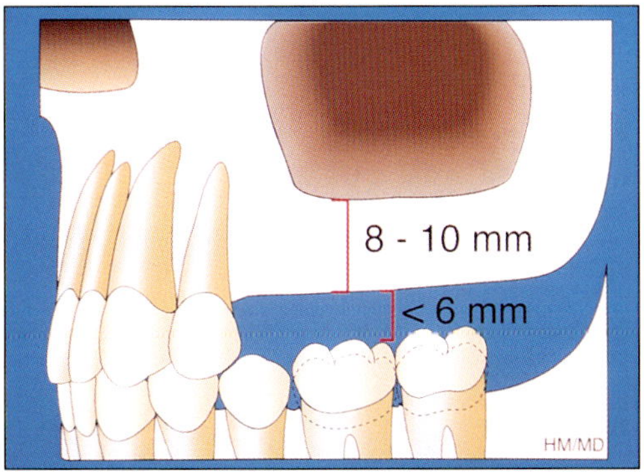

Fig 8-1 Limited bone volume and reduced prosthetic space.

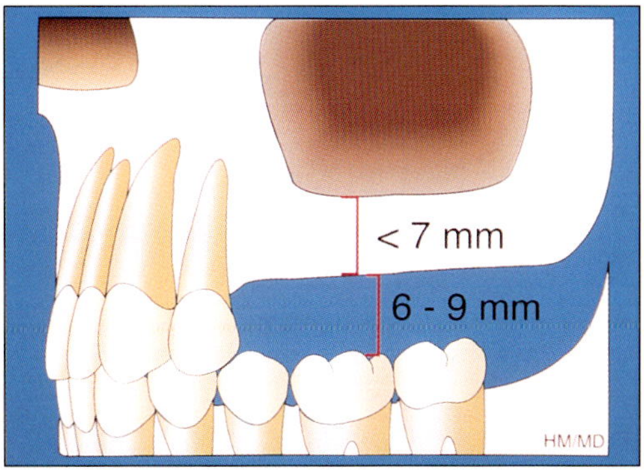

Fig 8-2 Insufficient bone volume and adequate prosthetic space.

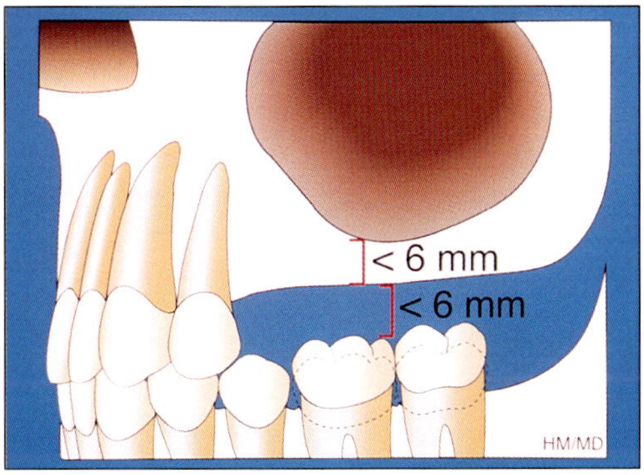

Fig 8-3 Insufficient bone volume and reduced prosthetic space.

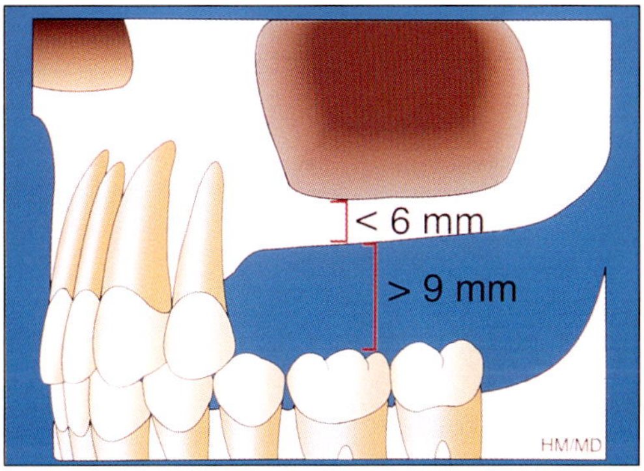

Fig 8-4 Insufficient bone volume and increased prosthetic space.

b. In the mandible

The prosthetic space has been preserved using a fixed or removable maxillary partial prosthesis. The mandibular teeth must be assessed.

3. Insufficient bone volume and reduced prosthetic space (Fig 8-3)

Treatment planning for this situation is more complex and related to the two regions. The interarch distance must be adjusted.

a. In the maxilla

Two options may be considered depending on the residual bone volume:

- placing tuberosity implants combined with implants in the premolar region[4,8]
- sinus filling procedure (subsinus graft)[8,9]

b. In the mandible

The curve of Spee must be restored using:

- coronoplasty if the curve is slightly disturbed
- in the severe cases, the ideal treatment consists of crown lengthening combined with a fixed prosthesis

Table 8-2 Prosthetic and surgical treatment according to the mandibular bone volume and available prosthetic space

Prosthetic space	Limited bone volume	Insufficient bone volume
Reduced	Prosthetic treatment in the maxilla: —Coronoplasty in presence of a slight tooth overeruption —Crown lengthening and fixed prosthesis if overeruption is extensive	Prosthetic treatment in the maxilla: —Coronoplasty in presence of a slight tooth overeruption —Crown lengthening and fixed prosthesis if overeruption is extensive
	Surgical treatment: —Multiple short standard implants —Large-diameter implants	Surgical treatment: —Short large-diameter implants —Inferior dental nerve repositioning
Adequate	Prosthetic treatment in the maxilla: —Preservation of the prosthetic space	Prosthetic treatment in the maxilla: —Preservation of the prosthetic space
	Surgical treatment: —Multiple short standard implants —Large-diameter implants —Inferior dental nerve repositioning	Surgical treatment: —Short large-diameter implants —Supracrestal implants (1 to 3 mm) combined with a GBR procedure
Increased	Prosthetic treatment in the maxilla: —Preservation of the prosthetic space if the curve of Spee is normal —Fixed prosthesis if the curve of Spee is altered	Prosthetic treatment in the maxilla: —Preservation of the prosthetic space if the curve of Spee is normal —Fixed prosthesis if the curve of Spee is altered
	Surgical treatment: —Multiple short standard implants —Large-diameter implants —Supracrestal implants (1 to 3 mm) combined with a GBR procedure	Surgical treatment: —Supracrestal implants (3 mm) combined with a GBR procedure —Onlay autogenous bone graft

GBR = guided bone regeneration.

4. *Insufficient bone volume and increased prosthetic space (Fig 8-4)*

In this situation, the treatment planning is complex. A significant interarch distance must be maintained.

a. In the maxilla

The treatment may consist of:

—autogenous onlay bone graft and sinus grafting if the height loss is combined with sinus pneumatization; the dental implants are placed in a second surgical stage[10]

—autogenous onlay bone graft combined with immediate or delayed implant placement if the sinus pneumatization is not significant

b. In the mandible

If the curve of Spee is not disturbed, the different treatment approaches are surgical. If the curve of Spee is disturbed, a prosthetic approach must be considered.

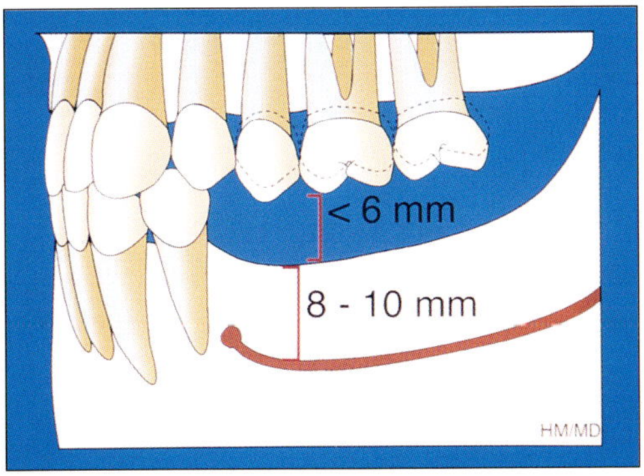

Fig 8-5 Limited bone volume and reduced prosthetic space.

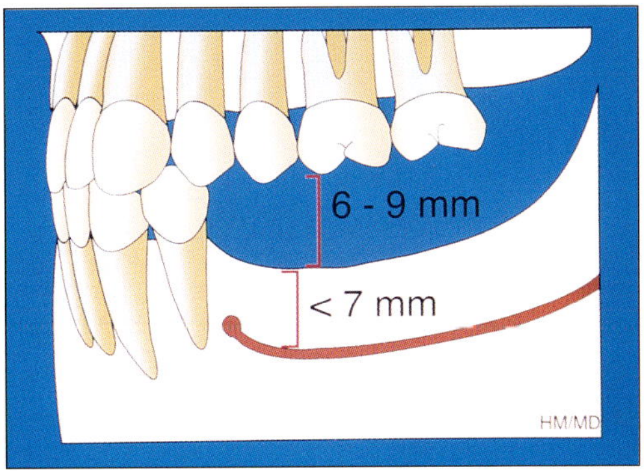

Fig 8-6 Insufficient bone volume and adequate prosthetic space.

B. Prosthetic space and mandibular bone volume (Table 8-2)

1. Limited bone volume and reduced prosthetic space (Fig 8-5)

a. In the mandible

Placing the implants above the inferior dental nerve is possible when 9 mm of residual bone height is available.[1]

b. In the maxilla

It is necessary to adjust the prosthetic space in order to obtain an adequate occlusal curve and an interarch distance greater than 5 mm. Concerning the maxillary teeth, the following approach must be performed:

—coronoplasty of the maxillary teeth if the overeruption is slight
—crown lengthening combined with endodontic treatment and a fixed prosthesis if the overeruption is significant

2. Insufficient bone volume and adequate prosthetic space (Fig 8-6)

a. In the mandible

Three options may be considered according to the residual bone volume:

—if the available space is 8 to 9 mm, a wide ridge allows the use of short large-diameter implants[11,12]
—if the available space is 7 mm, a 3-mm bone augmentation of the ridge height may be considered, using a titanium-reinforced membrane combined or not with an autogenous bone graft
—if the available space is less than 7 mm, inferior dental nerve repositioning may be considered; the risks of this procedure must be very seriously considered and explained to the patient

b. In the maxilla

The prosthetic space has been preserved using a fixed or removable mandibular partial prosthesis. The maxillary teeth must be assessed.

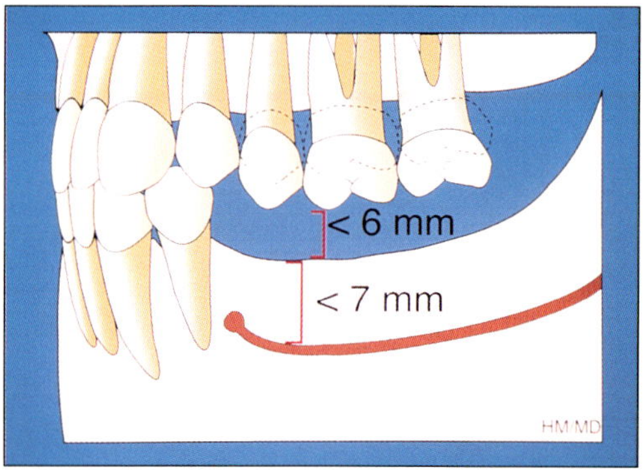

Fig 8-7 Insufficient bone volume and reduced prosthetic space.

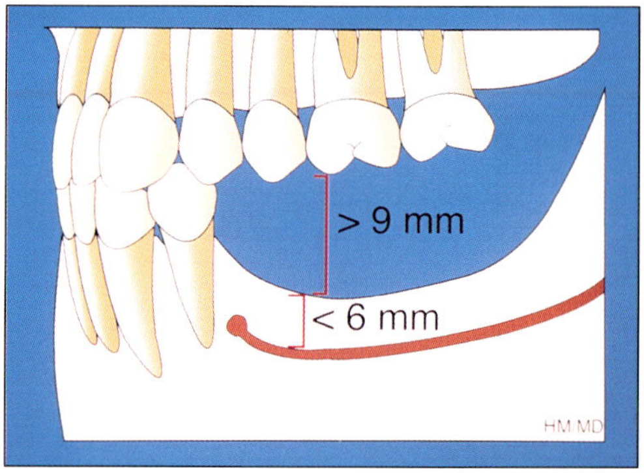

Fig 8-8 Insufficient bone volume and increased prosthetic space.

3. *Insufficient bone volume and reduced prosthetic space (Fig 8-7)*

The treatment is more complex and concerns the two regions. The interarch distance must be adjusted.

a. In the mandible

Three options may be considered according to the residual bone volume:

—an 8 to 6 mm bone height combined with a large ridge allows the use of short large-diameter implants[2,11]
—if the available space is 7 mm, a 3-mm bone augmentation of the ridge height may be considered, using a titanium-reinforced membrane combined or not with an autogenous bone graft
—if the available space is less than 7 mm, repositioning of the inferior dental nerve may be considered[13]; the risks of this procedure must be very seriously considered and explained to the patient

b. In the maxilla

The curve of Spee must be adjusted using:

—coronoplasty if the curve is slightly disturbed
—in the severe cases, the ideal treatment consists of crown lengthening combined with a fixed prosthesis

4. *Insufficient bone volume and increased prosthetic space (Fig 8-8)*

a. In the mandible

The following procedures may be performed:

—an autogenous onlay bone graft with a delayed implant placement
—an autogenous onlay bone graft with immediate implant placement in order to secure the graft
—placement of supracrestal implants (3 to 4 mm) combined with a guided tissue regeneration procedure in order to increase the alveolar ridge height (the amount of clinical follow-up documented to date is not significant)[1]

b. In the maxilla

If the curve of Spee is not disturbed, the different treatment approaches are surgical. If the curve of Spee is disturbed, a prosthetic approach must be considered.

References

1. Martínez H, Davarpanah M, Celletti R, Missika P. Edentement mandibulaire postérieur. Classification et thérapeutique. Actual Odontostomatol 1999;208: 441–453.
2. Martínez H, Zerbib R, Tarragano H, Missika P. Les implants au niveau postérieur du maxillaire: Critères de choix de la technique chirurgicale. Implant 1997;3:5–15.
3. Atwood DA. Bone loss of edentulous alveolar ridges. J Periodontol 1979;50:11–21.
4. Brånemark P-I, Adell R, Albrektsson T, Lekholm U, Lindstrom J, Rockler B. An experimental and clinical study of osseointegrated implants penetrating the nasal cavity and maxillary sinus. J Oral Maxillofac Surg 1984;43:497–505.
5. Bahat O. Osseointegrated implants in the maxillary tuberosity: Report of 45 consecutive patients. Int J Oral Maxillofac Implants 1992;7:459–467.
6. Martínez H, Davarpanah M. Déficit osseux sous-sinusien: Traitement chirurgical. Objectif Paro 1997;160:2–4.
7. Tatum H Jr. Maxillary and sinus implant reconstructions. Dent Clin North Am 1986;30:207–229.
8. Boyne PJ, James RA. Grafting of the maxillary floor with autogenous marrow and bone. J Oral Surg 1980;38:613–616.
9. Tulasne JF, Saade J, Riachi A. Greffe osseuse du sinus maxillaire et implants de Brånemark. Cah Prothet Implantol 1993;(special issue 2):101–116.
10. Keller EE, van Roekel NB, Desjardins RP, et al. Prosthetic surgical reconstruction of the severely resorbed maxilla with iliac bone grafting and tissue-integrated prostheses. Int J Oral Maxillofac Implants 1987;2:155–165.
11. Davarpanah M, Martínez H, Tecucianu JF, Etienne D, Kebir M. Les implants de large diamètre. Résultats chirurgicaux à 2 ans. Implant 1995;1:289–300.
12. Langer B, Langer L, Herrmann I, Erug M. The wide fixture: A solution for special bone situations and rescue for the compromised implant. Part 1. Int J Oral Maxillofac Implants 1993;8:400–408.
13. Jensen J, Nock D. Inferior alveolar nerve reposition in conjunction with placement of osseointegrated implants: A case report. Oral Surg Oral Med Oral Pathol 1987;63:263–268.

CHAPTER 9

Specific Surgical Procedures

M. Davarpanah/H. Martínez/R. Celletti/R. Lazzara

Rehabilitation of an edentulous space is an important challenge for the clinician. A solely prosthetic approach to management of alveolar bone loss frequently leads to esthetic and/or functional compromises. Today, specific surgical techniques extend implant options and optimize their final results:

—extraction and immediate implant placement
—tuberosity and pterygomaxillary implants
—partial intrasinus and nasal fossa implants
—sinus grafting
—onlay bone grafts
—dental nerve repositioning
—guided bone regeneration (GBR)
—osteotomies and bone grafts

These specific techniques deviate from the conventional surgical protocol. An appropriate knowledge of the indications and surgical techniques is essential for treatment success.

I. Extraction and immediate implant placement

In 1989, Lazzara[1] described the protocol for immediate implant placement following extraction (Fig 9-1). This author advocates the use of grafting materials and/or membranes. The implant must be the longest possible according to the residual bone volume in order to ensure an adequate primary stability.[2] Recently, large-diameter implants have been

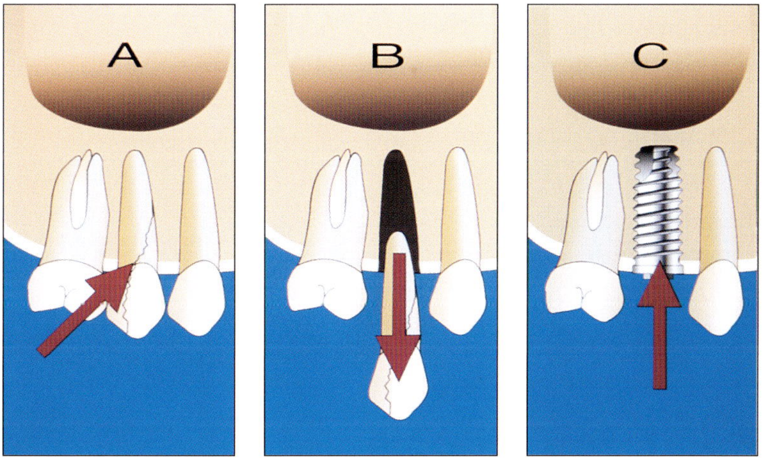

Figs 9-1a to 9-1c Diagrams illustrating extraction and immediate implantation.

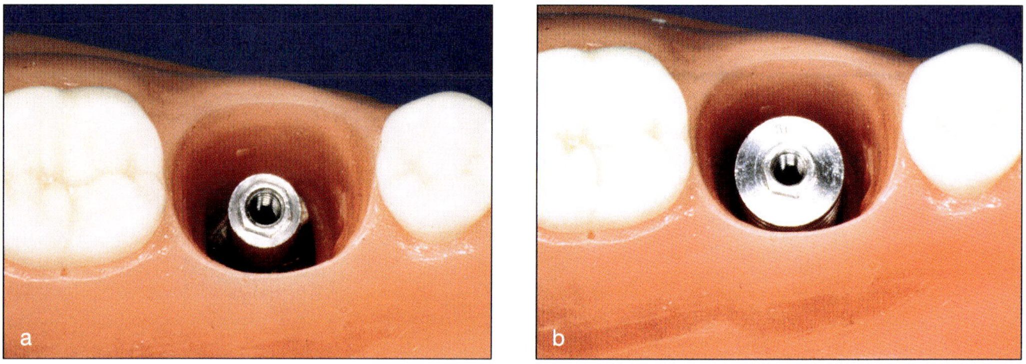

Fig 9-2 a = molar site and placement of a standard implant; note the significant difference between the extraction site diameter and the implant. b = a large-diameter implant fills the extraction site better.

recommended for immediate postextraction implantation. A large-diameter implant fills the extraction site more adequately.[3,4] This increase in diameter also allows better primary stability for the implant (Fig 9-2).[5]

A. Principles

1. *Indications*

The indications include:

—all tooth extraction (caries, fracture) free of any source of infection
—traumatic tooth avulsion with preservation of the bone capital
—endodontic complications indicating extraction
—root cracks
—rhizolysis of a deciduous tooth combined with agenesis of the permanent tooth
—internal or external root resorption
—postorthodontic root resorption

2. *Advantages*

The advantages of this technique are:

—limitation of the postextraction alveolar bone resorption
—reduced treatment time
—reduced number of surgical stages
—use of the dental axis
—good psychologic acceptance for the patient

3. *Disadvantages*

The disadvantages are of two types:

—difficulty in obtaining complete soft tissue closure at the implant site
—primary stability of the implant may sometimes be insufficient

4. *Contraindications*

There are several contraindications for this procedure:

—severe bone loss before or after extraction
—insufficient bone capital beyond the tooth apex, preventing implant stabilization
—presence of anatomic limitations (dental nerve, sinus)
—tooth extraction combined with severe source of infection

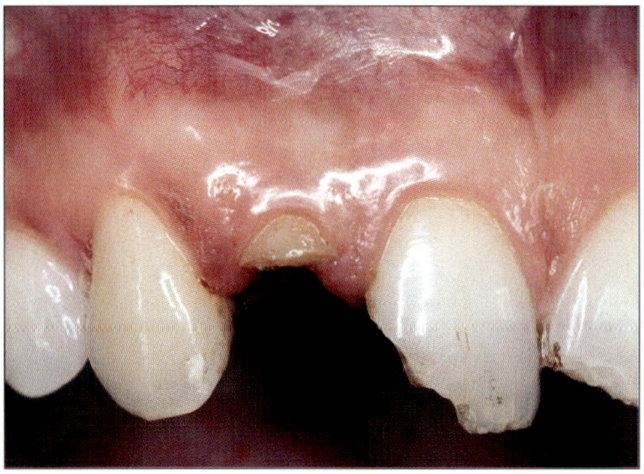

Fig 9-3 Clinical view of the maxillary right lateral incisor with palatal beveled fracture.

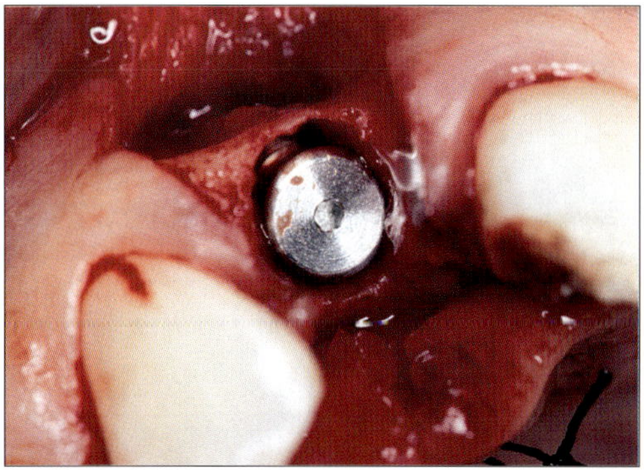

Fig 9-4 Extraction and immediate placement of a standard implant.

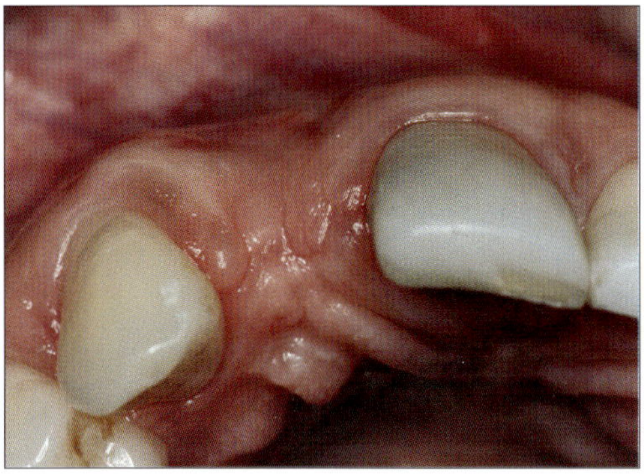

Fig 9-5 Occlusal view of the alveolar ridge at 6 months (before stage-two surgery). Note the tissue loss on the buccal aspect.

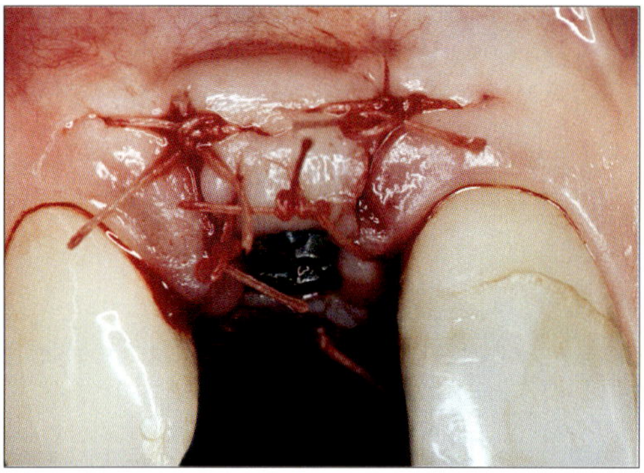

Fig 9-6 Implant exposure with the placement of a healing abutment and submerged connective tissue grafting.

5. *Technique*

The flap design must take in account the esthetic concerns and the importance of the primary implant site closure. An atraumatic tooth extraction procedure preserves the integrity of the alveolar bone walls. The alveolus must be completely debrided of all granulation tissue. Assessment of morphology and bone volume guides the treatment choice toward immediate or delayed implantation. Extraction followed by immediate implant placement is indicated in the presence of an insufficient number of bone walls. The primary stability of the implant must always be checked. In some cases, partial exposure of the implant surface imposes the use of bone grafts and/or membrane placement. Flap positioning must allow complete closure of the implant site (Figs 9-3 to 9-10).

Precise implant positioning is essential in the anterior regions. Indeed, excessive buccal implant emergence leads to an unesthetic result (long tooth and gingival margin displacement). On the other hand, an excessive lingual emergence must be compensated for

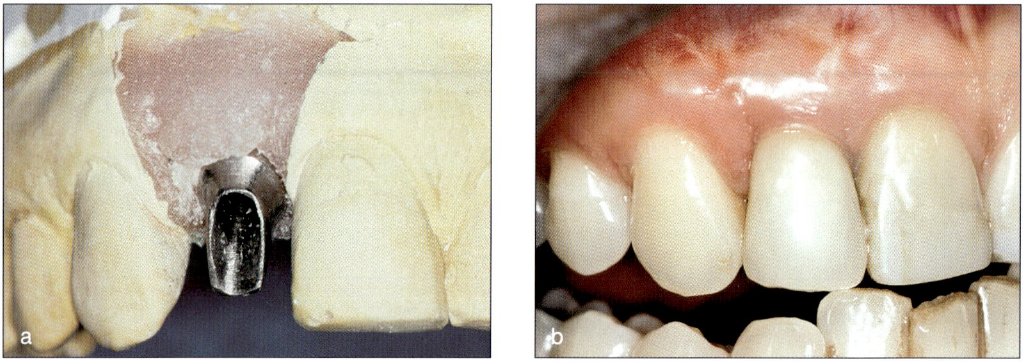

Fig 9-7 a = fabrication of the UCLA gold abutment at the laboratory; b = the provisional restoration cemented on the UCLA gold abutment will guide soft tissue healing.

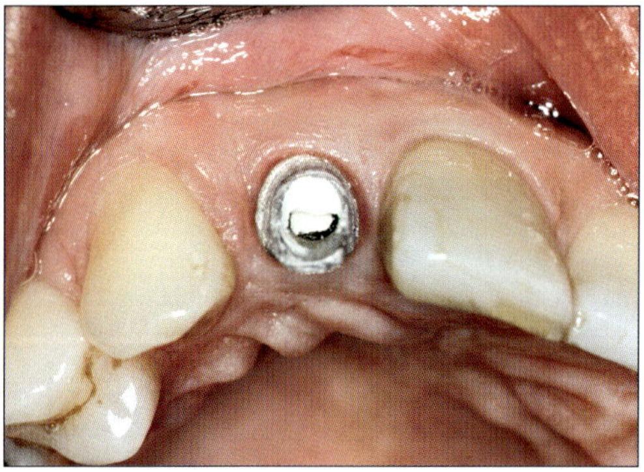

Fig 9-8 Occlusal view of the soft tissues after 3 months of temporization.

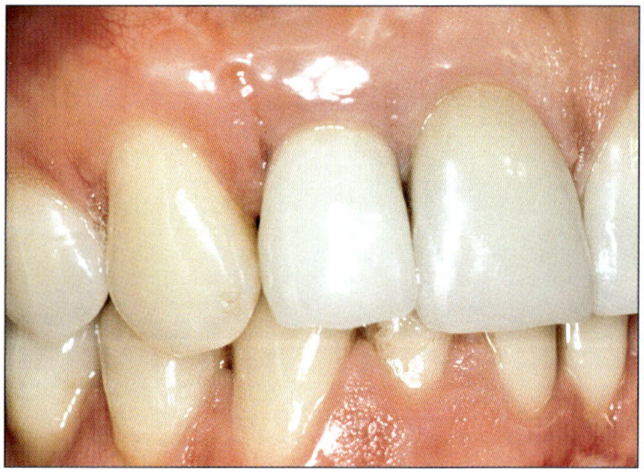

Fig 9-9 Clinical view of the final restoration (restoration, Dr P. Raygot).

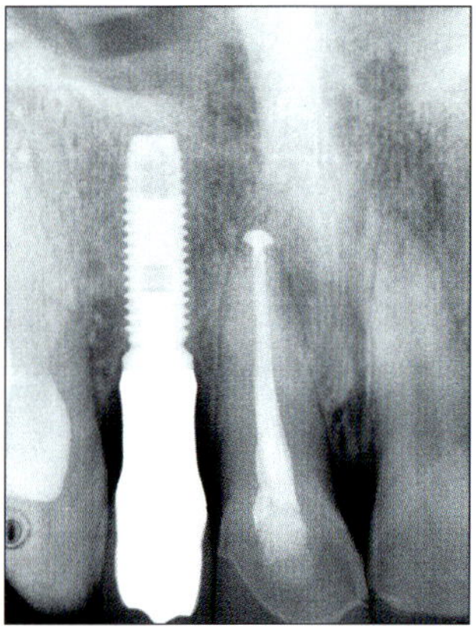

Fig 9-10 Control radiograph at 1 year.

by a prosthetic overcontour. The prosthetic buccal cantilever renders hygiene and peri-implant maintenance difficult.

All pressure resulting from the provisional restoration (removable, fixed, or bonded) during the osseointegration period must be avoided. All micromovements of the soft tissues covering the implants during the osseointegration period could contribute to implant failure.

B. Treatment alternative

1. *Implantation delayed for 6 to 8 weeks*

It is recommended to delay implant placement for 6 to 8 weeks under the following circumstances[6]:

- —in the presence of a severe source of infection in the extraction site
- —when it is difficult to obtain complete soft tissue closure over a membrane or a grafting material; 6 weeks of mucosa healing allows complete closure of the implant site and membrane coverage

2. *Implantation delayed for 6 to 8 months*

Implant placement 6 to 8 months following extraction is indicated in the presence of[6]:

- —a significant bone defect (cyst or tumor) associated with the extraction site
- —extensive bone loss indicating bone reconstruction
- —a residual bone volume that requires a bone graft prior to implant placement

II. Tuberosity and pterygomaxillary implants

A. Principles

In 1989, Tulasne[7] suggested the use of the pterygomaxillary bone mass for dental implant placement. This surgical procedure is indicated in the presence of a reduced infrasinus bone volume combined with pterygomaxillary bone volume sufficient to place an implant at least 13 mm long. The intracortical stabilization of the implant allows good results.[8]

Several authors have reported high success rates (92% to 98%) with pterygomaxillary implants (Table 9-1). In 1992, Tulasne[9] reported a success rate of 92% (from 0 to 7 years) for 66 tuberosity implants placed in 46 patients. The author emphasizes that most of the complications observed were mechanical. Bahat[10] published the results of 72 tuberosity implants placed in 45 patients. The author obtained a 93% success rate (mean 21 months). The use of long implants and reduced occlusal stresses allow these results. Khayat and Nader[11] obtained a 95% success rate for 65 tuberosity implants placed in 51 patients. The observation period was from 12 months to 4 years. For these authors, progressive loading of short implants is strongly recommended. Venturelli[14] reported only one failure out of 42 tuberosity implants. This author advocates a bicortical implant anchorage and a 6-month

Table 9-1 Surgical success rate of tuberosity implants

Author, year	Patients	Implants	Follow-up (mo)	Success (%)
Tulasne, 1992[9]	46	66	0–84	92
Bahat, 1992[10]	45	72	21 (mean)	93
Khayat and Nader, 1994[11]	51	65	0–48	95
Graves, 1994[12]	49	64	Not mentioned	89
Balshi et al, 1995[13]	44	51	1–63	86
Venturelli, 1996[14]	29	42	> 36	98
Fernandez Valeron and Fernandez Velazquez, 1997[15]	19	31	15–36	94

temporization period during loading. In 1997, Fernandez Valeron and Fernandez Velazquez[15] suggested the use of osteotomies for the preparation of tuberosity implant sites. These authors reported good results with a limited number of implants. Osteotomies allow condensation of the surgical bone site in order to enhance its density at the implant level.

B. Surgical technique

A mucoperiosteal incision performed on the crest of the pterygomaxillary notch up to the premolars, combined with releasing incisions, allows a large approach of the tuberosity region. The initial drilling point is often located 5 or 6 mm in front of the posterior edge of the tuberosity. The drilling axis is oriented obliquely, upwards, backwards, and inside.[9] The cortical bone must be reached and crossed through. This allows a bicortical stabilization of the implant (Figs 9-11 to 9-14).

Sufficient mouth opening is essential. The surgical procedure is delicate due to the presence of the posterior palatal artery. In order to avoid long-span fixed partial dentures, it is strictly recommended to associate a pterygomaxillary implant with two implants placed in front of the sinus.

III. Implants partially penetrating the sinus or the nasal fossa

This procedure, advocated in 1984 by Brånemark et al,[16] is indicated in the presence of an available 8- to 10-mm bone height under the sinus and the nasal fossae (Fig 9-15). At sinus level, the sinus membrane is slightly lifted with the implant. The consistency of this membrane normally allows its separation from the cortical layer without tearing or perforating. The implant is submerged to the selected depth. A bicortical anchorage is thus obtained (Figs 9-16 to 9-18). Radiographically, apical new bone formation is often visible after 1 year of healing. However, breaking through or tearing of the sinus membrane may occur. If the sinus is perfectly sound, the intrasinus implant is well tolerated. Hence, the created passage is obliterated by the implant. At the nasal fossa level, slight nose bleeding may occur 24 hours after implant placement.

IV. Sinus grafting

The sinus lift procedure and its grafting is a surgical technique that was described by Boyne and James in 1980.[17] These authors suggest the use of autogenous iliac bone grafts. Different autogenous bone donor sites have been proposed (calvarium, chin). Other authors advocate the use of different types of bone grafting materials (allografts, xenografts, heterografts, composite grafts).[18] Implant placement may be performed during the same surgical stage in the presence of a minimal height, thus facilitating the primary stability of the implant.

A. Sinus grafting and immediate implant placement

This technique is indicated when the available bone height ranges between 5 and 8 mm (Fig 9-19). A bone graft is performed. Different grafting materials (autogenous bone, xenografts, allografts, alloplastic or composite grafts) are used.[19-21] The results published with this procedure show a good short-term success rate (Table 9-2).

The first surgical stage consists of performing a full-thickness incision on the crest or slightly moved to the palatal aspect. If the sinus shows a significant volume, the posterior vascular components must be respected when performing the primary incision. Two vertical releasing incisions ending the first incision allow a full-thickness flap elevation. The buccal aspect of the maxillary bone is thus exposed. Kent and Block[22,28] suggest

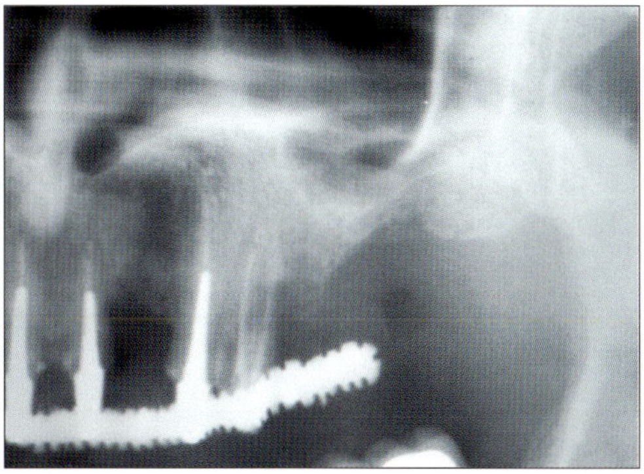

Fig 9-11 Panoramic radiograph showing a posterior edentulous maxilla. Implants are considered in the maxillary left first molar and in the tuberosity.

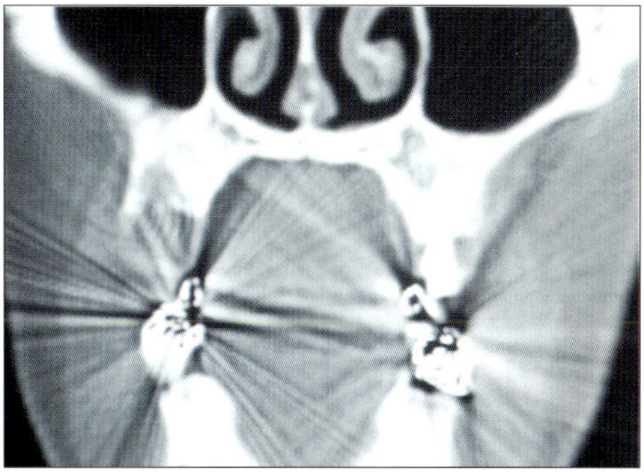

Fig 9-12 Scan showing adequate bone volume at the first molar.

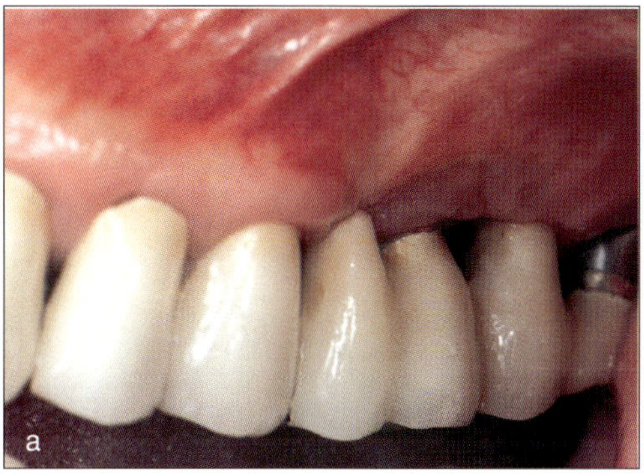

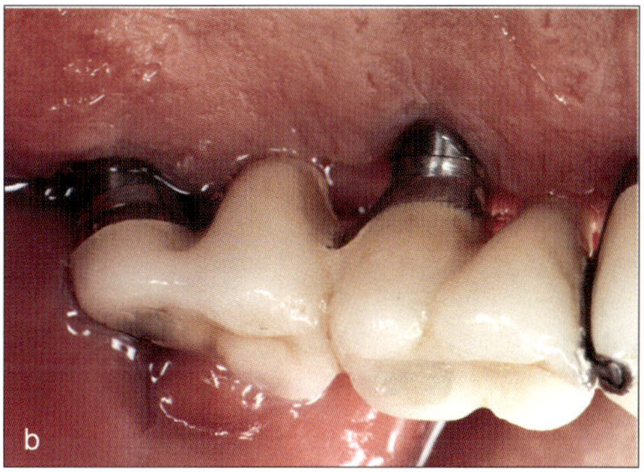

Figs 9-13a and 9-13b Buccal and palatal clinical views of the final prosthetic restoration (restoration, Dr P. Guilbert).

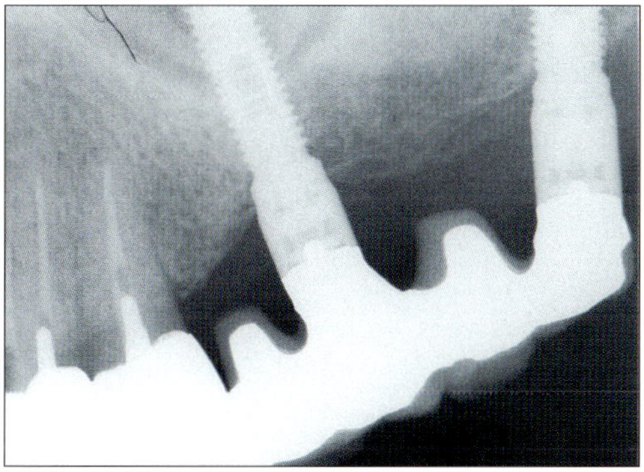

Fig 9-14 Control radiograph at 7 years.

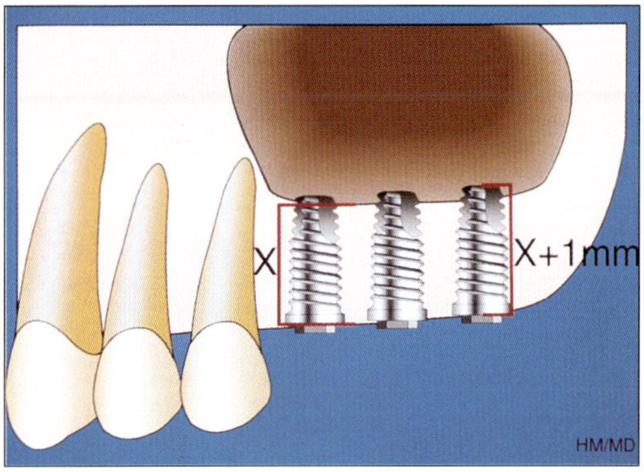

Fig 9-15 Diagram of implants partially penetrating the sinus.

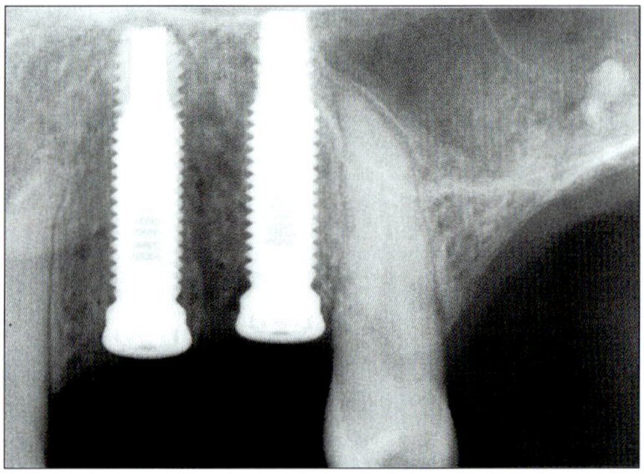

Fig 9-16 Radiograph showing the penetration of the distal implant beyond the subsinus cortical plate.

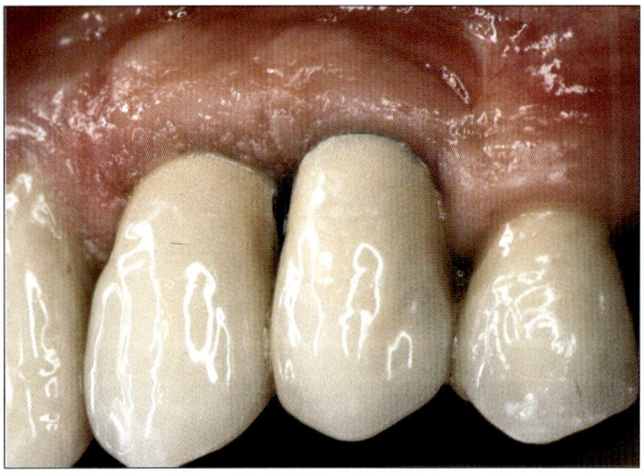

Fig 9-17 Clinical view of the final prosthetic restoration (restoration, Dr P. Raygot).

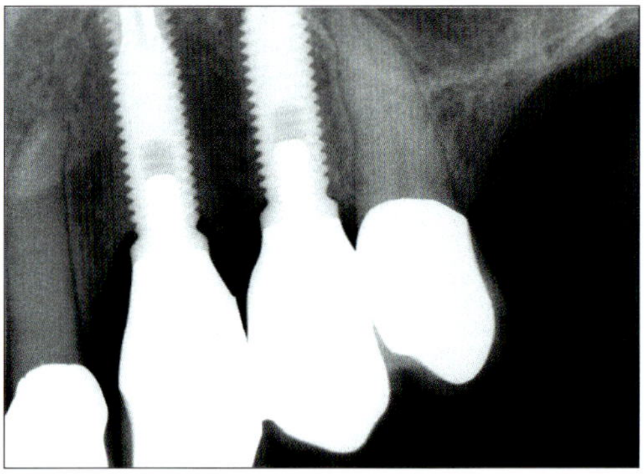

Fig 9-18 Control radiograph at 1 year.

Table 9-2 Surgical success rate with sinus grafting and immediate implant placement.

Author, year	Patients	Implants	Follow-up (mo)	Success (%)
Kent and Block, 1989[22]	11	54	12–48	100
Raghoebar et al, 1993[23]	25	93	6–36	93
Keller et al, 1994[24]	20	66	12–60	92
Zinner and Small, 1996[25]	50	215	7–60	98
Blomqvist et al, 1996[26]	49	171	14–58	83
Daelemans et al, 1997[27]	33	121	3–80	93

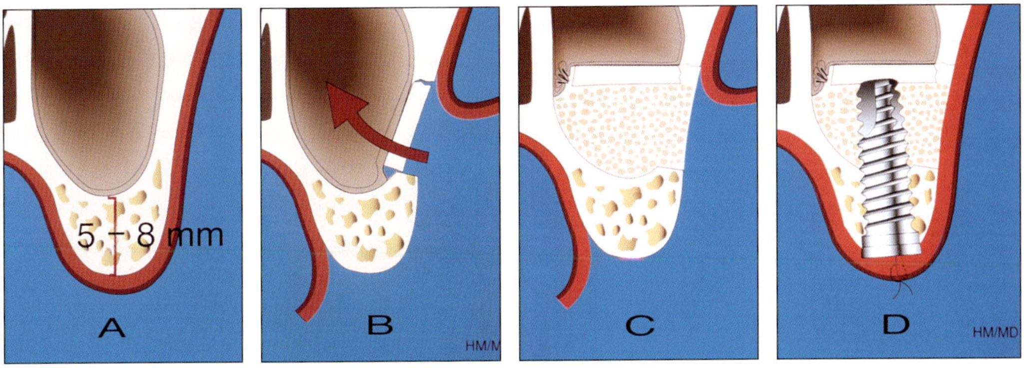

Figs 9-19a to 9-19d Sinus grafting and immediate implantation: a = 5 to 8 mm of subsinus bone volume available; b = performing and elevating the buccal bone flap; c = creating a new sinus floor and bone grafting; d = immediate implant placement.

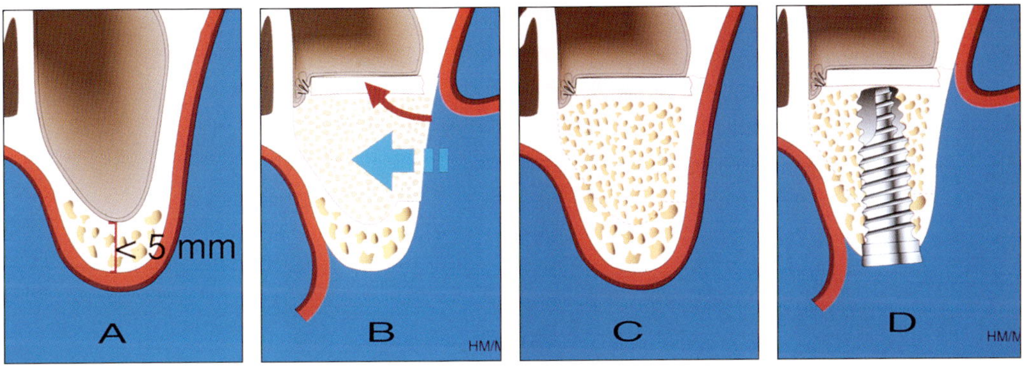

Figs 9-20a to 9-20d Sinus grafting and delayed implantation: a = available subsinus bone volume less than 5 mm; b = creating a new sinus floor and bone grafting; c = bone grafting after 6 months; d = implant placement.

different types of primary incisions according to the available height of attached gingiva.

A buccal osteotomy, using an upper hinged flap, is then performed to approach the sinus antrum. This osteotomy is performed using a bone bur. The flap presents either a rectangular or semicircular design. The sinus membrane appears with a white-grayish color. Membrane reflection is very delicate due to its adherence and fragility. Special curettes with variable curvatures are used. During this dissecting stage, membrane tearing may occur. The flap is pushed back inside and secured in a horizontal position. It represents the new sinus floor.

The cavity is carefully filled with the selected material. If a prior implant bone site preparation has been performed, the implant is subsequently placed. The full-thickness flap is repositioned and sutured hermetically.

B. Sinus grafting and delayed implant placement

When the available subsinus bone height is less than 5 mm, sinus elevation and grafting

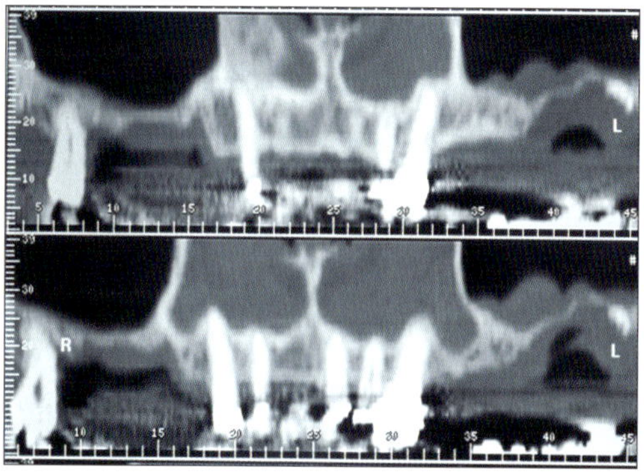

Fig 9-21 Panoramic scan showing a subsinus bone volume less than 3 mm.

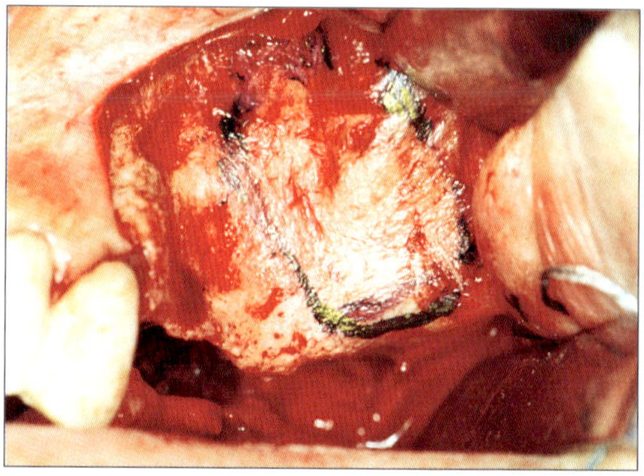

Fig 9-22 Clinical view after flap reflection and design of the buccal bone flap (surgery, Dr J.-F. Tulasne).

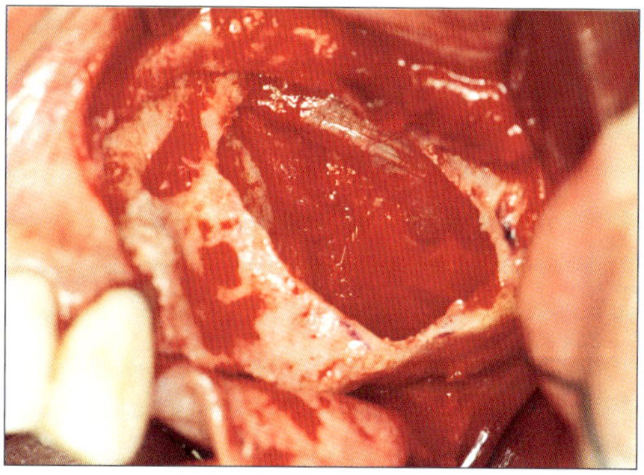

Fig 9-23 Clinical aspect after elevation of the buccal bone flap.

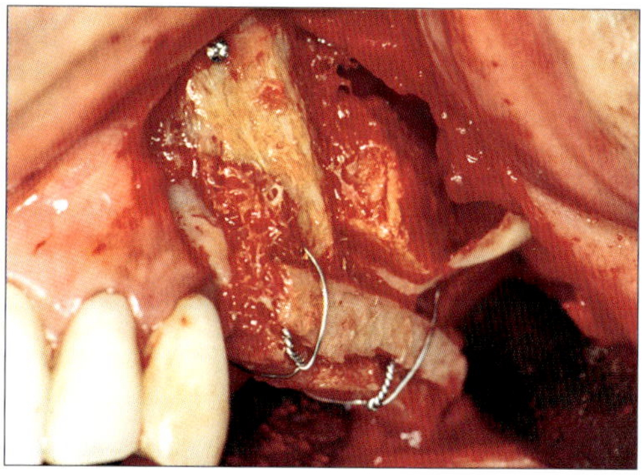

Fig 9-24 Placement of autogenous bone grafts (iliac harvest).

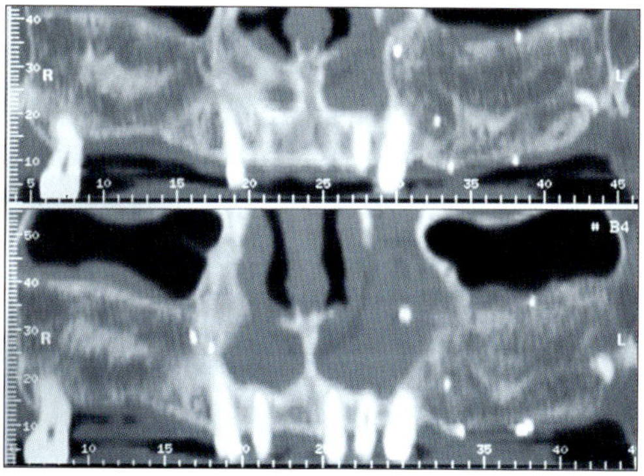

Fig 9-25 Control panoramic scan at 6 months after bone grafting. Note the adequate subsinus bone volume.

are indicated prior to implant placement. The implants are placed following a 6- to 8-month period of bone healing (Fig 9-20). The results obtained with this surgical approach are satisfactory (Table 9-3 and Figs 9-21 to 9-28).

Several modifications have been introduced to the initial technique described by Boyne and James.[17] Tulasne et al[31] prefer calvarium bone, which is the procedure used by Tessier[35] in craniofacial surgery since 1982. The author emphasizes that the postoperative effects are uneventful. The procedure includes creating a new sinus floor via the adaptation of a spongious cortical block. This bone

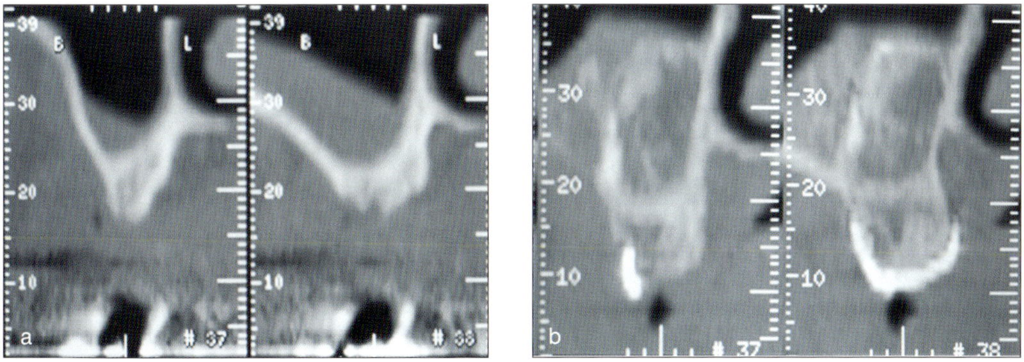

Figs 9-26a and 9-26b Oblique scans of the left maxillary region before and after performing the sinus grafting.

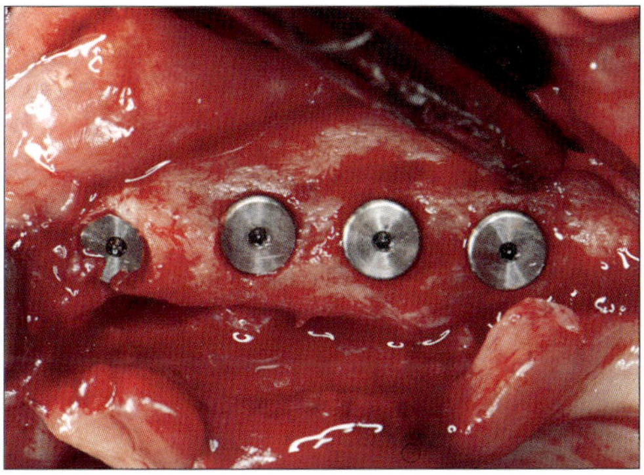

Fig 9-27 Placement of four implants in the left maxillary region.

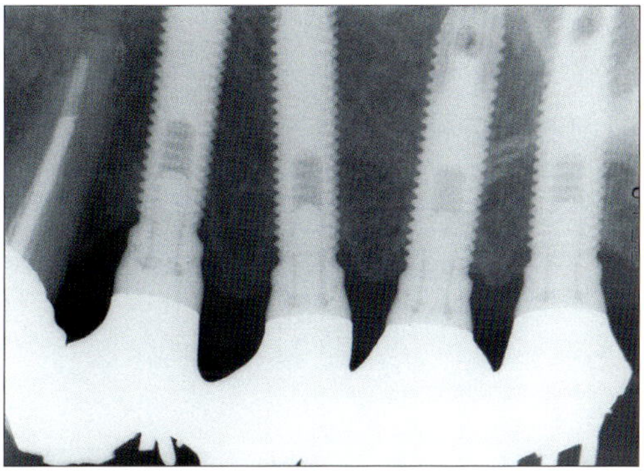

Fig 9-28 Control radiograph after 3 years of loading (Drs R. and S.-B. Cohen).

Table 9-3 Surgical success rate with sinus grafting and delayed implant placement.

Author, year	Patients	Implants	Follow-up (mo)	Success (%)
Hall and McKenna, 1991[29]	15	70	6–12	91
Tidwell et al, 1992[30]	48	203	12–32	93
Tulasne et al, 1993[31]	45	120	0–36	98
Chiapasco and Ronchi, 1994[32]	43	124	12–24	93
Zerbib et al, 1991[33]	142	465	≥ 6	95
Lundgren et al, 1996[34]	10	30	12–45	100

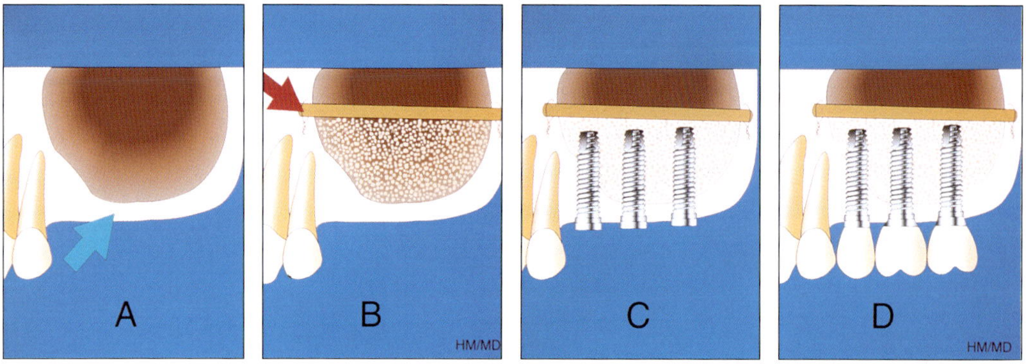

Figs 9-29a to 9-29d Sinus grafting technique proposed by J.-F. Tulasne: a = insufficient residual bone volume; b = creation of a new sinus floor using a spongious cortical block; c = implant placement after bone healing; d = prosthetic restoration.

block is perforated in order to facilitate the vascularization of the graft. The cortical side is placed against the sinus mucosa. The recessed fitting of the block inside the external wall of the maxilla and its osteosynthesis allow an ideal stabilization. A homogenous grafting using crushed spongious cortical bone inside a rigid cavity is thus performed (Fig 9-29). Results are promising. Tulasne et al[31] in 1993 reported the results obtained with 120 implants placed in 48 grafted sinus antra. Two failures out of 83 implants checked after 6 months or more of loading were reported. In 1991, Zerbib et al[33] reported 22 implants lost out of 465 checked implants. Fifteen failures occurred during implant exposure, and seven failures after a few weeks of loading. Two implants out of 142 treated patients presented sinus infection, and the graft had to be removed. In five patients, additional grafting was performed because of severe graft resorption. Raghoebar et al[23] use an iliac monocortical bone block, which is placed facing the previously reflected buccal flap, in order to create a new sinus floor. The obtained space is filled with spongious bone. The implants may be placed during the same surgical stage if the residual bone volume allows a good primary stabilization of the implants. According to these authors, the bone block is stabilized using the implants. The advantage of this monocortical block is to delimit the cavity and to prevent bone particles from flowing into the sinus in the case of sinus membrane perforation. Raghoebar et al report five lost implants (during the osseointegration period) out of 93 placed implants and 47 grafted sinuses. The observation period was 6 to 36 months.

V. Onlay bone grafts

Insufficient bone volume in relation to the anatomic limitations (maxillary sinus, nasal fossae, inferior dental canal) contraindicates the use of dental implants. Onlay bone grafts are indicated in the presence of insufficient bone height and/or width (Fig 9-30). They can be performed in the maxilla or in the mandible.[36-43] The aim of this treatment is to increase the height and/or the width of the residual ridge (Figs 9-31 to 9-38). The prosthetic space must also be assessed in order to have a favorable clinical implant:crown ratio and the best possible esthetic result.

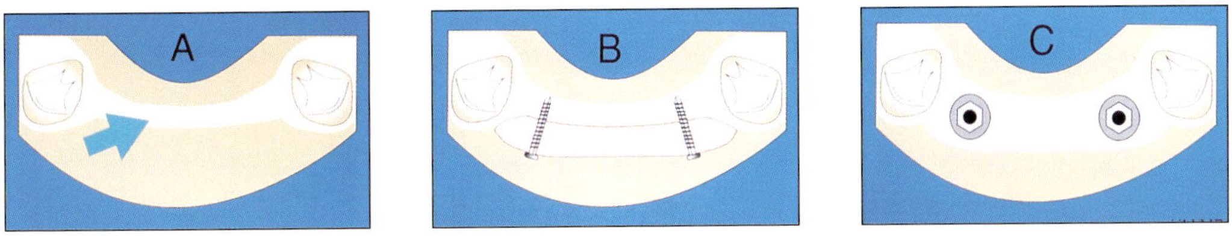

Figs 9-30a to 9-30c Apposition bone grafting technique: a = thin ridge; b = buccal apposition graft; c = implant placement after bone healing.

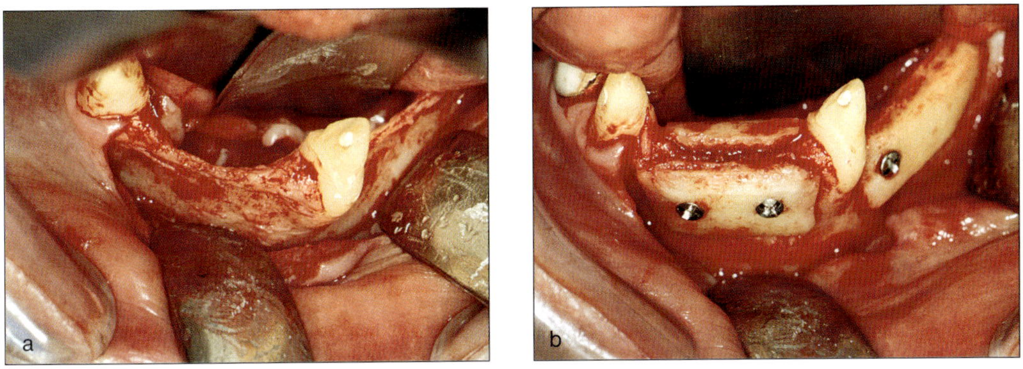

Figs 9-31a and 9-31b Occlusal views of a thin mandibular ridge before and after apposition of three blocks of calvarium spongious cortical bone (surgery, Dr J.-F. Tulasne).

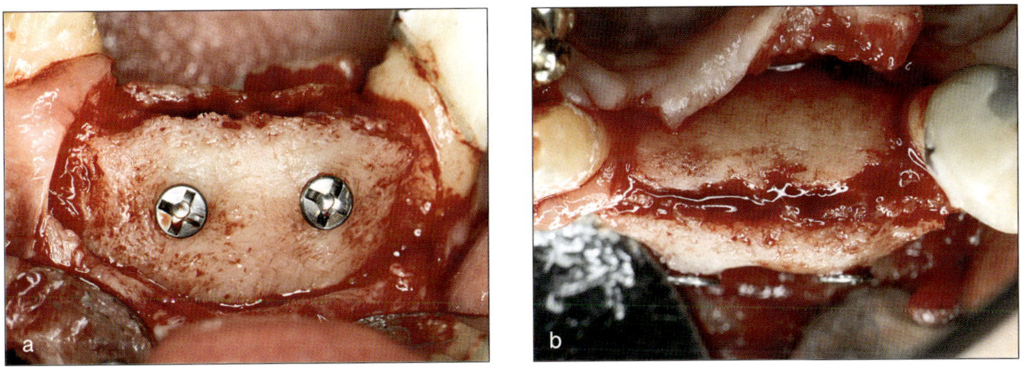

Figs 9-32a and 9-32b Buccal and occlusal views after 8 months of healing.

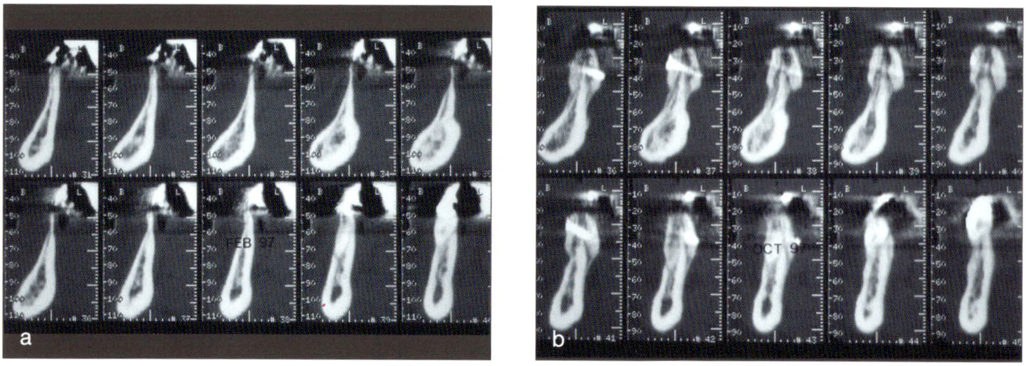

Figs 9-33a and 9-33b Oblique scans before surgery and after 8 months of healing.

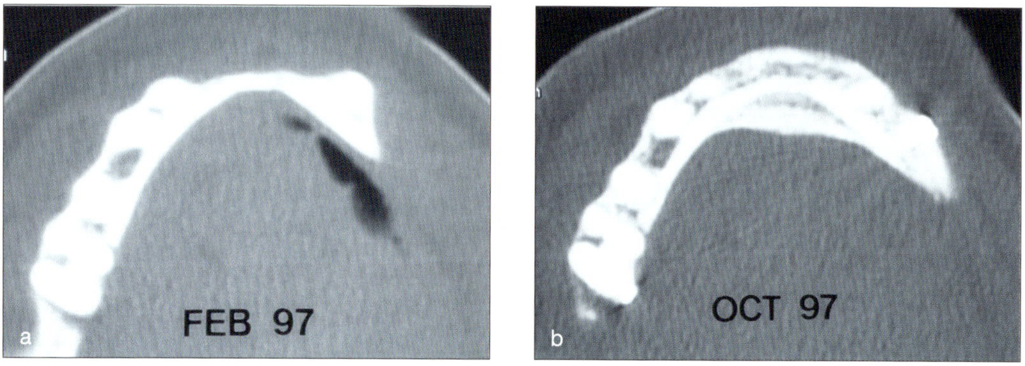

Figs 9-34a and 9-34b Axial scans before surgery and after 8 months.

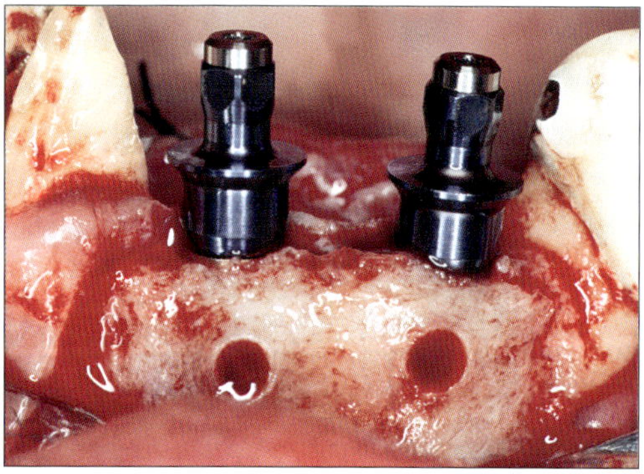

Fig 9-35 Placement of two implants in the symphysis after removal of the osteosynthesis screws.

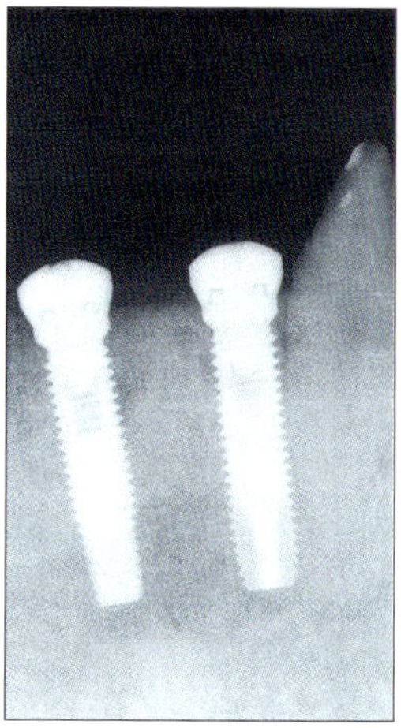

Fig 9-36 Control radiograph at 6 months, after placing healing abutments.

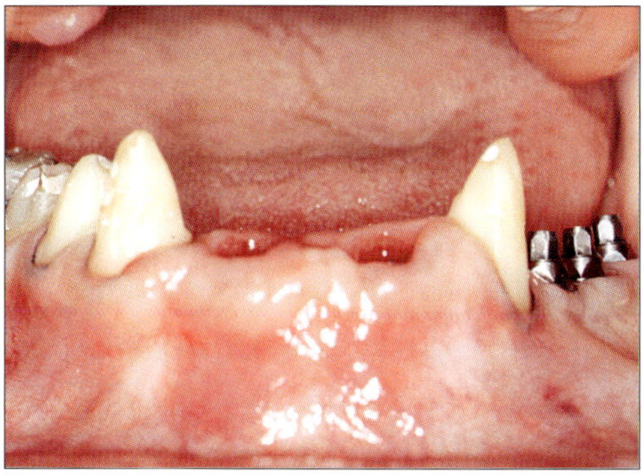

Fig 9-37 Clinical view after 6 weeks of soft tissue healing.

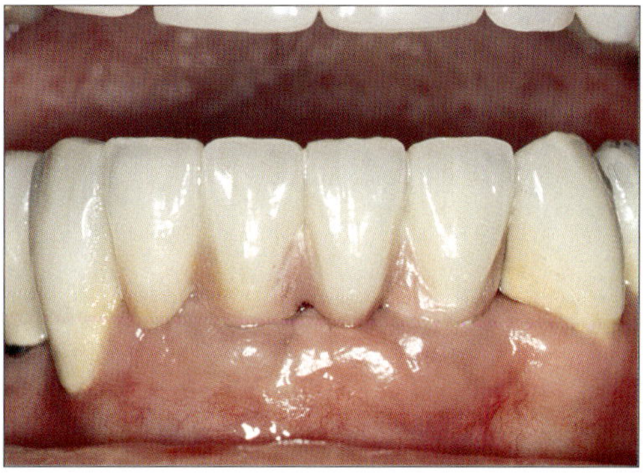

Fig 9-38 Final prosthetic restoration (restoration, Dr G. Audi).

In 1980, Breine and Brånemark[44] advocated the use of autogenous bone grafts with the placement of dental implants. The first results obtained using this technique, in the case of a centripetal resorption pattern in long-term edentulous patients, show that it leads to very thin alveolar ridges. A buccal onlay bone graft is the treatment of choice. The loss of bone height may be treated using an onlay bone graft on the ridge. The implant placement may be performed at the same surgical time or after 6 months of healing. Use of both onlay and inlay bone grafts (buccal and crestal) is indicated when bone resorption is combined.

A. Harvesting (donor) site

The most frequent donor sites used in implant surgery are the iliac crest, the calvarium, and the chin (Fig 9-39). Each site presents advantages and disadvantages (Table 9-4).

1. Iliac donor site

When a significant bone volume is necessary, the donor site of choice is the iliac crest. The advantages of the iliac donor site are:

—a significant bone volume can be harvested
—the two bone types (cortical and spongious) are present

The disadvantages of this donor site are:

—the procedure requires two surgical sites
—the postoperative effects are often painful
—the hospitalization period is longer
—a skin scar is present

A skin incision of 3 to 5 cm is performed at the iliac crest. Once the subcutaneous place is crossed, the periosteum is incised and reflected. The graft design is performed using a bone bur. Bone chisels allow mobilization of the cortical block. Following the cortical bone harvesting, spongious bone is harvested using a curette. The periosteum and the subcutaneous and cutaneous planes are then sutured.

2. Calvarium donor site

When a significant cortical bone volume is required, the calvarium is the donor site of choice. The advantages of this donor site are:

—a significant bone volume can be harvested
—the postoperative effects are seldom painful

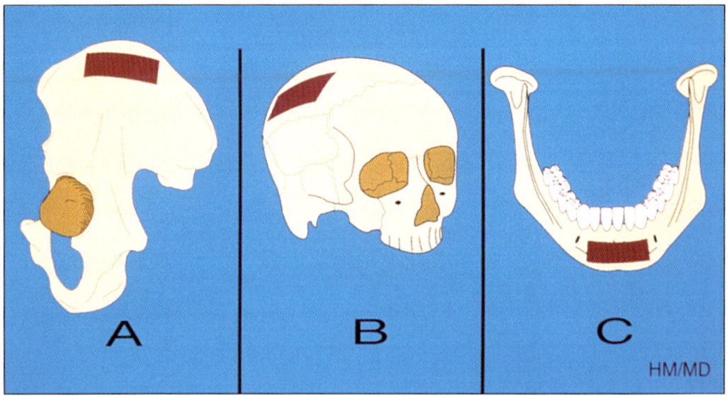

Fig 9-39 Autogenous bone harvesting sites: A = iliac crest; B = calvarium; C = mandibular symphysis.

Table 9-4 Advantages and disadvantages of different bone harvesting sites (modified according to Tulasne et al[45])

Harvesting site	Bone type	Available bone volume	Postsurgical pain	Scar	Hospital care period
Iliac crest	Cortical +++ Spongious +++	Abundant	Severe	Slightly visible	8 days
Calvarium	Cortical +++ Spongious ++	Variable	Minor	Invisible	2–3 days
Symphysis	Cortical ++ Spongious +	Poor	Minor	Invisible	Ambulatory or 2 days

+, ++, +++ indicate quantity of bone present, in increasing amounts.

—the postoperative scar is normally invisible (for patients with no baldness)

The disadvantages of this donor site are:

—the procedure requires two surgical sites
—the hospitalization period is at least 2 days

A skin incision of 7 to 9 cm is performed on the calvarium at the parietal bone. The flap dissection is performed. The periosteum is then incised and completely reflected. The graft design is performed using a bone bur, and the bone chisels move the cortical block before its harvesting. Closure of the periosteum and the subcutaneous and cutaneous planes is performed.

3. *Chin donor site*

The symphysis region is an intraoral donor site of choice. The advantages of this site versus an extraoral site are[46]:

—surgery time is shorter
—easy access
—more rapid healing
—absence of visible scars
—the postsurgical effects are well tolerated
—surgery may be performed under local anesthesia

The disadvantages of this donor site are:

—a limited quantity of bone to harvest
—risk of loss of sensitivity on the mandibular incisors

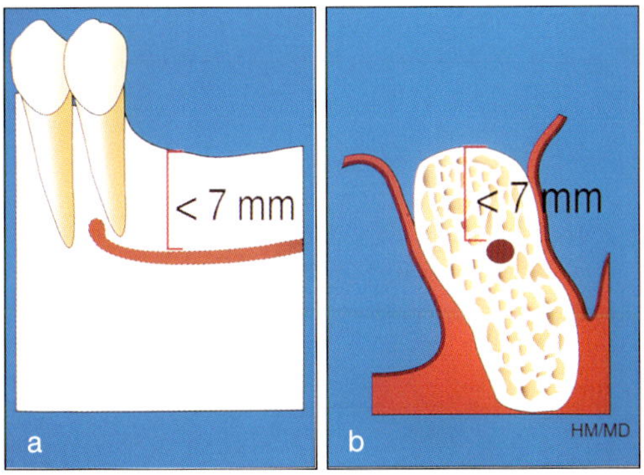

Figs 9-40a and 9-40b Diagrams illustrating insufficient mandibular bone volume above the alveolar dental canal.

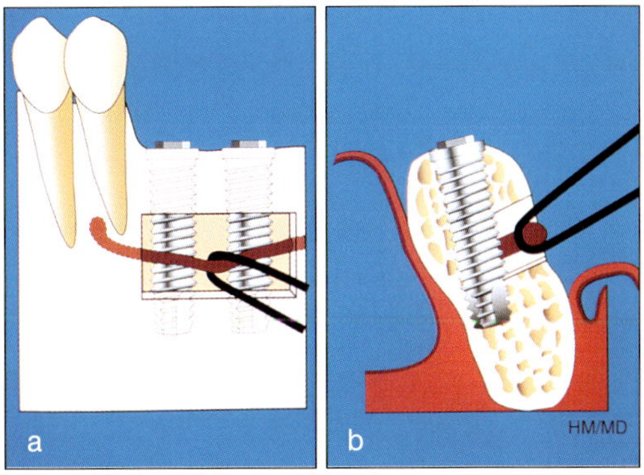

Figs 9-41a and 9-41b Diagrams illustrating inferior dental nerve repositioning and implant placement.

Following local and regional anesthesia (Spix's spine), a linear incision is performed on the mucosa between the respective distal aspects of the two canines. Reflection of a full-thickness flap gives access to the symphysis bone. Osteoectomy is performed using a bone bur. The upper limit must be located 5 mm under the teeth apices. The depth of the bone graft depends on the width of the symphysis and on the bony defect to be treated. The use of osteotomes allows mobilization and harvesting of the graft. The graft is then adapted to the recipient site. The donor site may be filled using a bone substitute or bone hemostatic wax. The flap is repositioned and sutured using a resorbable suturing material.

B. Graft adaptation and fixation

The block of spongious cortical bone must be perfectly trimmed in order to adapt to the previously prepared recipient site. Cortical perforations are performed on the recipient site using a bone bur, allowing an enhanced vascularization of the graft. The graft is secured using titanium fixation screws. The use of ligatures may be required in some cases. The contours of the adapted graft must be carefully checked in order to avoid any risk of mucosa perforation. The empty spaces located between the graft and the recipient site are filled in using the previously harvested spongious bone. The flap is repositioned; sometimes periosteal incisions are required to ensure full closure of the recipient site. The wearing of provisional prostheses must be avoided during the first 10 days. The interface of the prosthesis is relieved, thus avoiding all pressure on the grafted site.

VI. Inferior dental nerve repositioning

Insufficient bone height above the inferior dental canal contraindicates the use of dental implants. Assessment of the residual bone volume and available prosthetic space determines the treatment choice.

The combination of inadequate bone volume and insufficient prosthetic space is an indication for inferior dental nerve repositioning (Figs 9-40 and 9-41). In 1987, Jensen and Nock[47] described the dental nerve repositioning procedure combined with the placement of dental implants. Other authors[48–52] have suggested modifications to the initial procedure.

Table 9-5 Total sensitivity recovery after dental nerve transposition

			Total sensitivity recovery					Sensitivity
Author, year	**Patients**	**Sites**	**1–15 d**	**2–8 wk**	**3–5 mo**	**6–9 mo**	**9 mo**	**alteration**
Jensen et al, 1994[49]	6	10	–	–	6	–	3	1
Haers and Sailer, 1994[54]	9	17	Not mentioned			13		
Rosenquist, 1994[53]*	72	100	21 (100)	56 (100)	?	?	68 (72)	4 (72)
Hirsch and Brånemark, 1995[55]	18	24	3	3	Not mentioned			3
Sethi, 1995[56]	8	14	3	2	3	1	–	5
Kan et al, 1997[57]	15	21	Not mentioned			11		

*Number of checked sites in parentheses.

A. Technique

A regional block anesthesia is performed at Spix's spine, completed with a buccal and lingual local anesthesia. A mandibular scan allows location of the dental canal pathway. The incision line is located on the crest. Releasing incisions favor the exposure of the alveolar ridge buccal aspect. The mental foramen emergence is exposed, and the vascular and nerve bundle must be delicately manipulated. Repositioning of the mental nerve emergence was suggested by Rosenquist.[50] A buccal osteotomy allows freeing and moving of the vascular and nerve bundle. Several suggestions have been described to perform this osteotomy. The nerve is moved laterally and protected during the implant site preparation. An autogenous bone layer placed on the buccal aspect recovers the implant surface and avoids contacting the nerve. The buccal flap is repositioned and carefully sutured.

B. Contraindications

According to Rosenquist,[53] this technique presents specific contraindications:

—a residual ridge bone height less than 3 mm
—the combination of thick buccal cortical bone with a thin vascular and nerve bundle
—at-risk patient, susceptible to hemorrhages and infections (relative contraindication)
—difficult access to the surgical site (relative contraindication)

Valentini et al[52] add to these contraindications:

—very corticalized bone rendering difficult the protection of the vascular-nervous bundle
—insufficient patient motivation
—excessively lingual position of the inferior dental canal (relative contraindication)

C. Complications

The main disadvantage is the risk of a permanent loss of sensitivity in the case of nerve trunk sectioning. Sensitivity disorders progressively disappear following a delicate management of the dental nerve. However, sensitivity aftereffects (anesthesia, paresthesia, and dysesthesia) frequently occur. The irreversibility of these disorders is unpredictable (Table 9-5). This treatment option must not be considered a routine solution. Kan and coworkers[57,58] report a 52% alteration of the labio-

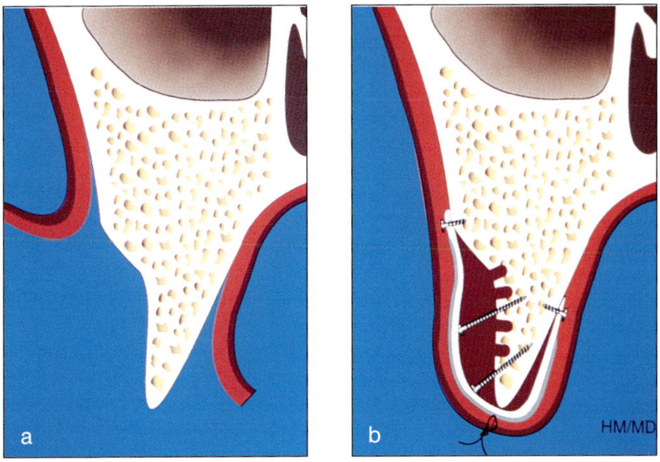

Fig 9-42a Diagram of a very thin ridge.

Fig 9-42b Illustration of the GBR technique with fixation screws.

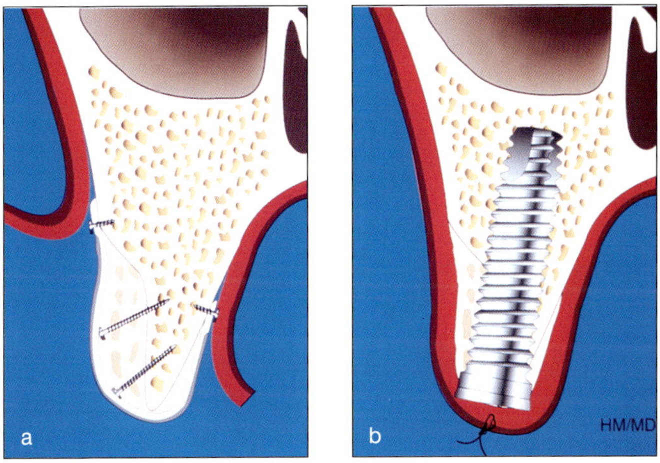

Fig 9-43a Diagram illustrating new bone formation.

Fig 9-43b Implant placement according to an ideal axis.

mental sensitivity. Rosenquist[53] presents a 94% rate of sensitivity normalization over 72 sites controlled at 18 months. According to this author, sensitivity recovery is very slow. A full normalization is obtained in 21% and 77% of the cases, respectively, at 1 week and 6 months.

Risk for mandibular fracture is increased in patients presenting severe bone resorption and/or poor-density bone. Kan et al[58] report the case of a spontaneous mandibular fracture 3 weeks after dental nerve repositioning and the placement of three implants. The position of the dental canal and the bone quality and quantity must be precisely assessed before making a decision for surgical intervention.

VII. Guided bone regeneration

GBR may be a treatment option for treating bone defects associated or not with implants (Figs 9-42 and 9-43). Its biologic principle is based on the concept of cell selectivity allow-

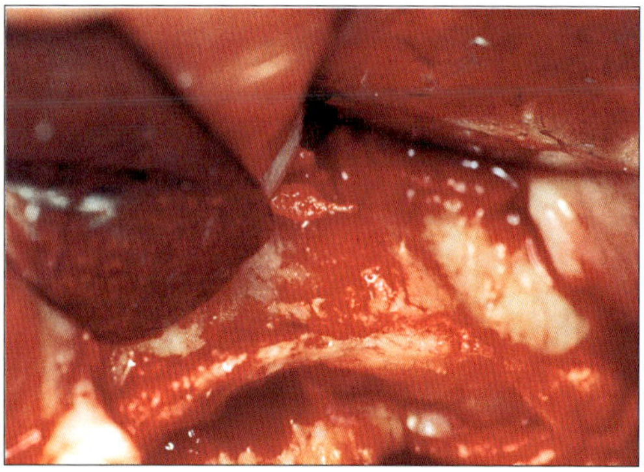

Fig 9-44 Residual knife-edged alveolar ridge in the maxilla.

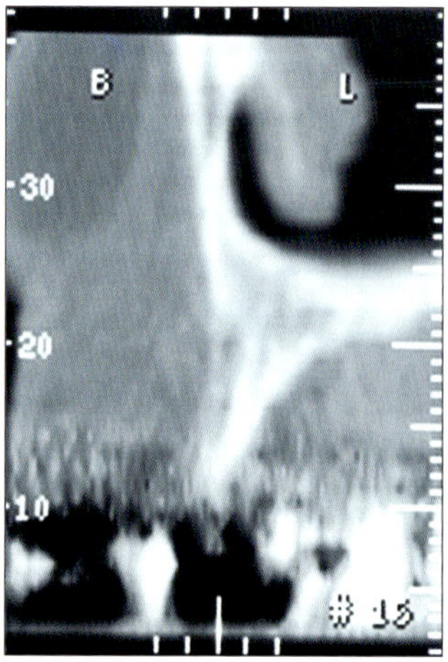

Fig 9-45 Oblique scan showing the thin alveolar ridge.

ing new bone formation. This concept was demonstrated by Murray et al[59] by performing mechanical isolation, using a plastic chamber, of a bone defect created inside the iliac bone of a dog. After healing, the inside of the chamber was filled with newly formed bone. Peri-implant GBR in the mandible was first studied in the dog by Becker and Becker.[60] Buccal dehiscences about 4 mm high were created before placing the implants. The test sites were covered using a membrane. A 1.37-mm mean bone gain was observed, versus 0.25 mm for the control group. Histologic assessment confirms new bone formation. Several publications have confirmed the efficacy of this technique in humans.[1,8,60–62]

A. The physical barrier (membrane)

The conventional membranes used are fabricated out of expanded polytetrafluoroethylene (e-PTFE), an inert and nonresorbable material. Gore-Tex augmentation material (GTAM) membranes are composed of two distinct parts: an internal part, more rigid with a limited porosity, excluding epithelial and connective cells from the bone healing process; and a more flexible external part, allowing perfect adaptation on the edges of the bone defect.[63] Other types of membranes fabricated out of other materials have been proposed to treat these bone defects. However, they lack sufficient clinical follow-up.

The space created using the physical barrier (membrane) allows the stabilization of a blood clot.[64] Starting from this clot, proliferation of differentiated cells leads to newly formed bone.[65,66]

B. Indications

Indications for GBR in implantology are:

—peri-implant dehiscences and fenestrations
—residual peri-implant bone defects
—immediate extraction and implantation
—localized bone ridge enlargement

C. Technique

Incision lines must allow complete coverage of the membrane. Granulation tissue debride-

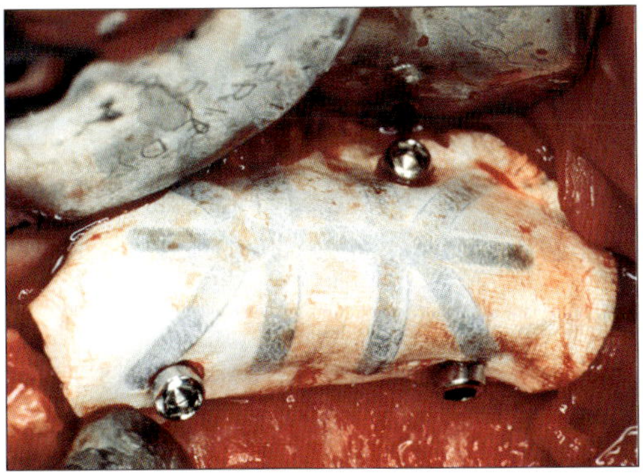

Fig 9-46 Placement of a titanium-reinforced Gore-Tex membrane secured with four fixation screws.

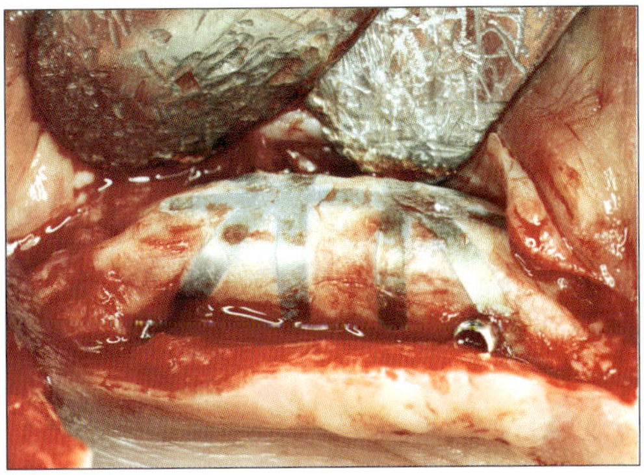

Fig 9-47 Clinical view of the membrane after 10 months of healing.

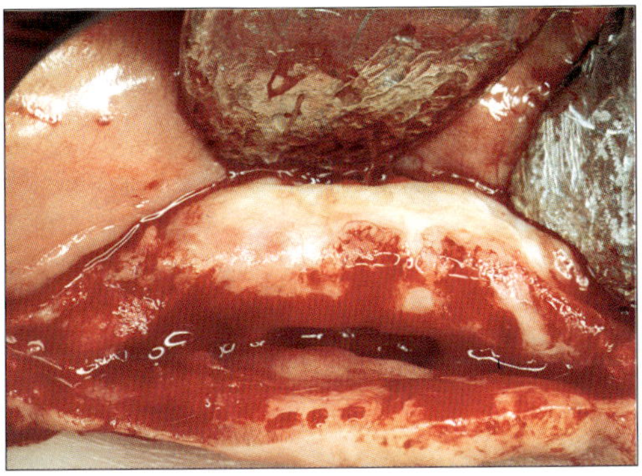

Fig 9-48 Note the excellent tissue regeneration after membrane removal.

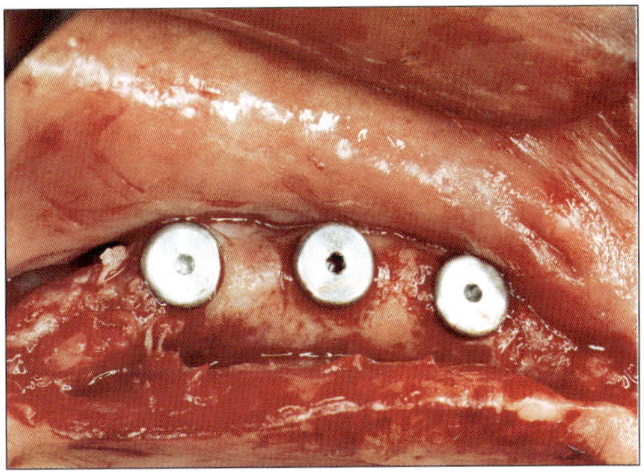

Fig 9-49 Implant placement.

ment is performed before placing the implant. The latter must be perfectly stable before membrane placement. A blood clot will fill the defect space to allow bone regeneration. Membrane type selection depends on the size and morphology of the defect. The membrane must cover the defect at least 3 mm beyond its limits without folding. The membrane must be perfectly stable before flap closure. Peri-implant defects are filled with the blood clot. Defect space maintenance may be performed using autogenous or allogeneous bone, alloplastic material, space-making screws, or a titanium-reinforced membrane. Securing the membrane using the implant cover screw reduces the space available in regard to the implant. A healing period ranging from 7 to 9 months is necessary before membrane removal (Figs 9-44 to 9-49).

The GTAM membrane must be removed as soon as one of the following complications occurs:

—infection
—soft tissue inflammation
—flap necrosis
—flap perforation
—pain

This therapy may also be performed combined with an autogenous bone graft. It seems that the membrane prevents partial resorption of the bone graft during healing.

Titanium-reinforced GTAM membranes allow maintenance of a larger space for the implant. GBR allows 4 mm of bone gain on the buccolingual aspect and 3 mm on the apicocoronal aspect. If bone reconstruction greater than these criteria is needed, it is preferable to use autogenous bone grafts.

D. Reflections

In 1995, Mellonig and Nevins[67] analyzed the results obtained with guided bone regeneration combined with implants.[68–70] They suggest three assessment groups.

1. Implants placed in extraction sites

Results show a high success rate for implants placed in an extraction site and combined with GBR. However, most publications consist of clinical case reports. It is recommended to use bone grafts combined with the membrane to treat large defects.

2. Peri-implant defects (dehiscence-fenestration)

The use of membranes to treat peri-implant defects enhances the regeneration process. Combining grafting materials is necessary for large defects. This material prevents membrane collapse. The best results are obtained using autogenous bone. Alloplastic grafts are less recommended. Premature membrane exposure leads to complications and may compromise the final result.

3. Localized ridge enlargement

The different clinical case reports allow the conclusion that localized ridge enlargement (vertical or horizontal) is a reliable treatment choice (4 mm wide and 3 mm high).[71,72] GBR performed using a mechanical support or combined with bone grafts allows similar bone reconstruction. Premature membrane exposure may jeopardize the GBR result.

VIII. Osteotomy and bone grafts

A. Sinus elevation

In 1994, Summers[73,74] developed a surgical technique using osteotomies. This technique is advocated in the presence of a 5- to 6-mm subsinus bone height combined with poor-density bone. Elevation of the subsinus floor by several millimeters is obtained following a progressive implant site preparation. The primary aim of this therapy is to preserve and enlarge the available bone volume. The bone is compacted laterally and apically around the implant site owing to the progressive enlargement of the osteotome diameters.

The use of different grafting materials and autogenous bone has also been suggested to enlarge bone volume. In 1994, Summers[74] reported a 96% success rate (from 0 to 5 years) for 143 implants placed in 46 patients. However, the implant choice and success criteria are not described. Horowitz[75] reports the placement of 47 (ITI) implants in 18 patients using the osteotome technique; that author obtained a 97% success rate. However, the number of implants placed during this short-term study (2 to 15 months, mean 5 months) is low.

B. Modified osteotome technique

In 1998, Lazzara[76] proposed the modified osteotome technique, which is based on the combined use of osteotomes, drills, and screwed implants (Figs 9-50 and 9-51). Neither the osteotome nor drill must penetrate

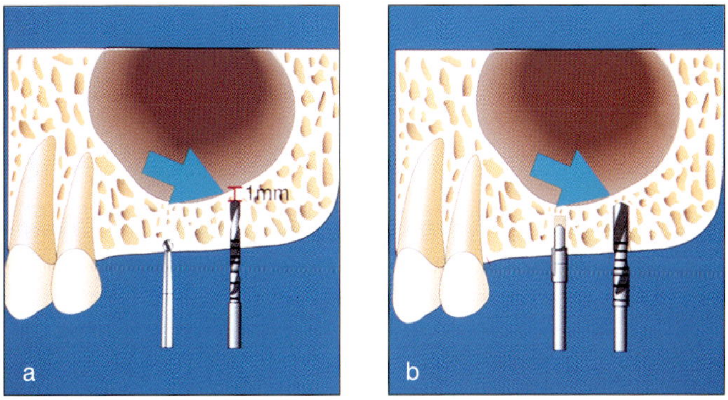

Fig 9-50a and 9-50b Preparation of implant sites with the modified osteotome technique.

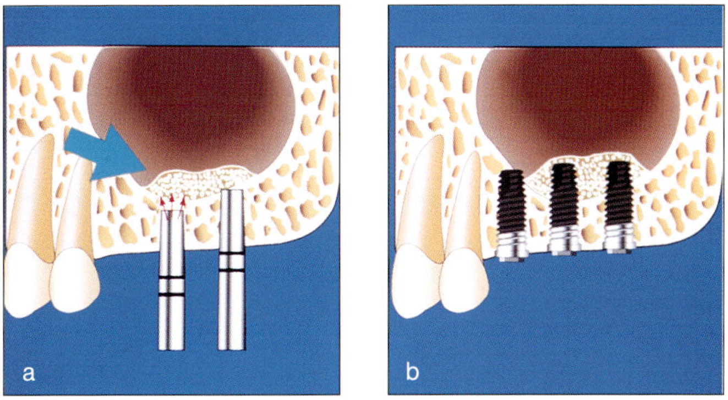

Figs 9-51a and 9-51b a = bone grafting is performed using osteotomes; b = view after implant placement.

the sinus antrum. This technique is indicated in the presence of a large ridge (greater than 6 mm) with a subsinus bone volume greater than 5 mm. A radiographic analysis (panoramic, long-cone, and computed tomographic scans) allows accurate assessment of anatomy and available subsinus bone volume (Figs 9-52 to 9-66).

The different steps of this technique are:

—Implant site preparation starts with the 2-mm drill. The drilling must remain 1 mm under the sinus floor. The surgical template specifies the prosthetic imperatives.
—At this stage, a periapical control radiograph is performed using a positioned direction indicator. The aim of this radiograph is to check the integrity of the subsinus cortical layer. It is important to recall that no instrument must penetrate the sinus antrum.
—The intermediate drill is only used for 2 to 3 mm. The 3-mm drill finishes the implant site preparation for a standard-diameter implant. Again, the drilling must stay 1 mm away from the sinus floor.
—A resorbable grafting material is introduced in the surgical site before using a No. 3 Summers osteotome. This material will act as a "stress-breaking cushion" in order to delicately fracture the sinus floor.
—At this stage, the integrity of the sinus membrane is checked (absence of condensation on the mirror when the patient is asked to blow with the nose closed). In the case of a sinus membrane perforation, two treatment options may be considered: either stopping

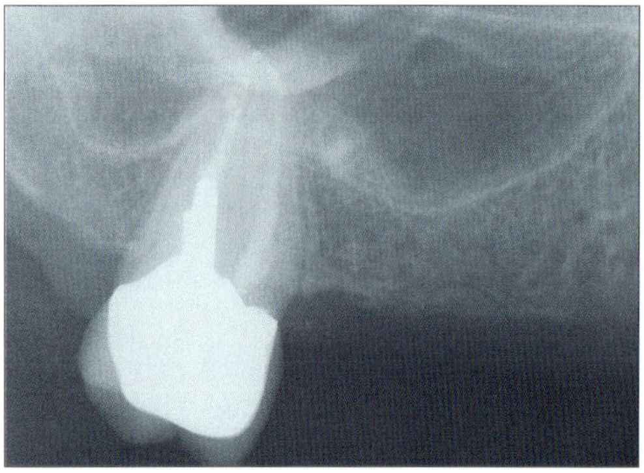

Fig 9-52 Radiograph demonstrating insufficient subsinus bone volume.

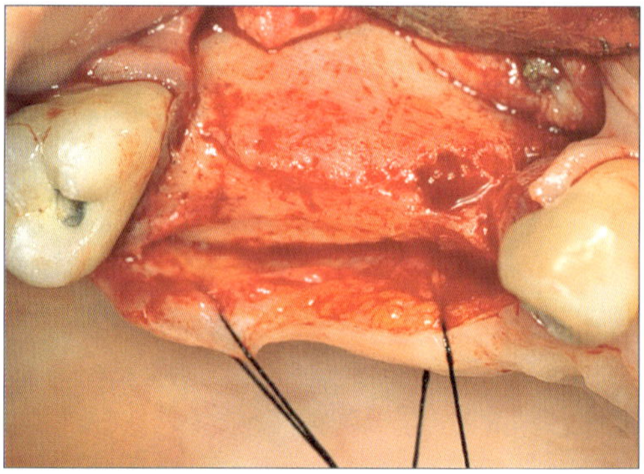

Fig 9-53 Clinical view after soft tissue flap reflection.

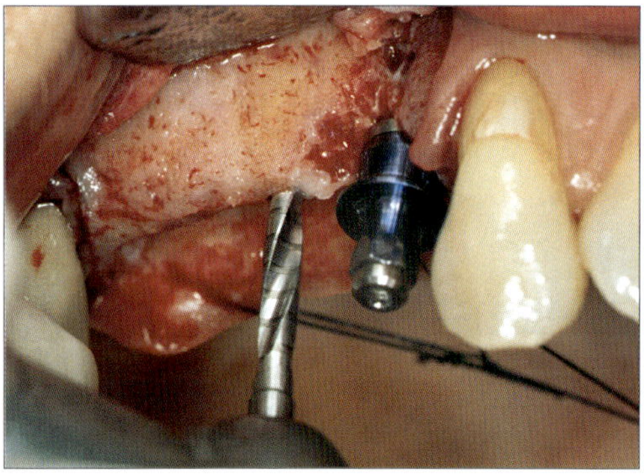

Fig 9-54 An implant is placed in the position of the maxillary right first premolar in a conventional manner. In the position of the second premolar, implant site preparation (modified osteotome technique) using a 2-mm drill.

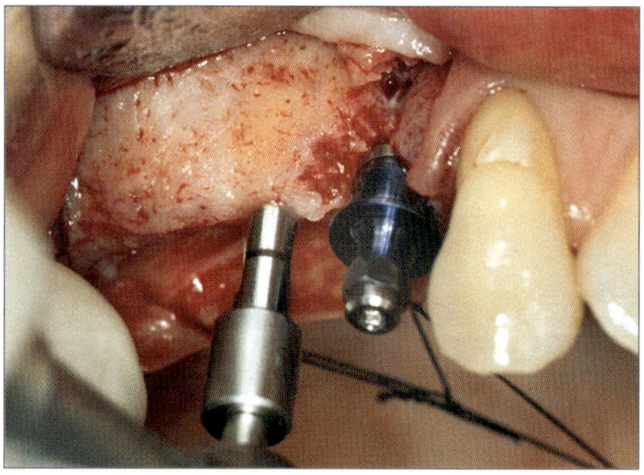

Fig 9-55 Use of an intermediate drill to widen the implant site up to 3 mm.

the surgery to continue it after 4 weeks of healing or performing a Caldwell-Luc buccal approach (conventional bone grafting technique).

–Autogenous bone harvesting combined or not with a resorbable grafting material is progressively introduced on the overall height of the implant site.

–Autogenous bone is condensed using an osteotome that must never penetrate the sinus antrum. The bone harvesting may be performed at the tuberosity, the ramus, or the chin. Each penetration of the osteotome and packing of the implant site incrementally allows increase of the implant height by 1 mm.

–Using a countersink drill is indicated only in the presence of a thick cortical layer or when the temporization is performed using a removable prosthesis.

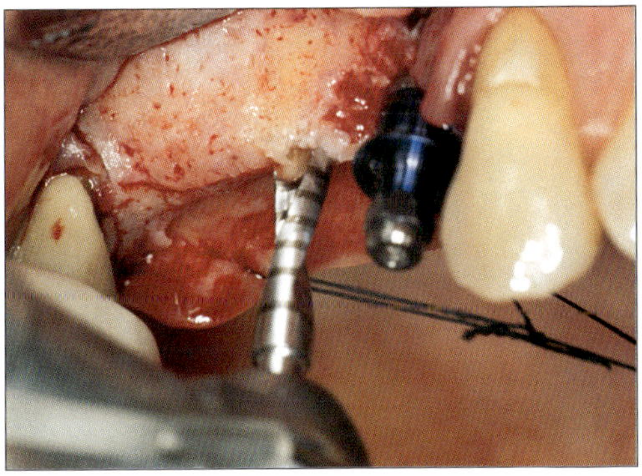

Fig 9-56 Implant site drilling using the 3-mm drill; the preparation must always stay 1 mm under the sinus floor.

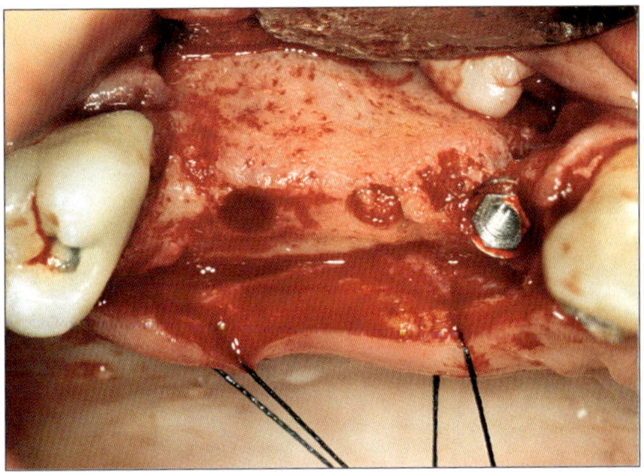

Fig 9-57 Placement of a resorbable bone grafting material.

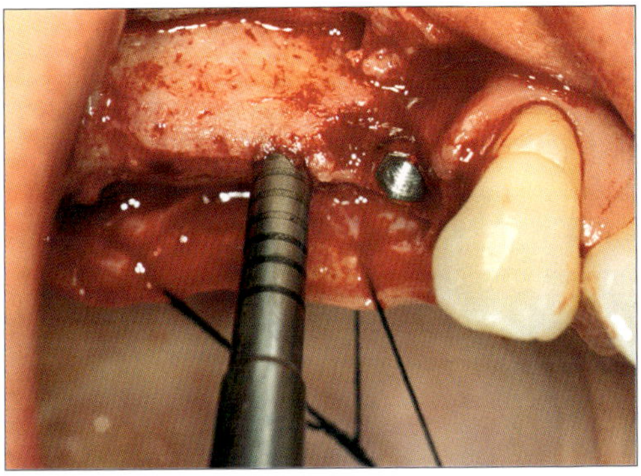

Fig 9-58 A No. 3 Summers osteotome allows careful fracture of the sinus floor. The integrity of the sinus membrane must be checked.

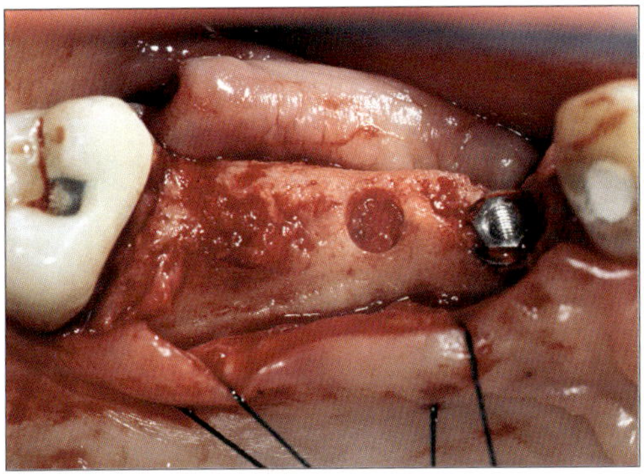

Fig 9-59 Occlusal view after progressive packing of autogenous bone into the implant site.

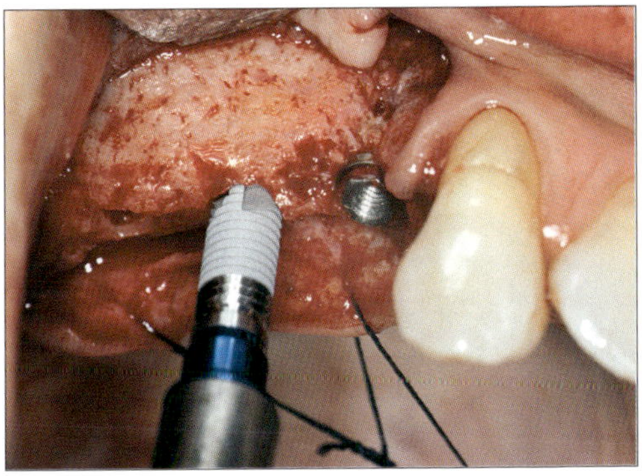

Fig 9-60 Placement of an Osseotite implant.

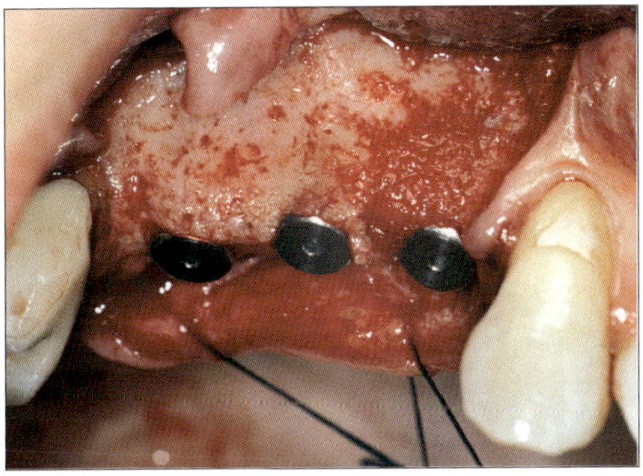

Fig 9-61 Final clinical view. The two distal implants have been placed according to the modified osteotome technique.

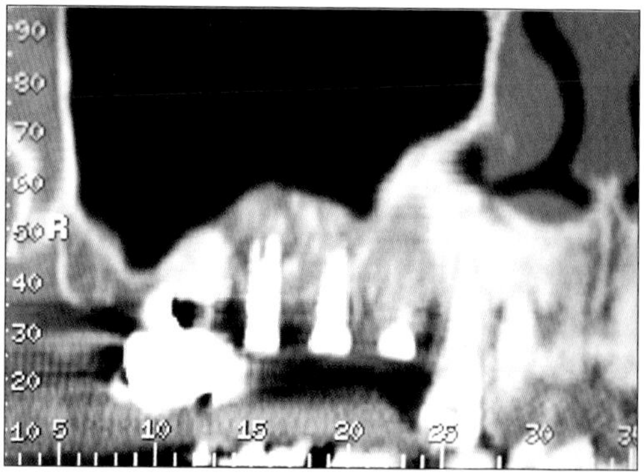

Fig 9-62 Control panoramic cut. Note the bone fill around the implant apices.

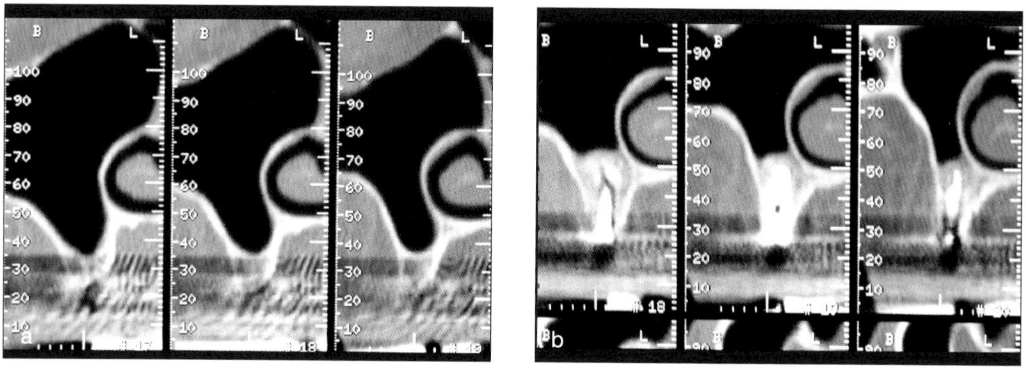

Figs 9-63a and 9-63b Presurgical and control oblique scans.

C. Preparation technique for a future implant site

In the presence of a subsinus bone volume of less than 4 mm, it is advocated that implant placement be delayed by 6 to 7 months following the bone grafting[77]:

- —A 2-mm-diameter drill allows location of the surgical site using a surgical template.
- —A 5-mm-internal-diameter trephine allows performance of the osteotomy by isolating a bone cylinder, which is dislocated using a No. 4 Summers osteotome. The sinus membrane is elevated with the bone cylinder, which acts as a stress-breaking cushion. The integrity of the sinus membrane must be checked. In the case of sinus membrane perforation, surgery will have to be stopped.
- —Autogenous bone is progressively placed until the required bone volume is obtained.
- —The implant placement will occur 6 to 7 months following bone healing.

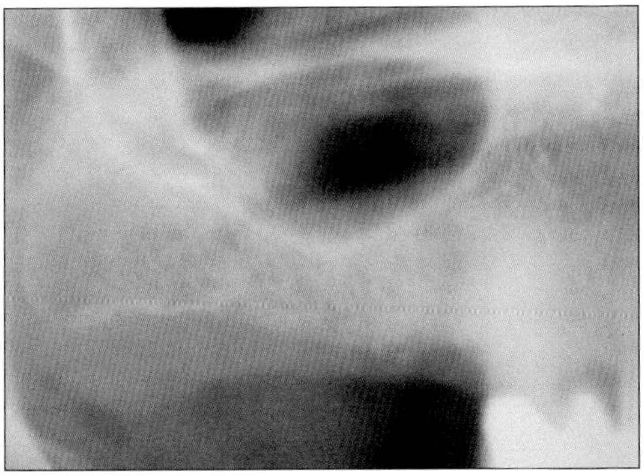

Fig 9-64 Radiograph of a posterior edentulous maxilla with a 5-mm subsinus bone volume in the position of the maxillary right first molar.

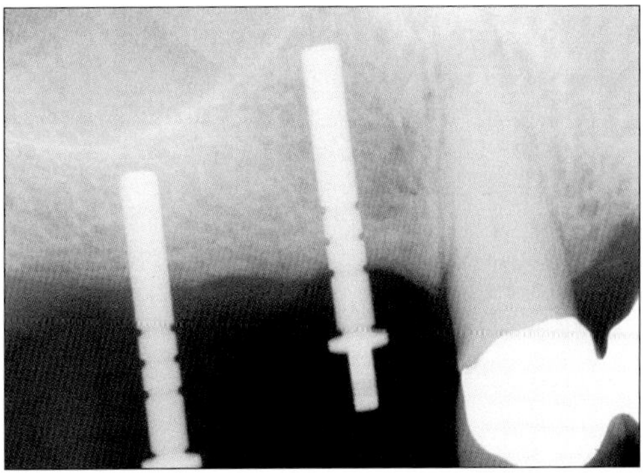

Fig 9-65 Control radiograph allows location of the sinus floor.

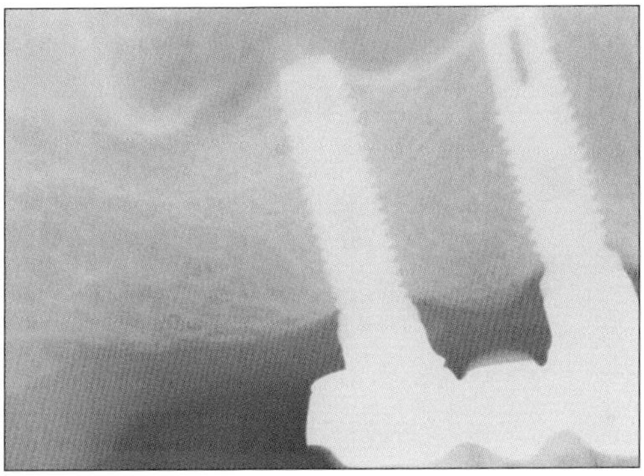

Fig 9-66 Radiograph at 1 year. Note the perfect osseointegration of the implants and the subsinus bone gain.

References

1. Lazzara RJ. Immediate implant placement into extraction sites: Surgical and restorative advantages. Int J Periodontics Restorative Dent 1989;9:333–343.
2. Gelb DA. Immediate implant surgery: Three-year retrospective evaluation of 50 consecutive cases. Int J Oral Maxillofac Implants 1993;8:388–399.
3. Davarpanah M, Martínez H, Tecucianu JF, Etienne D, Kebir M. Les implants de large diamètre. Résultats chirurgicaux à 2 ans. Implant 1995;1:289–300.
4. Graves SL, Jansen CE, Siddiqui AA, Beaty KD. Wide diameter implants: Indications, considerations and preliminary results over two-year period. Aust Prosthodont J 1994;8:31–37.
5. Langer B, Langer L, Herrmann I, Erug M. The wide fixture: A solution for special bone situations and rescue for the compromised implant. Part 1. Int J Oral Maxillofac Implants 1993;8:400–408.
6. Bert M, Missika P. Implantologie Chirurgicale et Prothétique. Paris: CdP, 1996.
7. Tulasne JF. Implant treatment of missing posterior dentition. In: Albrektsson T, Zarb GA (eds). The Brånemark Osseointegrated Implant. Chicago: Quintessence, 1989:103–115.
8. Bahat O. Treatment planning and placement of implants in the posterior maxillae: Report of 732 consecutive Nobelpharma implants. Int J Oral Maxillofac Implants 1993;8:151–161.

9. Tulasne JF. Implants ptérygo-maxillaires. Expérience sur 7 ans. Cah Prothet 1992;(special issue 1):39–48.
10. Bahat O. Osseointegrated implants in the maxillary tuberosity: Report of 45 consecutive patients. Int J Oral Maxillofac Implants 1992;7:459–467.
11. Khayat P, Nader N. The use of osseointegrated implants in the maxillary tuberosity. Pract Periodontics Aesthet Dent 1994;6:53–61.
12. Graves SL. L'implant ptérygoïdien. Une solution de restauration à la partie postérieure du maxillaire. Int J Periodontics Restorative Dent 1994;14:513–523.
13. Balshi TJ, Lee HY, Hernandez RE. The use of pterygomaxillary implants in the partially edentulous patient: A preliminary report. Int J Oral Maxillofac Implants 1995;10:89–98.
14. Venturelli A. A modified surgical protocol for placing implants in the maxillary tuberosity: Clinical results at 36 months after loading with fixed partial dentures. Int J Oral Maxillofac Implants 1996;11:743–749.
15. Fernandez Valeron J, Fernandez Velazquez J. Placement of screw-type implants in the pterygomaxillary-pyramidal region: Surgical procedure and preliminary results. Int J Oral Maxillofac Implants 1997; 12:814–819.
16. Brånemark P-I, Adell R, Albrektsson T, Lekholm U, Lindstrom J, Rockler B. An experimental and clinical study of osseointegrated implants penetrating the nasal cavity and maxillary sinus. J Oral Maxillofac Surg 1984;43:497–505.
17. Boyne PJ, James RA. Grafting of the maxillary floor with autogenous marrow and bone. J Oral Surg 1980;38:613–616.
18. Valentini P, Abensur D. Elévation du plancher du sinus maxillaire à l'aide d'os lyophilisé déminéralisé et d'os bovin (Bio-Oss) et mise en place d'implants: Étude clinique sur 20 patients. Int J Periodontics Restorative Dent 1997;17:233–241.
19. Small SA, Zinner ID, Panno FV, Shapiro HJ. Augmentation of the maxillary sinus for implants: Report of 27 patients. Int J Oral Maxillofac Implants 1993;8: 523–528.
20. Smiler DG, Johnson PW, Lozada JL. Sinus lift and endosseous implants. Dent Clin North Am 1992; 36:151–186.
21. Tatum H Jr. Maxillary and sinus implant reconstructions. Dent Clin North Am 1986;30:207–229.
22. Kent JN, Block MS. Simultaneous maxillary sinus floor bone grafting and placement of hydroxylapatite-coated implants. J Oral Maxillofac Surg 1989;47: 238–242.
23. Raghoebar GM, Brouwer TJ, Reintsema H, van Oort RP. Augmentation of the maxillary sinus floor with autogenous bone for the placement of endosseous implants: A preliminary report. J Oral Maxillofac Surg 1993;51:1198–1203.
24. Keller EE, Eckert SE, Tolman DE. Mandibular ridge augmentation with simultaneous onlay iliac bone graft and endosseous implants: A preliminary report. J Oral Maxillofac Surg 1994;52:438–447.
25. Zinner ID, Small SA. Sinus lift graft using the maxillary sinuses to support implants. J Am Dent Assoc 1996; 127:51–57.
26. Blomqvist JE, Alberius P, Isaksson S. Retrospective analysis of one-stage maxillary sinus augmentation with endosseous implants. Int J Oral Maxillofac Implants 1996;11:512–521.
27. Daelemans P, Hermans M, Godet F, Malevez C. Augmentation osseuse du sinus maxillaire par greffe autogène avec pose immédiate d'implants: Étude rétrospective sur 5 ans. Int J Periodontics Restorative Dent 1997;17:27–39.
28. Kent JN, Block MS. Augmentation of the maxillary sinus floor with autogenous bone for placement of endosseous implants: A preliminary report. J Oral Maxillofac Surg 1993;51:1203–1205.
29. Hall HD, McKenna SJ. Bone graft of the maxillary sinus floor for Brånemark implants. Oral Maxillofac Surg Clin North Am 1991;3:869–874.
30. Tidwell JK, Blijdorp PA, Stoelinga PJ, Brouns JB, Hinderks F. Composite grafting of the maxillary sinus for placement of endosteal implants: A preliminary report of 48 patients. Int J Oral Maxillofac Surg 1992;21:204–209.
31. Tulasne JF, Saade J, Riachi A. Greffe osseuse du sinus maxillaire et implants de Brånemark. Cah Prothet 1993;(special issue 2):101–116.
32. Chiapasco M, Ronchi P. Sinus life and endosseous implants: Preliminary surgical and prosthetic results. Eur J Prosthodont Restorative Dent 1994;3:15–21.
33. Zerbib R, Ouhayoun JP, Freyss G. Apports osseux et chirurgie implantaire. J Parodontol 1991;10:177–188.
34. Lundgren S, Moy P, Johansson C, Nilsson H. Augmentation of the maxillary sinus floor with particulate mandible: A histologic and histomorphometric study. Int J Oral Maxillofac Implants 1996;11: 760–766.
35. Tessier P. Autogenous bone graft taken from the calvarium for facial and cranial applications. Clin Plast Surg 1982;9:531–537.
36. Isaksson S, Alberius P. Maxillary alveolar ridge augmentation with onlay bone grafts and immediate endosseous implants. J Craniomaxillofac Surg 1992; 20:2–7.

37. Jensen J, Krantz Simonsen E, Sindet-Pedersen S. Reconstruction of the severely resorbed maxilla with bone grafting and osseointegrated implants: A preliminary report. J Oral Maxillofac Surg 1990;48: 27–32.
38. Keller EE, van Roekel NB, Desjardins RP, et al. Prosthetic surgical reconstruction of the severely resorbed maxilla with iliac bone grafting and tissue-integrated prostheses. Int J Oral Maxillofac Implants 1987;2:155–165.
39. Keller EE. Reconstruction of the severely atrophic edentulous mandible with endosseous implants: A 10-year longitudinal study. J Oral Maxillofac Surg 1995;53:305–320.
40. Lindstrom J, Brånemark P-I, Albrektsson T. Mandibular reconstruction using the preformed autologous bone graft. J Plast Reconstr Surg 1981; 15:29–36.
41. Lindstrom J, Symington JM. Osseointegrated dental implants in conjunction with bone grafts. Int J Oral Maxillofac Implants 1988;3:31–39.
42. Misch CM, Misch CE, Resnik RR, Ismail YH. Reconstruction of maxillary alveolar defects with mandibular symphysis grafts for dental implants. Int J Oral Maxillofac Implants 1992;7:360–366.
43. Wesseling KH, Neukamm FW, Scheller H, et al. Clinical aspects of osseointegrated implants in the extremely resorbed edentulous lower and upper jaw. Z Zahnarztl Implantol 1992;7:51–55.
44. Breine U, Brånemark P-I. Reconstruction of alveolar jaw bone. An experimental and clinical study of immediate and preformed autologous bone grafts in combination with osseointegrated implants. Scand J Plast Reconstr Surg 1980;14:23–48.
45. Tulasne JF, Amzalag G, Sansemat JJ. Implants dentaires et greffes osseuses. Cah Prothet 1990;71: 81–102.
46. Antoun H, Misch C, Diestsh F, Feghali M. Augmentation de crête par greffe osseuse prélevée à la symphyse mentonnière. J Parodontol Implant Orale 1995;14:285–294.
47. Jensen O, Nock D. Inferior alveolar nerve repositioning in conjunction with placement of osseointegrated implants: A case report. Oral Surg Oral Med Oral Pathol 1987;63:263–268.
48. Friberg B, Ivanoff CJ, Lekholm U. Inferior alveolar nerve transposition in combination with Brånemark implant treatment. Int J Periodontics Restorative Dent 1992;12:441–449.
49. Jensen J, Reiche-Fischel O, Sindet-Pedersen S. Nerve transposition and implant placement in the atrophic posterior mandibular alveolar ridge. J Oral Maxillofac Surg 1994;52:662–668.
50. Rosenquist B. Fixture placement posterior to the mental foramen with transpositioning of the inferior alveolar nerve. Int J Oral Maxillofac Implants 1991;7:45–50.
51. Smiler DG. Repositioning the inferior alveolar nerve for placement of endosseous implants: Technical note. Int J Oral Maxillofac Implants 1993;8:145–150.
52. Valentini P, Abensur D, Missika P. La latéralisation du nerf alvéolaire en implantologie: Techniques chirurgicales et résultats préliminaires. J Parodontol 1994; 13:335–341.
53. Rosenquist B. Implant placement in combination with nerve transpositioning: Experience with the first hundred cases. Int J Oral Maxillofac Implants 1994; 9:522–531.
54. Haers PE, Sailer HF. Neurosensory function after lateralisation of the inferior alveolar nerve and simultaneous insertion of implants. Oral Maxillofac Surg Clin North Am 1994;7:707–716.
55. Hirsch JM, Brånemark P-I. Fixture stability and nerve function after transposition and lateralization of the inferior alveolar nerve and fixture installation. Br J Oral Maxillofac Surg 1995;33:276–281.
56. Sethi A. Repositionnement du nerf dentaire mandibulaire en dentisterie implantaire: Rapport préliminaire. Int J Periodontics Restorative Dent 1995;15:475–481.
57. Kan JY, Lozada JL, Goodacre CJ, et al. Endosseous implant placement in conjunction with inferior alveolar nerve transposition: An evaluation of neurosensory disturbance. Int J Oral Maxillofac Implants 1997; 12:463–471.
58. Kan JY, Lozada JL, Boyne PJ, et al. Mandibular fracture after endosseous implant placement in conjunction with inferior alveolar nerve transposition: A patient treatment report. Int J Oral Maxillofac Implants 1997;12:655–659.
59. Murray G, Holden R, Roachlau W. Experimental and clinical study of new growth of bone in a cavity. Am J Surg 1957;93:385–387.
60. Becker W, Becker BE. Guided tissue regeneration for implants placed into extraction sockets and for implant dehiscences: Surgical techniques and case reports. Int J Periodontics Restorative Dent 1990;10:377–391.
61. Dahlin C, Lekholm U, Lindhe A. Gain osseux induit par la presence d'une membrane. Etude clinique de 10 fixtures en titane après mise en charge fonctionnelle de un à trois ans. Int J Periodontics Restorative Dent 1991;11:273–281.
62. Nyman S, Lang N, Buser D, Brägger U. Bone regeneration adjacent to titanium implants using guided tissue regeneration: A report of two cases. Int J Oral Maxillofac Implants 1990;5:9–14.

63. Davarpanah M, Tecucianu JF, Slama M, Celletti R. Régénération osseuse en implantologie: Utilisation des membranes Gore-Tex GTAM. J Parodontol 1991;10:169–176.
64. Buser D, Brägger U, Lang NP, Nyman S. Regeneration and enlargement of jaw bone using guided tissue regeneration. Clin Oral Implants Res 1990;1: 22–32.
65. Jovanovic SA, Spiekermann H, Richter JE. Bone regeneration around titanium implants in dehisced defect sites: A clinical study. Int J Oral Maxillofac Implants 1992;7:233–245.
66. Jovanovic SA, Schenk RK, Orsini M, Kenney EB. Supracrestal bone formation around dental implants: An experimental dog study. Int J Oral Maxillofac Implants 1995;10:23–31.
67. Mellonig JT, Nevins M, Régénération guidée de défauts osseux associés à des implants. Evaluation du résultat fondé sur la preuve. Int J Periodontics Restorative Dent 1995;15:169–185.
68. Mellonig JT, Triplet J. Guided tissue regeneration and endosseous dental implants. Int J Periodontics Restorative Dent 1993;13:109–119.
69. Simion M, Baldoni M, Zaffe D. Jaw bone enlargement using immediate implant placement associated with a split-crest technique and guided tissue regeneration. Int J Periodontics Restorative Dent 1992;12:463–473.
70. Simion M, Trisi P, Piattelli A. Vertical ridge augmentation using a membrane technique associated with osseointegrated implants. Int J Periodontics Restorative Dent 1994;14:497–511.
71. Simion M, Jovanovic SA, Trisi P, Scarano A, Piattelli A. Vertical ridge augmentation around dental implants using a membrane technique and autogenous bone or allografts in humans. Int J Periodontics Restorative Dent 1998;18:9–23.
72. Tinti C, Parma-Benfenati S, Polizzi G. Vertical ridge augmentation: What is the limit? Int J Periodontics Restorative Dent 1996;16:221–229.
73. Summers RB. A new concept in maxillary implant surgery: The osteotome technique. Compend Contin Educ Dent 1994;15:152–162.
74. Summers RB. The osteotome technique: Part 3—Less invasive methods of elevation of the sinus floor. Compend Contin Educ Dent 1994;15:698–710.
75. Horowitz I. Use of xenograft bone with aspirated bone marrow for treatment of cystic defects of the jaws. Head Neck 1989;11:516–523.
76. Lazzara RJ. Technique d'ostéotome modifiée. Personal communication, Congrès de la Société Française de Parodontologie, Marseille, 1998.
77. Summers RB. The osteotome technique: Part 4—Future site development. Compend Contin Educ Dent 1995;16:1090–1099.

CHAPTER 10

Nonsubmerged Implant Techniques

P. Bouchard/H. Martínez/M. Davarpanah/G. Alcoforado

In 1969, Brånemark et al[1] defined osseointegration as a direct bone-implant contact. According to these authors, complete submerging of the implant is one of the essential factors for implant success.[2] This submerging avoids premature implant loading, infection risk, and apical migration of epithelial cells on the implant surface. The standard protocol therefore imposed two surgical stages.

Schröeder et al[3] suggested the term "functional ankylosis" to define the direct link of bone tissue with the implant surface. According to them, complete submerging of the implant is not a major condition to obtain functional ankylosis. Numerous studies have reported very good success rates with implants placed in one surgical stage (Table 10-1).

I. Nonsubmerged implants

A. History

In the 1970s, Schröeder et al,[3] in association with the Straumann Institute, developed a one-stage endosseous implant (Figs 10-1 to 10-5). Histologic and clinical studies performed on animals and humans confirm the achievement of osseointegration. Several implant designs were successively marketed in the 1970s and 1980s.[10] In 1985, the ITI group proposed a new implant system based on the different results obtained.

The aim of this new proposition is to:

- integrate, within a single system, the previously developed ITI implants
- simplify the surgical protocol
- extend the indications

Table 10-1 Middle- and long-term results using the ITI system

Author, year	Follow-up (y)	Implants	Edentulous type	Success (%)
Buser et al, 1992[4]	5	126	Partial, single unit	95
Wedgwood et al, 1992[5]	3	461	Complete	96
Bernard et al, 1995[6]	3	100	Partial	99
Wismeyer et al, 1995[7]	6.5	218	Complete	97
Versteegh et al, 1995[8]	7	135	Complete	64
Buser et al, 1997[9]	8	2,359	Partial, single, complete	91

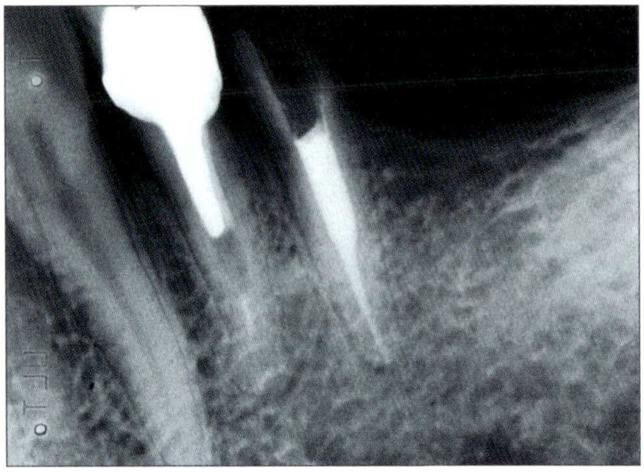

Fig 10-1 Preoperative radiograph in a 50-year-old patient. Two ITI implants are to be placed in the positions of the mandibular left first and second molars.

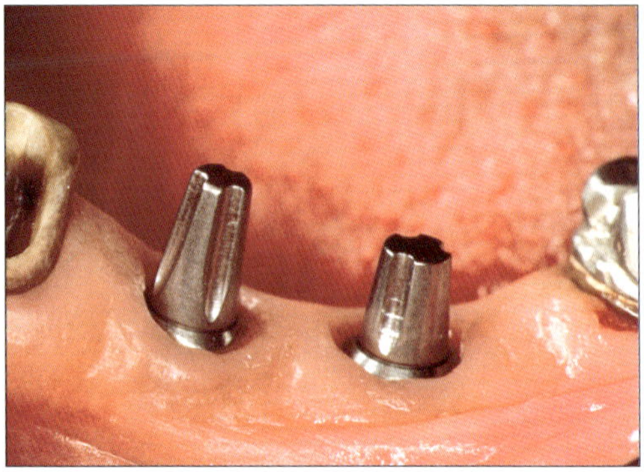

Fig 10-2 Clinical view 4 months after implant placement: two solid abutments of 5.5 and 4 mm are connected.

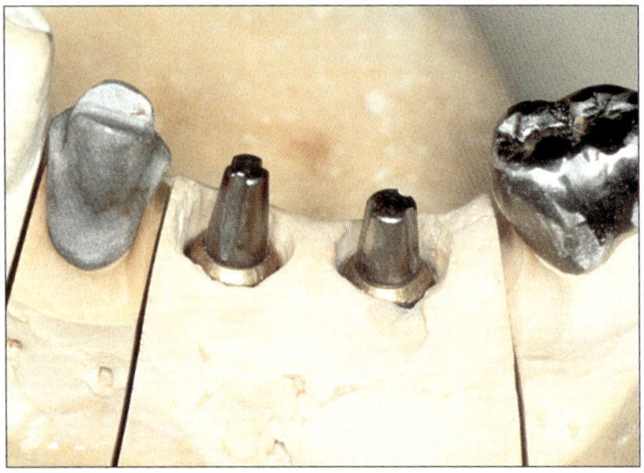

Fig 10-3 View of prosthesis fabrication. Each component is independent (laboratory, Frédéric Auger).

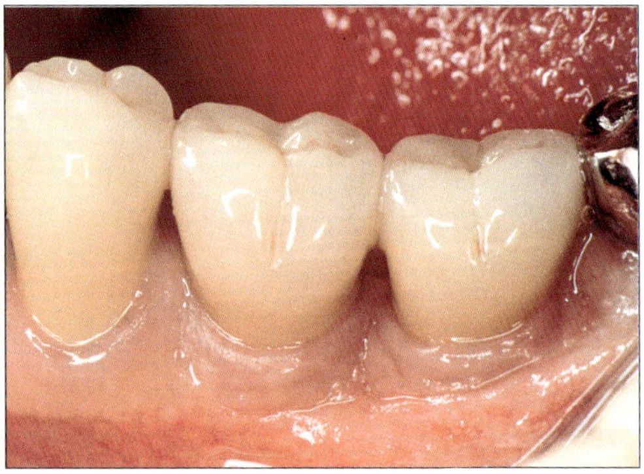

Fig 10-4 Clinical view of the final restoration at 1 year. Note the perfect tissue integration at the cervical level.

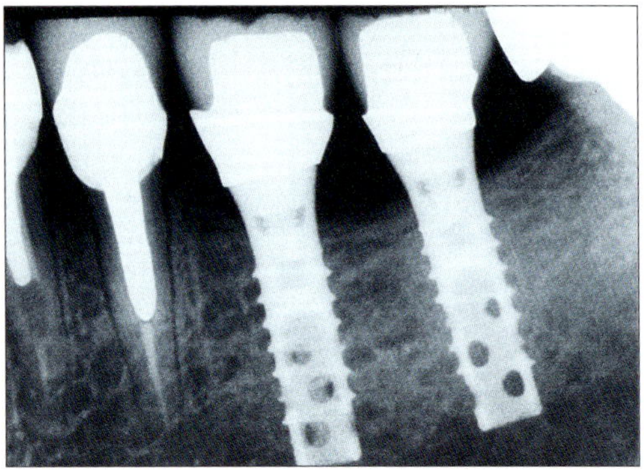

Fig 10-5 Control radiograph at 1 year.

Three types of implants were then proposed:

—solid screw
—hollow screw
—hollow cylinder

B. Principles

Despite the evolution of the system and the new implant designs offered, four basic concepts have remained unchanged for more than 20 years:

—nonsubmerged system
—one-step surgery
—commercially pure titanium implant (grade 4)
—titanium plasma-sprayed (TPS) surface

C. Implant design

The coronal part of the nonsubmerged implant (3 mm of height) offers a coronal countersink (1.8 mm) and an internal threading designed to receive the prosthetic parts. The transmucosal component presents a polished surface. This type of surface limits bacterial plaque adhesion, allowing good mucosal adaptation. The implant body is coated with TPS (rough surface). This surface processing allows an increase of the bone-implant contact surface. Today, different implant diameters (3.3 and 4.8 mm) are offered to answer different clinical situations.

D. Prosthetic abutment

The abutment presents a 6-degree taper. The 8-degree Morse cone allows connection to the implant. Screwing the abutment on the implant is performed using a torque wrench at 35 Ncm. The abutment allows fabrication of cemented restorations.

E. Peri-implant tissues: Histology

Several studies have confirmed the integration of nonsubmerged ITI implants.

1. Epithelium

The peri implant epithelium is nonkeratinized. It is thinner apically and continues as an epithelium in close contact with the smooth implant surface.[11] The most apical epithelial cells are separated from the bone crest by a connective tissue mantle adapted to the implant surface.[12–14]

2. Connective tissue

A connective tissue layer separates the epithelium from the top of the bone crest.[15] In the presence of a keratinized mucosa and a rough surface, a direct contact of perpendicular fibers with the implant surface has been observed.[11] This connective fiber distribution is not observed when keratinized tissue is absent or in the presence of a smooth implant surface. A bundle of dense fibers parallel to the implant surface and inserted in the crestal bone then ensures a functional barrier.[13]

3. Bone tissue

A direct contact between the bone and the implant surface has been demonstrated using the nonsubmerged implants.[3,14] According to Buser and coworkers,[4,13,16] the percentage of direct bone-implant contact is increased in the presence of a rough surface.

F. Advantages and disadvantages of the nonsubmerged implants

1. Advantages

- Simplification of the surgical protocol
- Improvement of the primary stability com-

pared to submerged implants because of the cervical countersink[17]
- Simplification of the prosthetic protocol owing to the solid abutments
- Reduced number of surgical stages by eliminating stage-two surgery, which offers three advantages:

—improvement of patient comfort
—reduced cost
—elimination of peri-implant bone resorption risks consecutive to the second surgical stage

2. Limitations

a. Esthetic risk

Despite the existence of two implant neck heights (1.8 and 2.8 mm) and four diffferent healing caps (2, 3, 4, and 5 mm), postoperative recession of the peri-implant tissues is difficult to predict, especially in the presence of thin or lacking gingiva. In this situation, there is a risk for implant neck exposure after healing. If soft tissue management must be considered in a second stage, the technique thus loses its main advantage, ie, no second surgery. After abutment loading, the prosthetic management of the transitional phase may turn out to be more complex, especially for the solid abutments.

b. Bacterial risk

The healing caps have a transmucosal emergence during the osseointegration period. Poor oral hygiene during this phase may contraindicate this type of implant.

c. Mechanical risk

During the osseointegration period, pressure from the interface of the provisional removable denture on the healing caps must be strictly avoided.

d. Surgical risk

Guided bone regeneration (GBR) procedures offer little indication for this type of implant. The need for a second-stage surgery for membrane removal negates the one-step procedure benefit.

3. Reflections

The best indications for nonsubmerged implants are posterior edentulous patients with good oral hygiene or when esthetics are not a major concern. When implantation becomes complex (bone grafting, GBR), the use of nonsubmerged implants must be very carefully considered. The one-step technique is a simple procedure to apply in simple cases. It may therefore be considered as a first choice in the treatment planning. For complex, esthetic, or functional cases, today the two-step technique offers more adaptibility from a surgical as well as prosthetic point of view.

II. One-step submerged implants

The good results obtained with the nonsubmerged implants have led to questions regarding the need for submerging, ie, two surgical steps using surbmerged systems. In a multicenter study, Buser et al[9] reported 13 primary failures of 2,359 nonsubmerged implants. These good results cannot be extrapolated to the submerged implants because the implant design and surface properties are different. However, several study groups have published good short-term results using submerged implants (Brånemark system) placed in one surgical step[10] (Table 10-2).

A. Surgical protocol

A surgical phase similar to the conventional protocol, and advocated by Brånemark et al,[1] has been performed. Following implant placement, the healing abutments, normally used at second-stage surgery, are screwed onto the implants before suturing.

B. Preliminary results

The obtained short-term results are satisfactory (see Table 10-1). The one-step submerged implants offer success rates similar to those reported using the conventional two-step technique. These interesting multicenter results must be confirmed for a larger number of cases.

C. Advantages and limitations

Placing submerged implants in a one-step procedure offers the same advantages and limitations as for the nonsubmerged implants. However, the lack of published literature for poor-density bone situations and the insufficient follow-up of this treatment option must be mentioned.

III. New propositions

In 1988, the 3i firm (Implant Innovations) proposed a new nonsubmerged implant (TG Osseotite). This new implant design (Figs 10-6 to 10-13) offers the advantages of a nonsubmerged implant and those of the Osseotite implant (hybrid design) (Figs 10-14 to 10-19).

A. Implant design

Two types of implant design are marketed according to the height of the soft tissues (1.8 and 2.8 mm). The implant neck (nonsubmerged part) is countersunk, and the platform is 5 mm in diameter. The 8-degree Morse cone on the internal aspect of the neck allows a perfect adaptation of the screwed abutment. The coronal part presents a smooth surface up to the third thread of the implant. This surface limits bacterial plaque adhesion and enhances good mucosal adaptation. Starting from the third thread, the implant body presents a rough surface (acid etched). This surface processing allows an increase in the implant anchoring surface.

Table 10-2 Short-term results using submerged implants placed in one-step surgery

Author, year	No. of implants	No. of failures	% failures
Ericsson et al, 1994[18]	32	2	6.3
Henry and Rosenberg, 1994[19]	24	0	0.0
Bernard et al, 1995[20]	10	0	0.0
Becker et al, 1997[21]	135	6	4.4
Collaert and De Bruyn, 1998[22]	211	6	2.8

B. Prosthetic abutments

Two prosthetic abutments are available: a straight inlay core and a hexagonal intermediate component. The straight abutment is indicated for cemented prosthesis fabrication. This abutment is screwed at 32 Ncm inside the implant and imposes an ideal implant positioning. An 8-degree Morse cone allows abutment connection and guarantees its rotation because of friction. The hexagonal abutment is indicated to fabricate screw-retained restorations. It is a gold cylinder to be cast on (gold UCLA principle). It allows fabrication of an inlay core according to an ideal prosthetic axis and a screw-retained restoration.

C. Clinical characteristics

- Combining two types of surface properties enhances soft tissue longevity around the implant neck (smooth surface) and offers better osseointegration (etched surface).

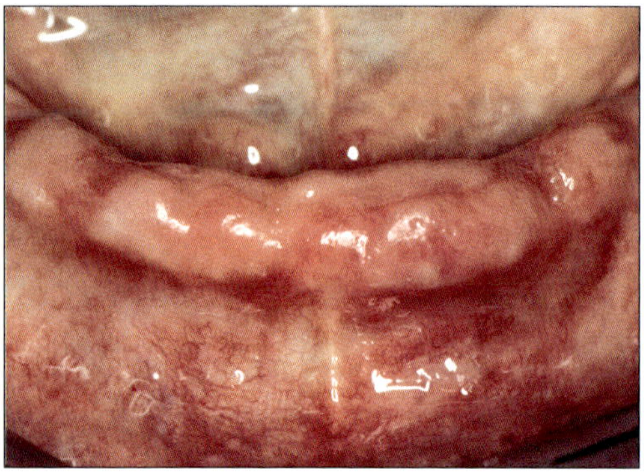

Fig 10-6 Seventy-year-old completely edentulous female patient. Preoperative clinical view in the mandible (case treated in association with Dr P. Viargues).

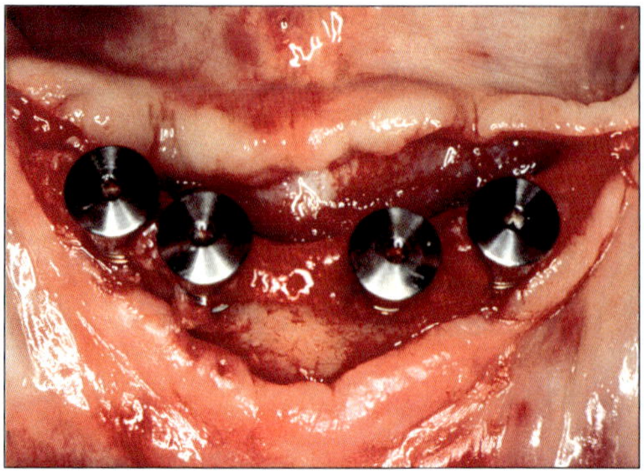

Fig 10-7 Four TG Osseotite implants in the mandible.

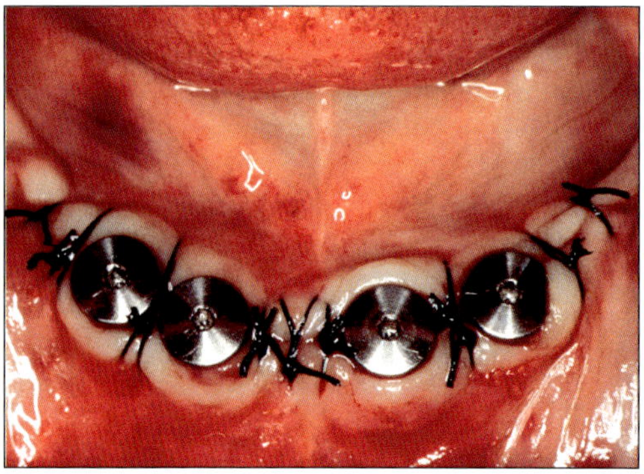

Fig 10-8 Clinical view after suturing.

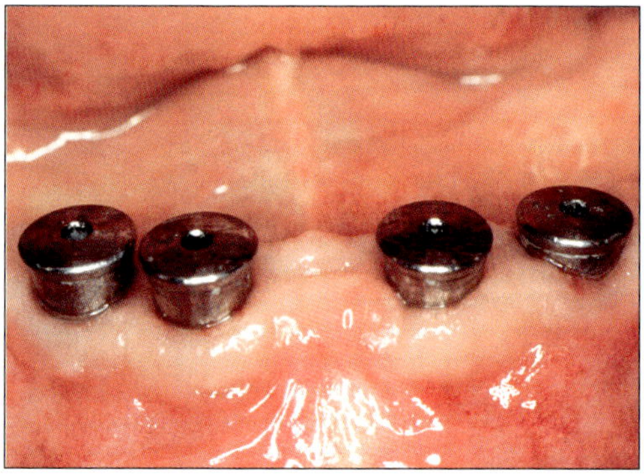

Fig 10-9 Clinical view at 5 months.

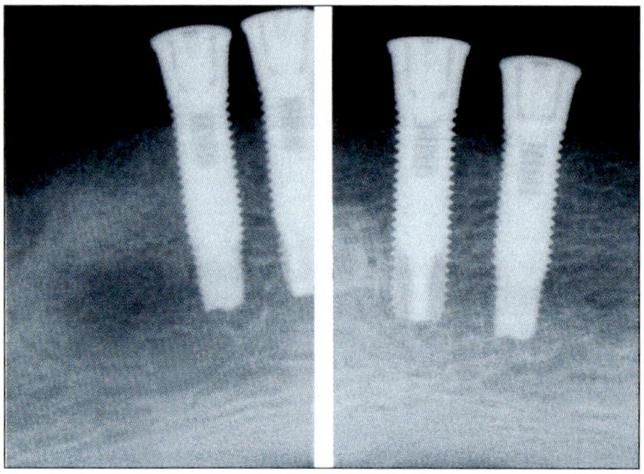

Fig 10-10 Radiographic views before loading.

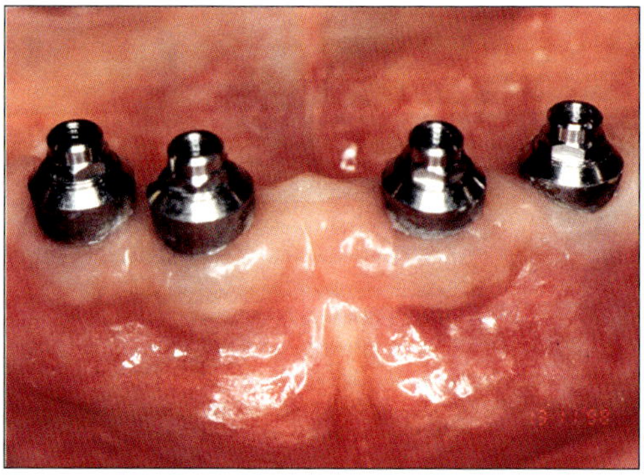

Fig 10-11 Clinical view after abutment connection.

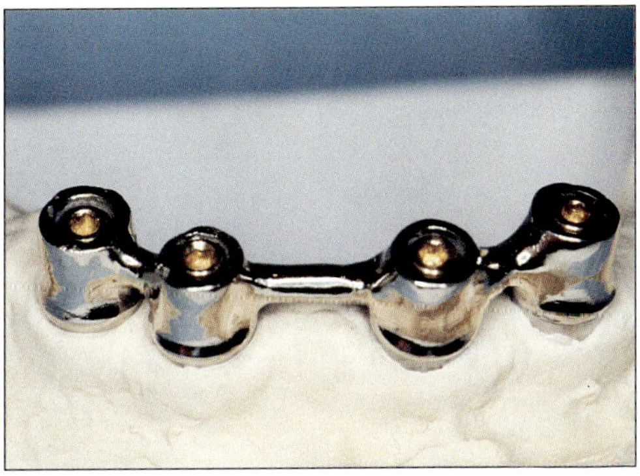

Fig 10-12 Bar fabrication at the laboratory over the four implants.

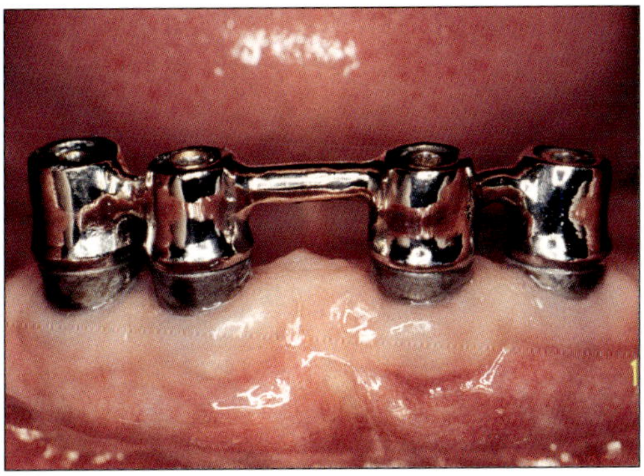

Fig 10-13 Clinical view after bar positioning.

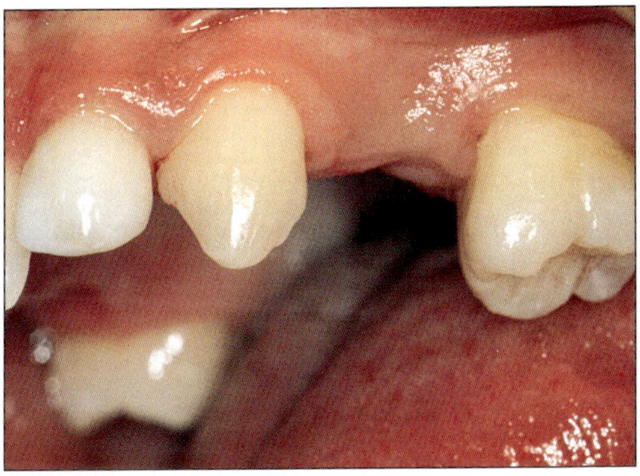

Fig 10-14 Twenty-year-old patient presenting agenesis of a premolar (case treated in association with Dr G. Kuhn).

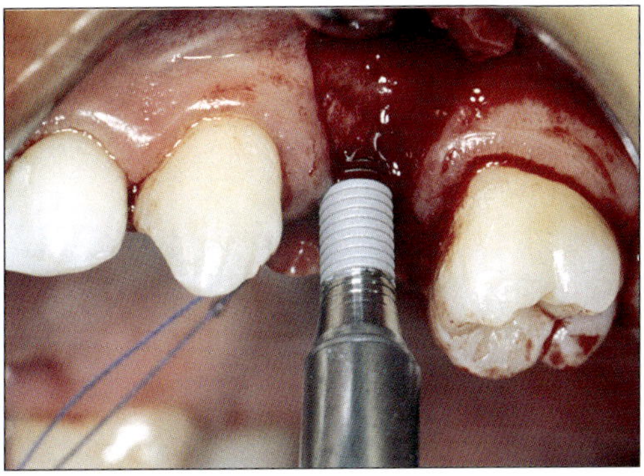

Fig 10-15 Direct placement of a TG Osseotite implant.

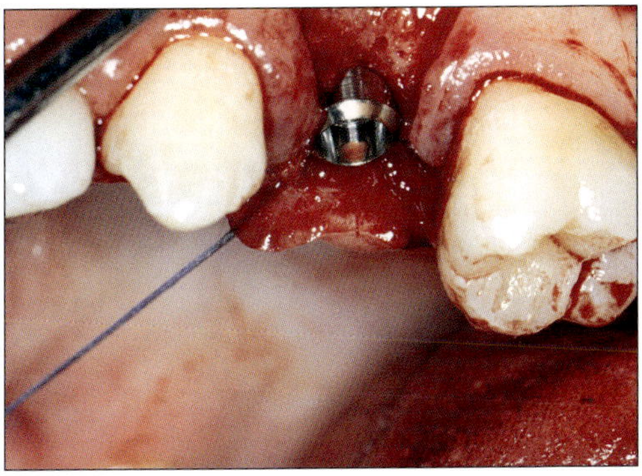

Fig 10-16 Positioned implant.

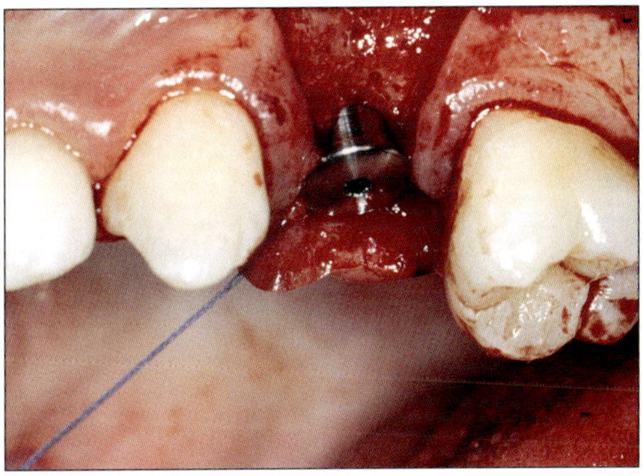

Fig 10-17 Healing screws in place.

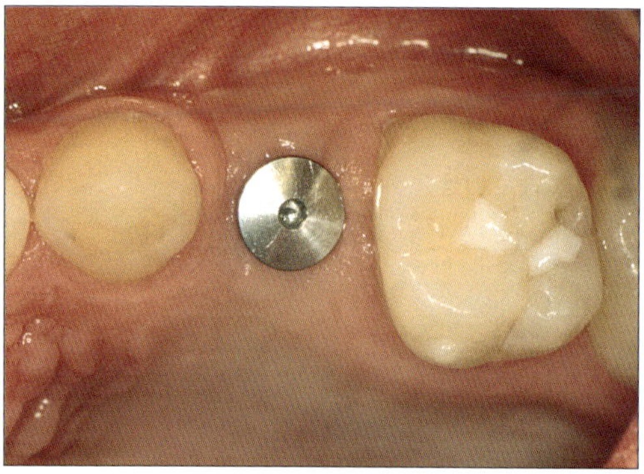

Fig 10-18 Clinical view at 4 months.

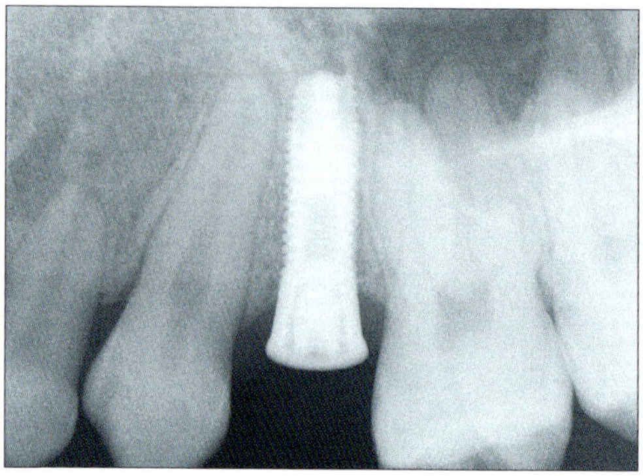

Fig 10-19 Control radiograph at 4 months.

- Optimization of bone healing is observed in the presence of spongy bone.
- Reducing the bone healing period offers the option of rapid loading.

D. Reflections

1. *Instrumentation*

The surgical material required for the nonsubmerged TG Osseotite implant placement is identical to that used for the submerged technique. The surgical ergonomics of the system are therefore excellent. The prosthetic instrumentation is practical.

2. *Implants*

They are self-tapping, which is not the case for the ITI system. This new implant presents a shorter interthread space, similar to the submerged implants, allowing an almost immediate bone engagement owing to the ICE end. The 8-degree Morse cone presents an internal stabilization chamber, allowing a 29% increase of the abutment's lateral stability.

The presence of a smooth titanium area at the neck limit, corresponding to about three threads, offers the advantage of a less rough surface than the plasma-sprayed or acid-etched surfaces. Bacterial plaque adhesion is therefore less likely. The importance of this adhesion is well known in peri-implantitis development.[23] During peri-implantitis treatment, detoxification of the implant surface using an air-polishing device has been suggested.[24]

Alteration of the implant surface appears less important on smooth titanium than on the plasma-sprayed surface.[25] The clinical follow-up is less extensive than for the ITI implants, which remain the standard in terms of one-step technique.

References

1. Brånemark P-I, Zarb GA, Albrektsson T. Tissue-Integrated Prostheses: Osseointegration in Clinical Dentistry. Chicago: Quintessence, 1985.
2. Adell R, Lekholm U, Rockler B, Brånemark P-I. A 15 year study of osseointegrated implants in the treatment of edentulous jaw. Int J Oral Surg 1981;10: 387–416.
3. Schröeder A, Pohler O, Sutter F. Gewebsreaktion auf ein Titan-Hohlzylinderimplantat mit Titan-Spritzschichtoberfläche. Schweiz Monatsschr Zahnheilkd 1976;86:713–727.
4. Buser D, Sutter F, Weber HP, Belser U, Schröeder A. The ITI dental system: Basics, indications, clinical procedures and results. Clin Dent 1992;52:1–23.
5. Wedgwood D, Jennings K, Critchlow H, et al. Experience with ITI osseointegration implants at five centers in the UK. Br J Oral Maxillofac Surg 1992;30:377–381.
6. Bernard JP, Belser UC, Szmukler S, Martinet JP, Attieh A, Saad PJ. Intérêt de l'utilisation d'implants ITI de faible longueur dans les secteurs postérieurs: Résultats d'une étude clinique de 3 ans. Med Buccale Chir Buccale 1995;1:11–18.
7. Wismeyer D, van Waas MA, Vermeeren J. Overdentures supported by ITI implants: A 6.5 year evaluation of patient satisfaction and prosthetic after care. Int J Oral Maxillofac Implants 1995;10:744–749.
8. Versteegh P, van Beek GJ, Slagter J, Ottervanger JP. Clinical evaluation of mandibular overdentures supported by multiple bar fabrication: A follow-up study of two implant systems. Int J Oral Maxillofac Implants 1995;10:595–603.
9. Buser D, Mericske-Stern R, Bernard JP, et al. Long-term evaluation of non-submerged ITI implants. Part 1: 8-year life table analysis of a prospective multi-center study with 2,359 implants. Clin Oral Implants Res 1997;8:161–172.
10. Buser D, Belser U, Lang NP. The original one-stage dental implant system and its clinical application. Periodontol 2000 1998;17:106–118.
11. Schröeder A, Vander Zypen E, Stich H, Sutter F. The reaction of bone, connective tissue and epithelium to endosteal implants with sprayed titanium surfaces. J Maxillofac Surg 1981;9:15–25.
12. Buser D, Schenk RK, Steinemann S, Fiorellini JP, Fox CH, Stich H. Influence of surface characteristics on bone integration of titanium implants. A histomorphometric study in miniature pigs. J Biomed Mater Res 1991;25:889–902.
13. Buser D, Weber HP, Donath K, Fiorellini JP, Paquette DW, Williams RC. Soft tissue reactions to non-submerged unloaded titanium implants in beagle dogs. J Periodontol 1992;63:225–235.
14. Listgarten MA, Buser D, Steinemann SG, Donath K, Lang NP, Weber HP. Light and transmission electron microscopy of the intact interfaces between non-submerged titanium-coated epoxy resin implants and bone or gingiva. J Dent Res 1992;71:364–371.
15. Bernard JP, Rousseau P, Buser D, Belser UC. Tissus mous péri-implantaires et techniques non enfouies. J Parodontol Implantol Orale 1994;13:7–14.
16. Buser D, Weber HP, Lang NP. Tissue integration of non-submerged implants: 1-year results of a prospective study with 100 ITI hollow-cylinder and hollow-screw implants. Clin Oral Implants Res 1990;1:33–40.
17. Ouhayoun JP, Itic J, Goffeaux JC, Bouchard P. Comparaison de deux systèmes implantaires enfouis et non enfouis. J Parodontol 1994;13:17–30.
18. Ericsson I, Randow K, Glantz PO, Lindhe J, Nilner K. Clinical and radiographical features of submerged and non-submerged titanium implants. Clin Oral Implants Res 1994;5:185–189.
19. Henry P, Rosenberg J. Single-stage surgery for rehabilitation of the edentulous mandible. Preliminary results. Pract Periodontics Aesthet Dent 1994;6:1–8.
20. Bernard JP, Belser UC, Martinet JP, Borgis SA. Osseointegration of Brånemark fixtures using a single-step operating technique. A preliminary prospective one-year study in the edentulous mandible. Clin Oral Implants Res 1995;6:122–129.
21. Becker W, Becker BE, Israelson H, et al. One-step surgical placement of Brånemark implants: A prospective multicenter clinical study. Int J Oral Maxillofac Implants 1997;12:454–462.
22. Collaert B, De Bruyn H. Comparison of Brånemark fixture integration and short-term survival using one-stage or two-stage surgery in completely and partially edentulous mandibles. Clin Oral Implants Res 1998;9:131–135.
23. Kébir M, Bouchard P. Diagnostic des lésions péri-implantaires postprothétiques. Considérations biologiques et biomécaniques. Cah Prothet 1996;94: 55–62.
24. Malet J, Bouchard P. Diagnostic clinique et traitements des lesions péri-implantaires postprothétiques. Rev Odontoestomatol 1996;25:449–458.
25. Chairay JP, Boulekbache H, Jean A, Soyer A, Bouchard P. Scanning electron microscopic evaluation of the effects of an air-abrasive system on dental implants: A comparative study between machined and plasma-sprayed titanium surfaces. J Periodontol 1997;68:1215–1222.

CHAPTER 11

Implants in the Young Patient

M. Davarpanah/H. Martínez/M. Kebir

In the young patient, dental implants may be considered for treatment of edentulism following tooth agenesis, premature loss of permanent teeth, or in the presence of congenital syndromes. The skeletal changes caused by growth and implant behavior, which is identical to that of an ankylosed tooth, often contraindicate this treatment option. However, several clinicians have reported the use of dental implants in the young patient. Understanding of maxillofacial growth allows specification of the few indications for implants in the young patient.

I. Skeletal growth

Growth of the maxilla is constant up to the teenage years.[1,2] It is very active during the first years. According to Delaire et al,[3] the face reaches about 80% of its adult size at 5 years of age. This growth process decreases rapidly to a minimal activity during the prepubescent period.[4] An important new growth peak occurs near the age of 17. The complete statural growth occurs 18 to 24 months earlier in the female. The duration of the pubertal growth peak is identical in both sexes. The size of the arches is larger in the male. This difference is due to an increased length and speed of the growth period at puberty. Complete growth in the female is almost achieved near 15 years of age. Inversely, for the male, it may continue up to the age of 19 or more. It is therefore easier to consider dental implants in a young female after the age of 15.

Few studies have observed the behavior of dental implants in growing bone. The implant is considered an ankylosed tooth. The clinical reports and animal studies have confirmed the absence of movement of implants in relation to the alveolar bone and the adjacent teeth. The implant behaves like an ankylosed deciduous tooth (Fig 11-1). Bone remodeling caused by growth would lead to progressive embedding of the implants. Indeed, an implant placed in the symphysis may find itself in a more lingual position because of the bone resorption and apposition processes of the maxillofacial growth.

A. Maxilla

The development of the midface (Fig 11-2) depends on:

–the growth at suture level
–the modeling growth originating from the periosteum (bone apposition and resorption)

Growth occurs simultaneously in the different dimensions of space.

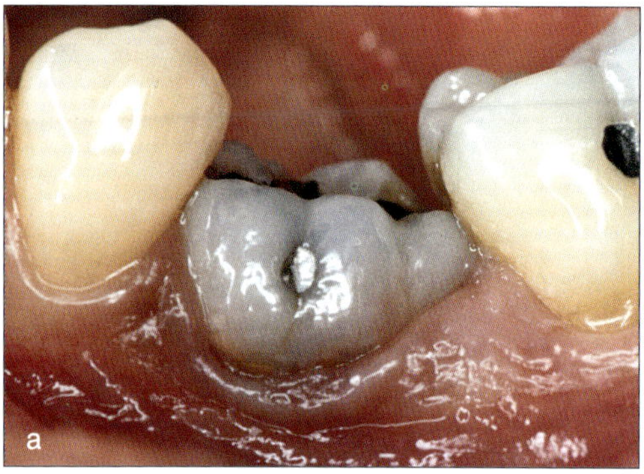

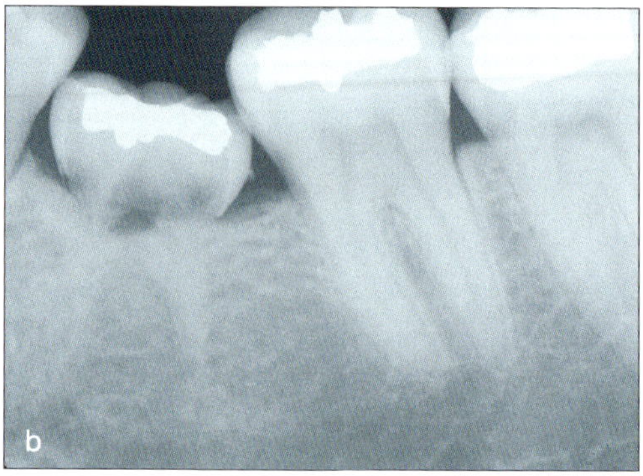

Figs 11-1a and 11-1b Clinical and radiographic views of an ankylosed deciduous molar. Note the normal eruption of the opposing teeth leading to an apparent submerging of the lacteal tooth.

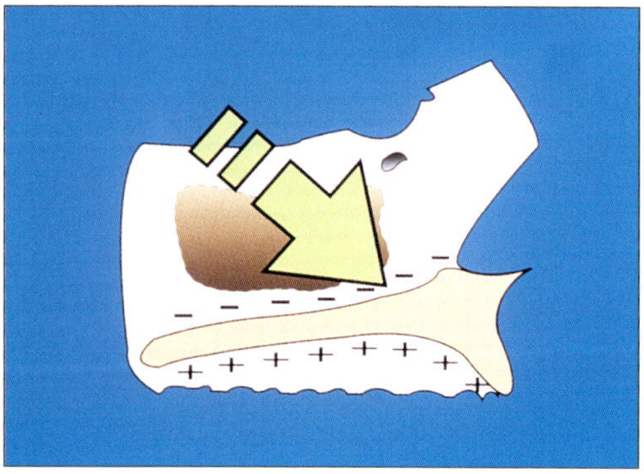

Fig 11-2 Diagram illustrating the apposition and resorption areas in the maxillary alveolar ridge during growth. The maxilla moves forward and downward.

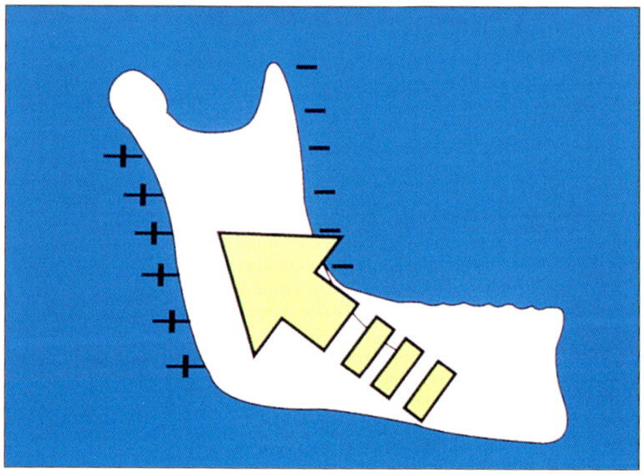

Fig 11-3 Diagram illustrating the mandibular displacement during growth. The growth in length of the mandible essentially depends on the resorption and the apposition of the ramus.

1. Anterior-inferior growth

The perimaxillary suture system allows growth to occur. The nasal septum induces a displacement of the maxilla downward and forward. This anteroinferior development may reach 3 cm between the age of 3 and the end of growth. According to Björk and Skieller,[5] this growth pattern is not linear, but curved, more sagittal during the juvenile period and more vertical during the teenage years. The anteroposterior growth also depends on the transversal growth of the maxilla.

2. Transversal growth

Widening of the maxilla depends on the sagittal and maxillomalar suture system. The transversal growth of the alveolar arch, and of its maxillary base, occurs at the transverse palatal suture level. This growth is about 3 cm from the age of 3 to the end of growth.

3. Vertical growth

Vertical growth of the maxilla is due to passive suture displacement and to the modeling growth of the alveolar ridge.

B. Mandible

The mandibular growth (Fig 11-3) mainly depends on:

—the growth of the condylar fibrocartilage
—the modeling growth originating from the periosteum (bone resorption and apposition)

Mandibular growth may be assessed in the three dimensions of space.

1. Growth in length

The growth in length depends mainly on the resorption of the anterior edge of the ramus and on the bone apposition in the posterior edge of the ramus. The body lengthens progressively as the ramus resorbs.

2. Growth in width

The growth in width depends on the growth in length because of the posterior divergent form of the mandibular arch. The modeling growth also participates in this enlargement.

3. Growth in height

Activity of the condylar cartilage mainly determines the vertical dimension.

II. Review of the literature

Starting in the 1950s, Björk and Skieller[5] studied the facial growth in humans (from age 4 to adult) using metal implants strategically positioned in the maxilla (zygomatic process, anterior aspect of the maxilla, and anterior nasal spine). Annual radiographic controls (from age 4 to 21) allowed assessment of bone growth in the three dimensions of space. Animal studies (12-week-old pigs)[6,7] have also allowed assessment of growth of the maxilla around implants and teeth. Implants do not follow tooth migration during growth. Alteration and/or deviation of tooth bud eruption is also observed around implants. In the posterior segments (implant in a premolar site), eruption of the teeth adjacent to the implants creates peri-implant intrabony defects.

Furthermore, implants are located in a more lingual position. In the anterior segments, implant movement is less important. However, changes in the mandibular angle during growth may modify the axis of symphysis implants. Several authors report some clinical cases using implants placed in the child and in the teenager.[7] Lack of follow-up for these patients limits the value of the information on the progress of these implants. Moreover, the difference in growth changes observed from one individual to another render the assessment of the importance of growth difficult.

Westwood and Duncan[8] report three clinical cases of dental implants placed in the teenager. During growth, a progressive submerging of two posterior implants in a 15-year-old boy was observed. A normal vertical alveolar bone around the adjacent teeth explains the formation of peri-implant intrabony defects.

Brugnolo et al[9] report three cases of maxillary single-unit implants placed in young patients (aged from 11.5 to 13 years). The treated cases were followed for a period of 2.5 to 4.5 years. The three implant-supported, single-unit crowns progressively positioned themselves in infraclusion (Fig 11-4). In one of these young patients, the maximum vertical growth observed was 3 mm (Figs 11-5 to 11-9).

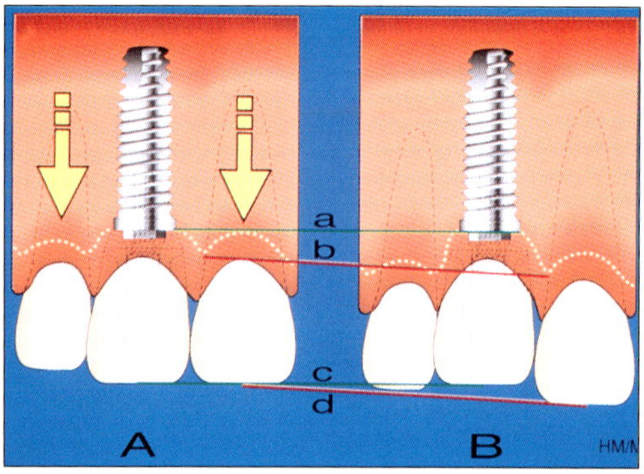

Fig 11-4 An implant placed during growth behaves like an ankylosed tooth. Physiologic vertical growth of the adjacent natural teeth leads to a shift of soft tissues, bone, and clinical crowns.

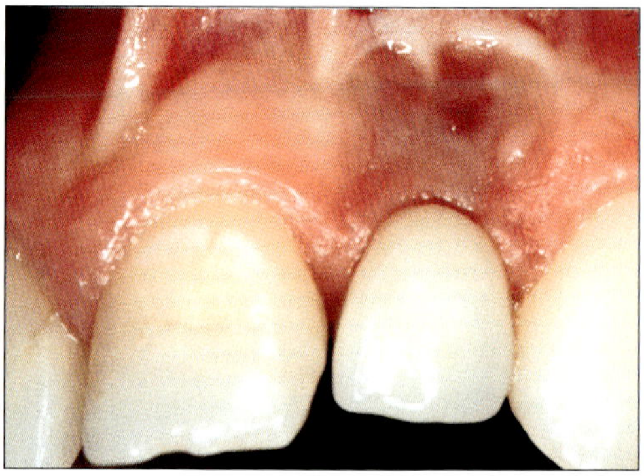

Fig 11-5 Clinical view of an implant-supported crown on the maxillary left lateral incisor in a 13.5-year-old patient. The implant was placed at the age of 11.5. A relapsing gingival abscess is observed on the buccal aspect of the tooth (clinical case of Dr G. Cordioli).

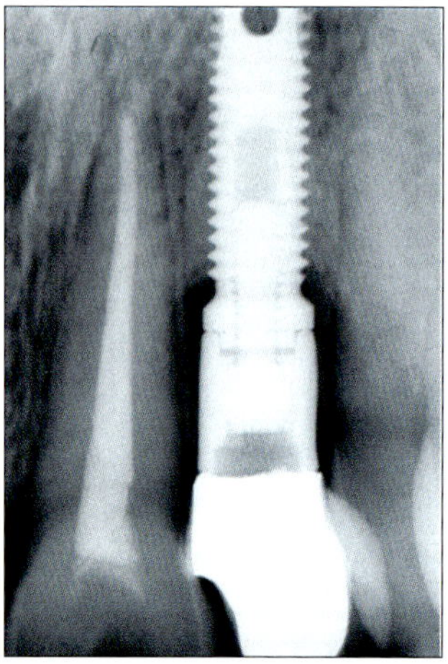

Fig 11-6 Note the significant peri-implant intrabony defect.

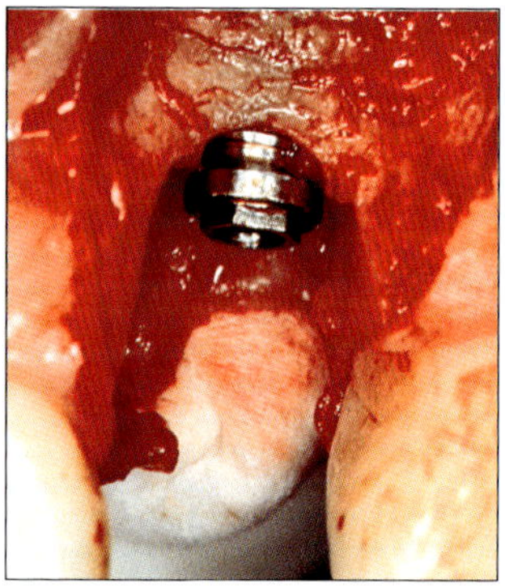

Fig 11-7 Clinical view after flap reflection and peri-implant granulation tissue removal. Note the very apical position of the implant in relation to the cementoenamel junction of the adjacent teeth.

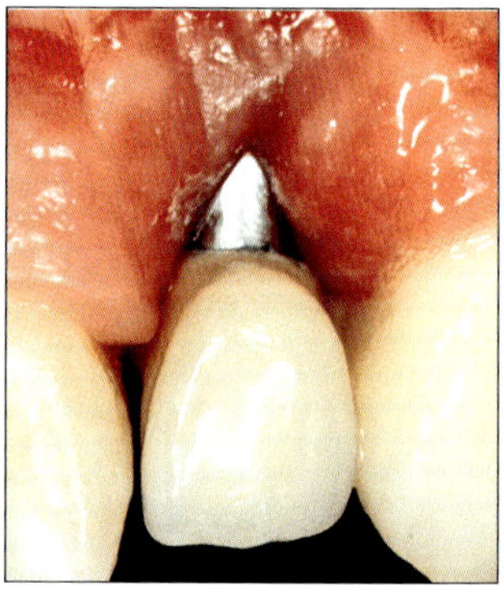

Fig 11-8 Postsurgical view at 4 months. Note the significant gingival recession.

Thilander et al[10] studied the evolution of 27 Brånemark implants placed in 15 teenagers. No implant was lost. An infraclusion of the implant-supported crown is found in all patients with incomplete growth. The increase of the observed vertical growth ranges from 0 to 1.6 mm for the incisors and from 0 to 0.6 mm for the canines and the premolars. A bone loss is observed on the adjacent teeth in the presence of an implant-root proximity.

Tschernitschek et al[11] retrospectively assessed the progress of 49 implants (34 in the anterior segments) in 25 children and teenagers. The authors advocate starting

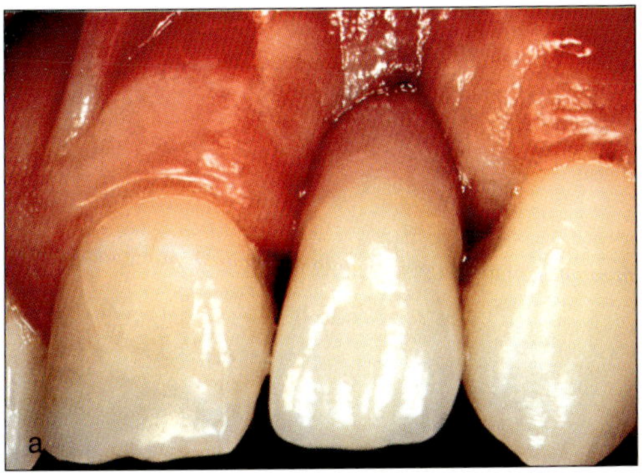

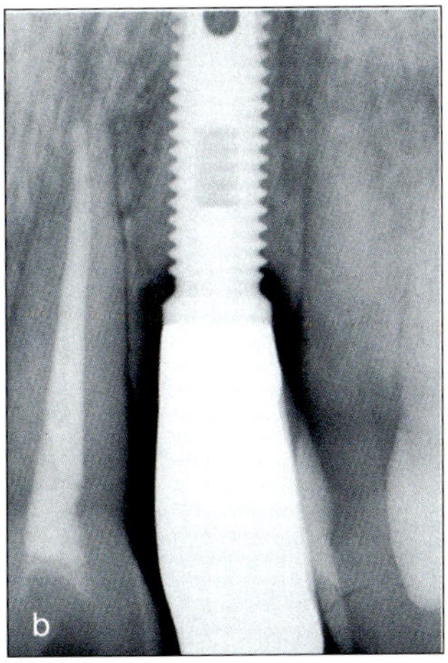

Figs 11-9a and 11-9b Clinical and radiographic views of the new implant-supported crown at the level of the lateral incisor. Note on the radiograph the importance of the crown height of the tooth, and the persisting intrabony defect.

implant treatment once the growth peak is achieved, namely around the age of 15 to 16 years for females and 17 to 18 years for males.

III. Treatment reflections

The different studies on growth and the clinical dental implant cases reported in the child and the teenager allow establishment of the prognosis of a dental implant placed in a young patient according to age and edentulism type.

Bone remodeling by apposition and resorption may give the impression of significant displacement of a maxillary implant placed in a child's anterior alveolar ridge (Fig 11-10). An implant placed at the age of 4 is ankylosed in the alveolus. With growth, the coronal part of the implant is progressively submerged and the apices exposed. This treatment option may have dramatic esthetic and functional consequences.

The bone changes that occur during growth are also important in the posterior regions. In the child, a posterior implant may lead to developmental disruptions in the neighboring structures. An implant placed at the beginning of mixed dentition offers little chance to be used at puberty. The use of implants during puberty is indeed less risky,

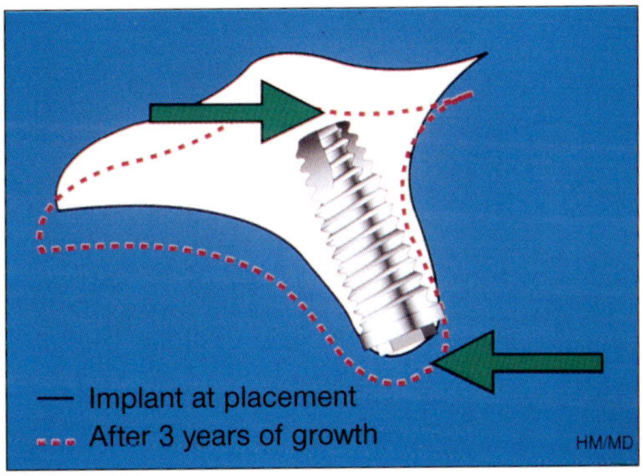

Fig 11-10 Diagram showing the growth (anteroinferior) of the anterior alveolar ridge around an implant placed in a young patient. The tissue changes give the impression of significant displacement of the implant.

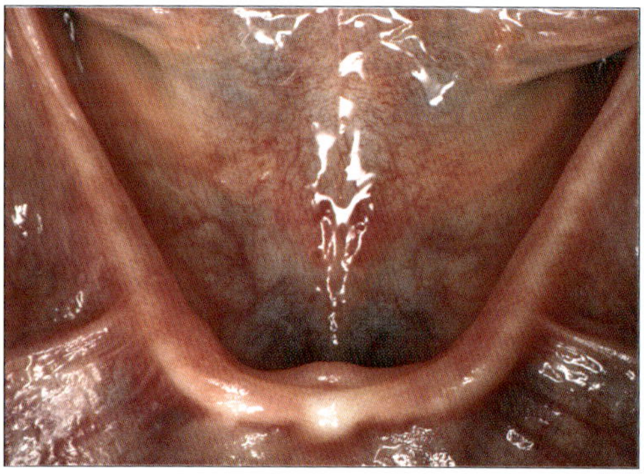

Fig 11-11 Clinical view of a 14-year-old patient affected by ectodermal dysplasia. Note the total absence of mandibular teeth.

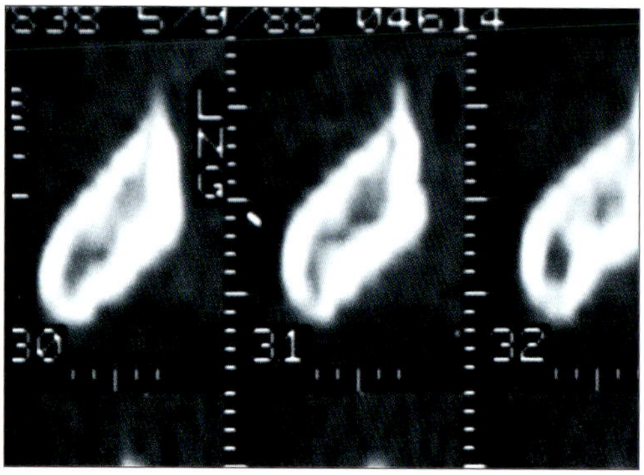

Fig 11-12 Oblique scans of the mandible. Note the residual bone volume in the symphysis allowing the placement of dental implants.

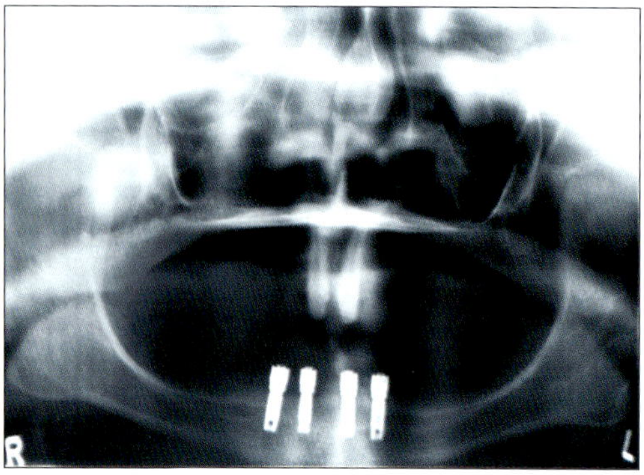

Fig 11-13 Radiographic control after stage-two surgery.

but tissue changes remain unpredictable. The vertical maxillary bone growth is more important in the incisors in relation to the canines and premolars. The use of fixed prosthesis splinting of implants must be avoided in the child. This type of prosthesis may lead to severe disturbances of transversal growth if the implants link two hemi-arches. The mandible is a unique bone with specific anatomy and growth dynamics that differ from the maxilla. Absence of sutures renders the placement of a mandibular implant less risky. The symphysis suture is completely closed several months after birth. The possibility for a growth site to be affected is nonexistent in the mandible. The use of mandibular implants in the child should be a temporary solution. Indeed, bone remodeling progressively modifies the implant position and axis.

The prognosis of symphysis implants in the young patient is more favorable than that of posterior implants. However, prosthetic rehabilitation must be modified as growth occurs.

IV. Ectodermal dysplasia

Ectodermal dysplasia is a genetic pathology that may occur through different syndromes. They are characterized by the involvement of at least two tissues originating from the ectoderm: tooth (oligodontia or anodontia), hair (trichodysplasia), nails (onychodysplasia), and sudoriferous and sebaceous glands (dyshidrosis or asteatosis). In the child, this pathology often leads to functional, esthetic, and psychologic problems.

Dental treatment must be part of a multidisciplinary approach in order to improve

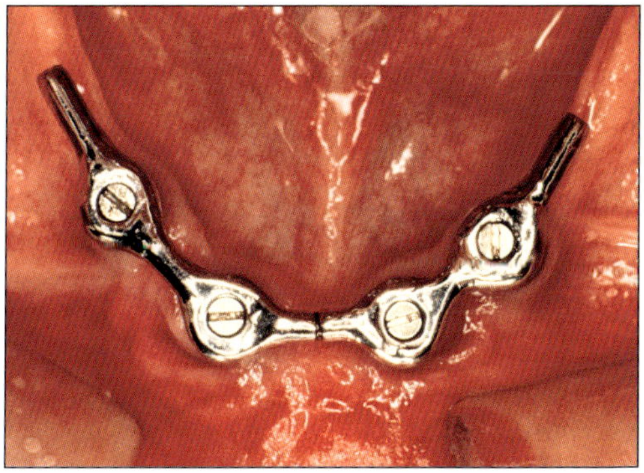

Fig 11-14 Positioning of a screw-retained bar on four mandibular implants.

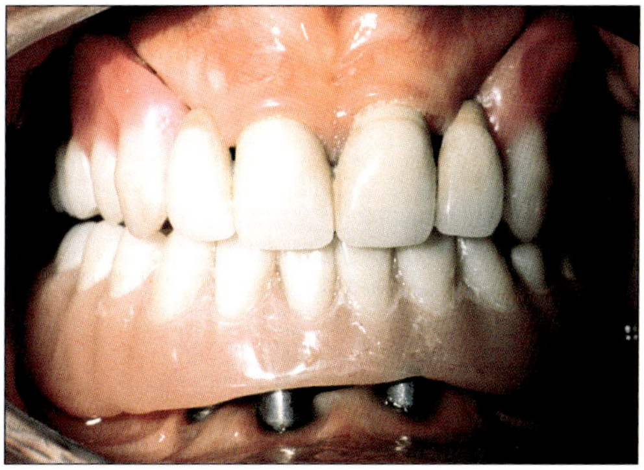

Fig 11-15 Clinical view of the final prosthetic result. The psychologic response of the patient is very favorable.

everyday life for these children. Different prosthetic options (removable, fixed, and implant supported) have been proposed. In extreme cases (anodontia), the implant choice must be considered. It is important to emphasize that the prosthesis must be checked and regularly readjusted. The maxillary growth must not be altered by a fixed prosthesis connecting the two hemi-arches. Several authors report the use of dental implants as anchoring means to fabricate removable or fixed prostheses in young patients affected with ectodermal dysplasia. A secondary submerging of the implants is observed in several cases. The psychologic response in these young patients is in all cases very favorable (Figs 11-11 to 11-15).

V. Recommendations

- Knowledge of maxillary growth is important before considering implants in the young patient.
- The risk of alteration in the maxillary growth, as well as the functional and esthetic facial complications, are considerable in the child.
- The long-term prognosis of an implant positioned in the child is very uncertain.
- It is advised to wait until the end of growth for the placement of dental implants in the young patient.
- Implants may be considered on average after 15 years in the female and after 18 years in the male.

The end of growth may be established in an empiric manner for the teenager when he or she has not changed shoe size for 18 months.

References

1. Cronin RJ, Oesterle LJ, Ranly DM. Mandibular implants and the growing patient. Int J Oral Maxillofac Implants 1994;9:55-62.
2. Cronin RJ, Oesterle LJ. Implant use in growing patients. Dent Clin North Am 1998;42:1-33.
3. Delaire J, Le Diascorn H, Lenne Y. La croissance de la face. Rev Odontoestomatol 1972;19:363-391.
4. Minsk L, Polson AM. Dental implant outcomes in post-menopausal women undergoing hormone replacement. Compend Contin Educ Dent 1998;19: 859-864.
5. Björk A, Skieller V. Growth of the maxilla in three dimensions as revealed radiographically by the implant method. Br J Orthod 1977;4:53-64.
6. Odman J, Grondahl K, Lekholm U, Thilander B. The effect of osseointegrated implants on the dento-alveolar development. A biometric and radiographic study in young pigs. Eur J Orthod 1991;13:279-286.
7. Thilander B, Odman J, Grondahl K, Lekholm U. Aspects of osseointegrated implants inserted in growing jaws. A biometric and radiographic study in young pigs. Eur J Orthod 1992;14:99-109.
8. Westwood RM, Duncan JM. Implants in adolescents: A literature review and case reports. Int J Oral Maxillofac Implants 1996;11:750-755.
9. Brugnolo E, Mazzocco C, Cordioli G, Majzoub Z. Résultats cliniques et radiographiques après la pose d'implants unitaires chez de jeunes patients. Cas cliniques. Int J Periodontics Restorative Dent 1996;16:421-433.
10. Thilander B, Odman J, Grondahl K, Friberg B. Osseointegrated implants in adolescents. An alternative in replacing missing teeth? Eur J Orthod 1994;16:84-95.
11. Tschernitschek H, Scheller H, Neukam W. Implantatversorgung bei Kindern und Jugendlichen. Implantologie 1996;4:311-318.

CHAPTER 12

Surface Properties

R. Lazzara/S. Porter/K. Beaty/M. Davarpanah/H. Martínez

Commercially pure titanium endosseous implants with a smooth surface have been in use for a longer period of time than any other type of implant (Fig 12-1). The excellent success rates obtained depend on the bone quality and volume. Indeed, for implants placed in type IV bone and in bone grafts (iliac bone), the reported failure rates are higher.[1] In this type of bone, rough-surfaced implants allow a higher bone-to-implant contact.[2]

Fig 12-1 Smooth surface of a commercially pure titanium implant. (Original magnification × 2000.)

I. Surface processing

Since the early 1980s, several groups have attempted to improve implant surface properties by adding new materials on the surface: titanium plasma spray (TPS) or hydroxyapatite (HA).[3,4] Other types of surface processing have also been suggested: sandblasting and acid etching ($HCl\text{-}H_2SO_4$, $HF\text{-}NO_3$). The aim of these technologies is to improve the quality of osseointegration and to increase the implant surface area. They are based on new concepts in terms of configuration and surface properties (Table 12-1).

Table 12-1 Characteristics of different types of implant surfaces[5]

Characteristic	Machined surface	TPS	HA	TiO sandblasted	Etched $HF\text{-}NO_3$	Etched $HCl\text{-}H_2SO_4$
Existing contaminants	No	Yes	Yes	No	No	No
Sprayed particles	No	Yes	Yes	Yes	No	No
Addition particles	No	Yes	Yes	No	No	No
Removal forces (torque)	Low	Mod High	High	Mod	Low Mod	High
Bone/implant contact	Low	Mod	High	Mod	Low Mod	High

Mod = moderate.

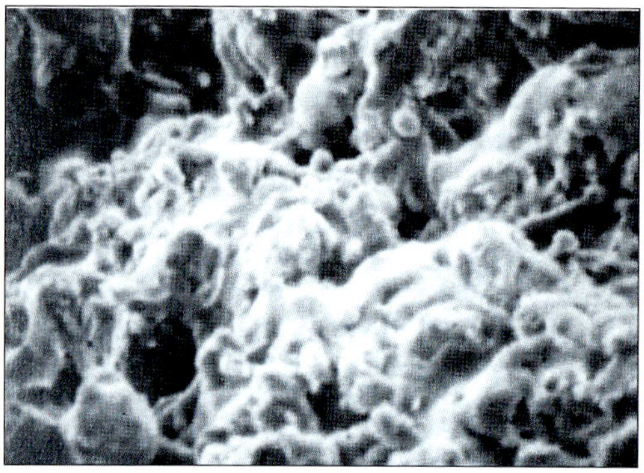

Fig 12-2 Implant surface coated with HA. Note the globular surface. (Original magnification × 2000.)

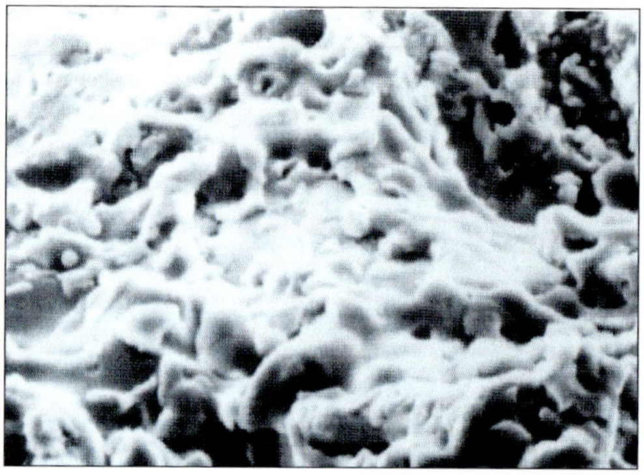

Fig 12-3 TPS implant surface. Note the globular surface. (Original magnification × 2000.)

A. Addition processing

The TPS and HA techniques alter the implant surface using additive processing. The aim is to optimize the biologic and physical characteristics of the bone-to-implant contact surface. The various techniques that have been reported for more than 20 years have not all provided a pure, uniform, and biologically stable surface. Indeed, long-term stability, as well as resistance to corrosion, of these surfaces is questioned. Surface erosion phenomena have been reported for the HA-coated implants.[3] Furthermore, the surface stratification of the implant using the TPS method demonstrates an irregular and globular surface.

The HA-coated implants and the TPS implants may have their rough surface exposed, thus favoring bacterial plaque retention (Figs 12-2 and 12-3). Development of peri-implantitis around this type of implant is enhanced by the presence of microscopic defects induced during fabrication. The microretentions exerted on the implant surface may lead to the release of the added particles. These particles may be observed in the surrounding tissues.[6]

B. Subtraction processing

The techniques using acid etching or sandblasting are subtractive processes that eliminate microscopic particles from the implant surface, thus creating an irregular morphology of the titanium (Figs 12-4 and 12-5). The subtractive methods increase the implant surface area without any contamination from added microparticles. The commercially pure titanium surface is preserved using this process. The probability for surface contamination and scattering of microparticles in the surrounding tissues is very low. However, for the sandblasted surfaces, the risk for existing powder remnants remains, although it is minimal. This type of mechanical processing may also alter the threading accuracy. For the etched surfaces, the risk for contamination is very low because no mechanical processing is performed at the surface.

Among the various studied surface-etching processes, the combination of HCl and H_2SO_4 seems to be the most reliable for obtaining a uniform rough surface (Fig 12-6). Topography analysis of an implant processed using this type of acid etching demonstrates peaks that are 0.3 to 1.5 μm apart (horizontal measurement) and from 1 to 2 μm in height

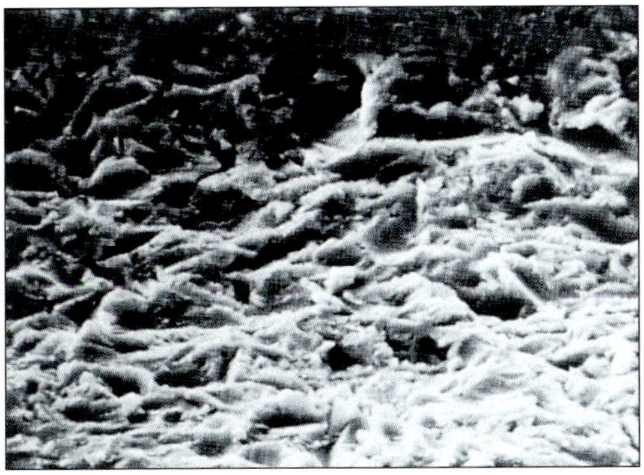

Fig 12-4 Implant surface processed using sandblasting. Note the presence of craters. (Original magnification × 2000.)

(vertical measurement). The knowledge of these dimensions is very important. Indeed, the bone matrix invades pores of 1 to 2 μm.

In a histochemical study performed on the rabbit, an inflammatory reaction around implants processed with TPS is demonstrated in the presence of giant cells at the bone-implant interface. Inversely, the smooth implants processed using the subtractive methods do not show this type of inflammatory reaction.[6]

II. Literature review: Different surface properties

Cell behavior is influenced by the physical characteristics and by the implant surface topography.[7] According to Predecki et al,[8] bone-healing kinetics depend on the mechanical fixation of cells at the implant surface. The surface irregularities must ideally form a right angle with the implant surface. Carlsson et al[9] report a higher removal torque for the rough-surfaced implants than for the smooth-surfaced implants after 6 weeks of implantation.

Buser et al[2] analyzed the percentage of direct bone-to-implant contact for different types of surfaces: sandblasted, HA coated, TPS, and acid etched. The highest bone-to-implant contact percentage is observed for the sandblasted and the acid-etched (HCl-H_2SO_4) surfaces. Davies and Dziedzic[10] also show a statistically significant increase of the osseointegration percentage for the acid-etched titanium implants (HCl-H_2SO_4), compared to the same implants with a smooth surface (Figs 12-7 and 12-8). This osseointegration quality is explained by the surface topography of titanium. Cordioli et al[11] obtained, in

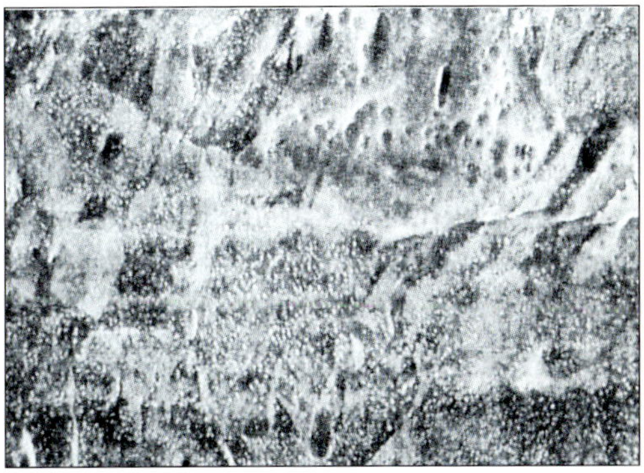

Fig 12-5 Implant surface etched using acid (HF-NO_3). Note the studded aspect. (Original magnification × 2000.)

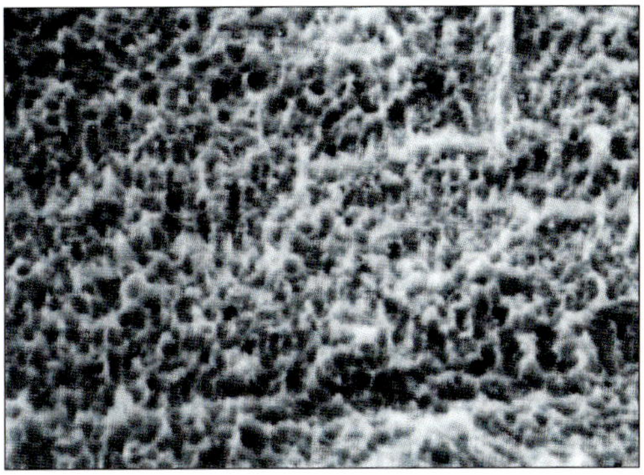

Fig 12-6 Implant surface etched using acid (HCl-H_2SO_4). Note the regularly rough surface (Osseotite). (Original magnification × 2000.)

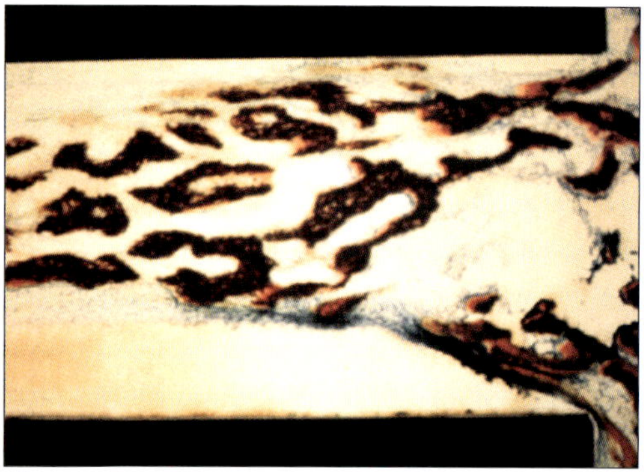

Fig 12-7 Histologic section, smooth-surfaced titanium chamber. Note the empty spaces near the implant. (Original magnification × 2000.)

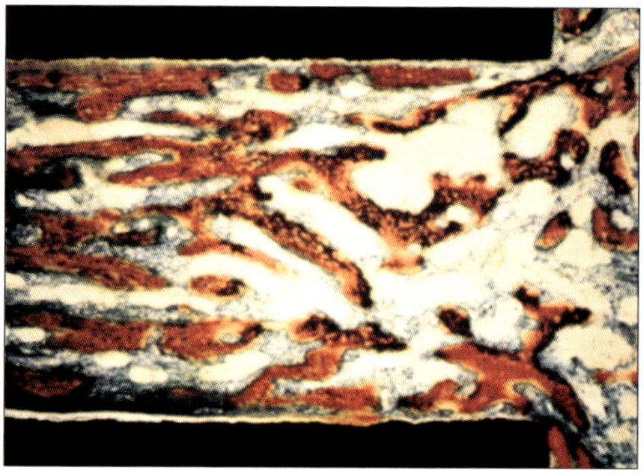

Fig 12-8 Histologic section, acid-etched titanium chamber (Osseotite). Note the close bone-implant contact. (Original magnification × 2000.)

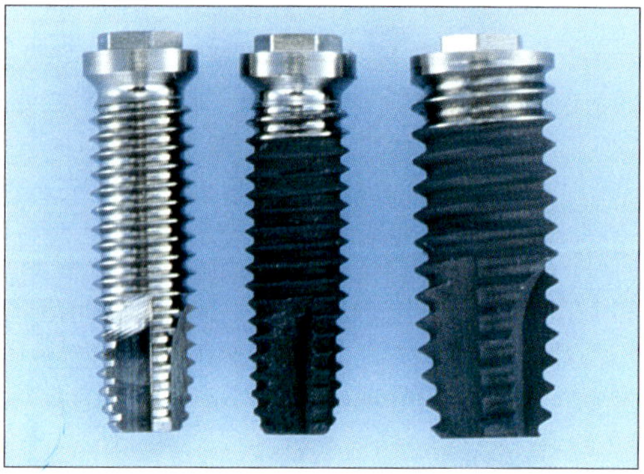

Fig 12-9 Hybrid implant: the acid-etched surface starts 3 mm from the implant neck. Note the comparison with the smooth implant surface.

the rabbit, a higher bone-to-implant contact with the acid-etched surface (Osseotite, 3i). These authors report 72.42% bone-implant contact for an acid-etched surface ($HCl-H_2SO_4$), 56.80% for the TPS implants, 54.80% for a sandblasted surface, and 48.60% for the smooth-surfaced implants. Lazzara et al[12] confirm these results in a histomorphometric study performed in humans. Two surfaces (smooth titanium and acid etched [$HCl-H_2SO_4$]) were assessed at 6 months in the posterior maxilla; 72.32% bone-implant contact was obtained using the smooth titanium implants.

III. Osseotite: A novel surface design

A rough implant surface enhances cell adhesion and fixation.[13] However, numerous studies have demonstrated the risks for mucositis and/or peri-implantitis using rough-surfaced implants. The long-term observations performed on smooth titanium implant surfaces report perfect soft tissue health. This surface property offers the greatest compatibility with the peri-implant mucosa.

A new implant surface preparation (hybrid design) was introduced in order to answer soft tissue as well as bone imperatives. The coronal part of the implant from the top to the third thread (3.0 mm) offers a smooth surface. Starting from the third thread up to the apex, the implant surface is acid etched ($HCl-H_2SO_4$). This combination of two types of surface properties ensures soft tissue longevity around the implant neck owing to the smooth surface and enhances osseointegration owing to the etched surface (Fig 12-9).

A. Advantages of the hybrid design

The advantages of this new implant surface preparation are:

- –increase of the bone-implant contact percentage
- –increase of the torque required to remove the implant
- –absence of surface contamination
- –absence of an additional layer
- –elimination of the risk for particle release or surface erosion
- –optimization of bone healing (etched surface)
- –maintenance of compatibility with the peri-implant mucosa (smooth surface)

B. Optimization of bone healing

Following an accurate implant positioning, a peri-implant space remains. Success for osseointegration depends on the type of tissue healing at the bone-implant junction.[14] The newly formed bone may fill this space via two phenomena: proximity osteogenesis and contact osteogenesis. The first phenomenon allows the formation of a peri-implant connective tissue matrix, or "fibrin plexus," originating from the bone border at the implant. In contact osteogenesis, new bone formation occurs in direct contact with the implant surface owing to the adherence of the fibrin plexus. Migration of the osteogenic cells on a fibrin matrix attached to the titanium surface allows a close adaptation of the bone tissue against the implant. The fibrin matrix formation originates from the initial blood clot. The wetting characteristics of the implant surface influence retention of the initial blood clot. An acid-etched surface (HCl-H_2SO_4) allows an excellent blood and serous fluid dispersion during implant placement. The microtopography created by this chemical process increases the wettability of commercially pure titanium.

- –At the contact of a smooth titanium surface, insufficient adhesion of the fibrin plexus favors the formation of cavities at the implant. These spaces determine the percentage of direct bone-implant contact.
- –Inversely, the presence of microscopic rugosities on the etched surface facilitates fibrin plexus retention. In a second stage, mineralization of the bone matrix will allow a greater bone-implant contact surface.
- –The histologic studies of Dziedzic et al[15] show an improvement of bone anchorage using etched surface implants compared to smooth-surfaced implants. The force required to extract the acid-etched implant (Osseotite) is 4 to 5 times higher than for the smooth-surfaced implant.

C. Clinical note

In the presence of insufficient bone quality (type IV), stabilization and the adhesion of the fibrin plexus become essential for implant success. Type IV bone has a low mineralization. Its morphology is structured by bone-free regions (cavities). In this type of bone, it is imperative for the space near the implant to be colonized by the fibrin plexus. The contraction of this plexus tends to reduce the fibrin-implant contact surface. Surface conditioning is therefore of great importance in the presence of poor-quality bone.

With self-tapping implants, the use of the tapper is eliminated during the surgical site preparation, resulting in a better implant adaptation.

D. Clinical results

Good short-term clinical results have been obtained using the acid-etched implant (HCl-H_2SO_4).[16,17] The preliminary report (following 12 months of loading) of a multicenter study shows a 98.6% success rate for 2,236 implants used for treating different types of edentulous cases.[16]

References

1. Jaffin R, Berman C. The excessive loss of Brånemark fixtures in type IV bone: A 5-year analysis. J Periodontol 1991;62:2–4.
2. Buser D, Schenk RK, Steinemann S, Fiorellini JP, Fox CH, Stich H. Influence of surface characteristics on bone integration of titanium implants. A histomorphometric study in miniature pigs. J Biomed Mater Res 1991;25:889-902.
3. Cheang P, Khor KA. Addressing processing problems associated with plasma spraying or hydroxyapatite coatings. Biomaterials 1996;17:537–544.
4. Luthy H, Strub JR, Schärer P. Analysis of plasma flame-sprayed coatings on endosseous oral titanium implants exfoliated in man: Preliminary results. Int J Oral Maxillofac Implants 1987;2:197–202.
5. Osseotite implant: Technology Report. Palm Beach Gardens, FL: Implant Innovations, 1997.
6. Piattelli A, Scarano A, Corigliano M, Piattelli M. Presence of multinucleated giant cells around machined, sandblasted and plasma-sprayed titanium implants: A histological and histochemical time-course study in the rabbit. Biomaterials 1996;17: 2053–2058.
7. Brunette DM. The effects of implant surface topography on the behavior of cells. Int J Oral Maxillofac Implants 1988;3:231–246.
8. Predecki P, Auslaender BA, Stephan JE. Attachment of bone to threaded implants by ingrowth and mechanical interlocking. J Biomed Mater Res 1972;6:401–412.
9. Carlsson LT, Rostlund B, Albrektsson B, Albrektsson T. Removal torques for polished and rough titanium implants. Int J Oral Maxillofac Implants 1988;3:21–24.
10. Davies JE, Dziedzic DM. Bone growth in metallic bone healing chambers. Faculty of Dentistry and Center for Biomaterials at the University of Toronto. Presented at the Fifth World Biomaterials Congress, Toronto, 1996.
11. Cordioli G, Majzoub Z, Piattelli A, Scarano A. Removal torque and histomorphometric study of four different titanium surfaces: An experimental study in the rabbit tibia. Int J Oral Maxillofac Implants 2000;15:668–674.
12. Lazzara R, Testori T, Trisi P, Porter S, Weinstein R. A human histologic analysis of Osseotite and machined surfaces using implants with 2 opposing surfaces. Int J Periodontics Restorative Dent 1999;19:117–129.
13. Bowers KT, Keller JC, Randolph BA, Wick DG, Michaels CM. Optimization of surface micromorphology for enhanced osteoblast responses in vitro. Int J Oral Maxillofac Implants 1992;7:302–310.
14. Masuda T, Salvi G, Offenbacher S, Felton D, Cooper L. Cell and matrix reactions at titanium implants in surgically prepared rat tibiae. Int J Oral Maxillofac Implants 1997;12:472–485.
15. Dziedzic DM, Beaty KD, Brown GR, Heylum T, Davies JE. Bone growth in metallic bone healing chambers. Faculty of Dentistry and Center for Biomaterials at the University of Toronto. Presented at the Fifth World Biomaterials Congress, Toronto, 1996.
16. Davarpanah M, Martínez H, Etienne D, Tecucianu JF, Porter SS, Lazzara RJ. Résultats préliminaires d'un nouvel implant à surface hybride. J Parodontol Implantol Orale 1999;1:51–60.
17. Sullivan D, Sherwood R, Mai T. Preliminary results of a multicenter study evaluating a chemically enhanced surface for machined commercially pure titanium implants. J Prosthet Dent 1997;78:379–386.

CHAPTER 13

Loading Concepts

H. Martínez/M. Davarpanah/R. Lazzara/K. Beaty

Two of the principles advocated by Brånemark et al[1] in order to obtain osseointegration are submerging of the implant and loading after 4 to 6 months of bone healing. The respect of these principles has allowed an increase in the success rate of endosseous implants.[2] The clinical application of these principles represents numerous constraints for the patient. In the completely edentulous, wearing of the removable denture is not allowed until 8 to 15 days following implant placement. The patient must then wear a transitional removable denture for 4 to 6 months (osseointegration period). This prosthesis is often difficult for the patient to accept from a functional and psychologic point of view. In 1990, Schnitman et al[3] suggested fabrication of an immediate transitional prosthesis. Different preliminary studies have reported interesting success rates using an immediate loading protocol. Early loading (2 months) is advocated by the present authors using rough-surfaced implants (acid etched).[4]

I. Principles for the conventional protocol

A delay of 4 months in the mandible and 6 months in the maxilla (for the submerged systems) is recommended before loading the implant. The implant is surrounded with nonmineralized tissue during the early stages of osseointegration. It is sensitive to loads and micromovements during the first weeks of bone healing. Bone cell differentiation may be disturbed by traumatic forces. The latter favor the creation of a fibrous interface, leading to implant failure.[5] According to Donath,[6] this connective tissue forms around an implant that presents poor primary stability. Furthermore, progressive loading is advocated in order to obtain good bone maturation.

II. Principles for immediate loading

Today, numerous histologic and clinical studies allow reconsideration of the conventional protocol developed by the Swedish school. Indeed, the results reported for nonsubmerged implants show an efficacy equivalent to that obtained using the submerged systems.[7,8] Recent studies performing one-stage implant surgery using Brånemark implants also show very good short-term results.[9–13]

Several clinical short-term reports suggest immediate implant loading.[14–17] This treatment concept offers very precise indications. Indeed, the reported clinical results show success rates that are inferior to those obtained using the conventional protocol. The different studies have a similar protocol: a high number of implants are placed in acceptable-quality bone (90% of the cases are reported in the completely edentulous, the majority of them in the mandible). Three to five implants support

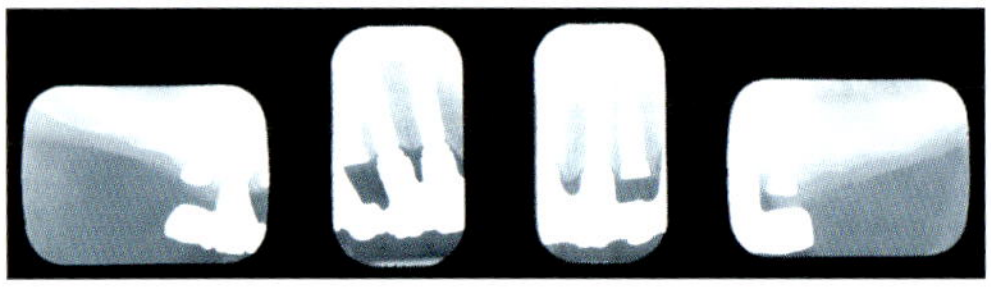

Fig 13-1 Immediate loading of an implant-supported fixed partial denture on five implants. A total of nine implants were placed in the maxilla, which presented type II bone quality (seven implants of 15 mm and two implants of 11.5 mm).

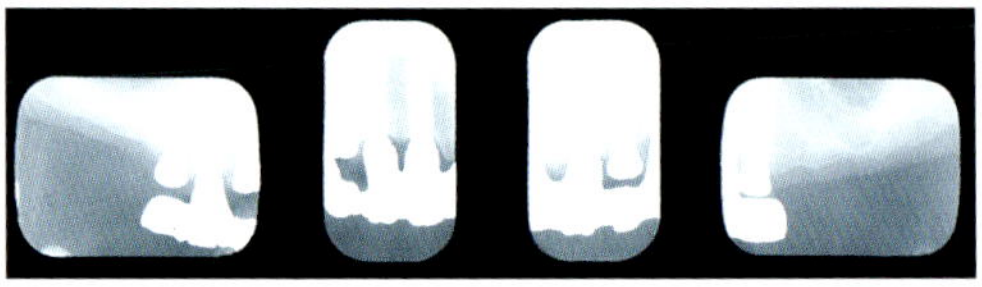

Fig 13-2 Radiograph after 6 months of loading and exposure of the last four implants. Note the absence of peri-implant bone loss.

the immediate prosthesis, and the other implants are submerged according to the conventional protocol. In most studies, selection of the supporting implants depends on their position in the arch and primary stability (Figs 13-1 and 13-2).

A. Advantages

This treatment option allows:

- immediate comfort for the patient
- avoidance of a removable denture during bone healing (the wearing of transitional removable prostheses is not well accepted by some patients from a social and functional point of view)

B. Contraindications

This technique includes some contraindications:

- low bone quality that limits good primary anchoring of the implants
- insufficient bone volume that limits the number and length of the implants
- patients with severe bruxism
- smoking patients

C. Review of literature

Several animal and human studies, as well as clinical reports published during the last few years, have allowed specification of the principles for immediate loading (Table 13-1). In 1992, Wohrle et al[18] presented the results at 5 years for 22 immediately loaded implants (Brånemark) out of 53 implants placed in the mandibles of eight patients. Thirty-one implants were therefore submerged according to the conventional protocol. The authors report three failures of immediate loading in the posterior regions. In 1997, the same group published their results at 10 years for 28 immediately loaded implants out of 63 implants placed in 10 patients.[16] The success rate was 86% (four implant failures) for the immediately loaded implants. It is very important to emphasize that only 14 implants, four of which were immediately loaded, out of 63 implants reported in the study were checked at 10 years.

Balshi and Wolfinger[19] show preliminary results for 40 immediately loaded implants out of 130 placed in the mandibles of 10 completely edentulous patients. The eight failures (80% success rate) reported by the authors were found in smokers or patients with bruxism or systemic disorders. Bone quality was type III for six of the failures and type IV in two failures. These authors report a 96% success rate for the delayed loading of 90 implants.

Tarnow et al[17] report the success rate from 1 to 5 years for 69 immediately loaded implants out of 107 implants placed in 10 completely edentulous patients (six man-

Table 13-1 Success rates with immediate and delayed loading

			Immediate loading			Delayed loading		
Author, year	Follow-up period (y)	No. of patients	No. of implants (site)	Failures	Success (%)	No. of implants	Failures	Success (%)
Wohrle et al, 1992[18]	1–5	8	22 (md)	3	86	31	0	100
Schnitman et al, 1997[16]	1–10	10	28 (md)	4	86	35	0	100
Balshi and Wolfinger, 1997[19]	1–2	10	40 (md)	8	80	90	4	96
Tarnow et al, 1997[17]	1–5	10	69 (md, mx)	2	97	38	1	97

Md = mandible; mx = maxilla.

dibles and four maxillae). This study presents a 97% success rate for the two groups (immediate or delayed loading). These authors advocate a transitional prosthesis reinforced using a metal splint fixed on at least five implants (length of at least 10 mm). This arch-form suprastructure positioned on a high number of well stabilized implants limits the risk for micromovement during bone healing. It is also important to emphasize that in most of the reported cases the opposing arch presented a complete removable denture.

D. Recommendations

Success for immediate loading depends on:

- Implant selection. Screw implants with a length of at least 10 mm are recommended. This type of implant offers an adequate mechanical retention. In the presence of a wide ridge, large-diameter implants increase the bone-implant contact surface and facilitate a bicortical anchorage.
- Implant distribution on the arch. Ideally, the immediately loaded implants must form a circular arc. This strategic distribution on the arch limits movements of the loaded implants.
- The number of placed implants. In order to treat an edentulous arch, a minimum of 10 implants is recommended, with the immediate loading of at least four implants in order to stabilize the transitional denture.
- Good stability of the loaded implants. Immediate loading of a maximum number of implants supporting a provisional prosthesis allows better distribution of occlusal forces.
- The bone quantity and quality. A minimum bone height (greater than 10 mm) and an adequate bone quality (type I or II) are ideally required in order to perform immediate loading.
- The type of transitional prosthesis. The prosthesis must include a metal structure that increases its rigidity. Cantilevers are prohibited because the loads can be considerable on the most distal implant. Furthermore, it is preferable to fabricate a screw-retained prosthesis.[17] The removal of a cemented prosthesis during the first months of healing may lead to implant failure. Indeed, the shearing forces exerted during prosthetic removal may jeopardize the osseointegration process.

Immediate loading is a very interesting option for the treatment of certain types of edentulous cases. However, the success rate reported by most groups is lower than that obtained using the conventional protocol. The treated groups, the number of implants placed, and the limited follow-up for this treatment option indicate that great prudence should be used in everyday practice.

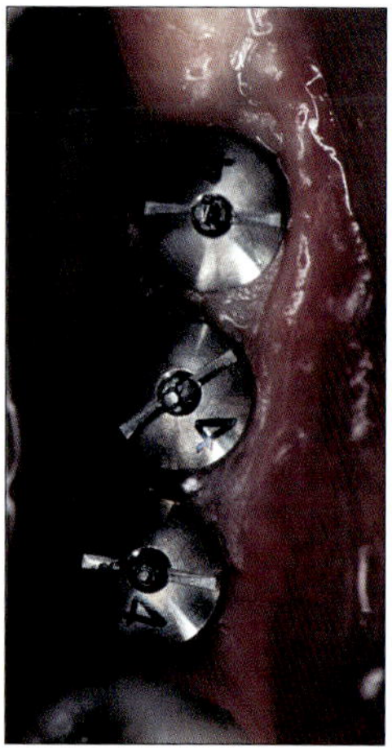

Fig 13-3 Occlusal view of three healing abutments (Osseotite).

Figs 13-4a and 13-4b **a** = Control radiograph 7 weeks after implant placement; **b** = control radiograph after 1 year of loading.

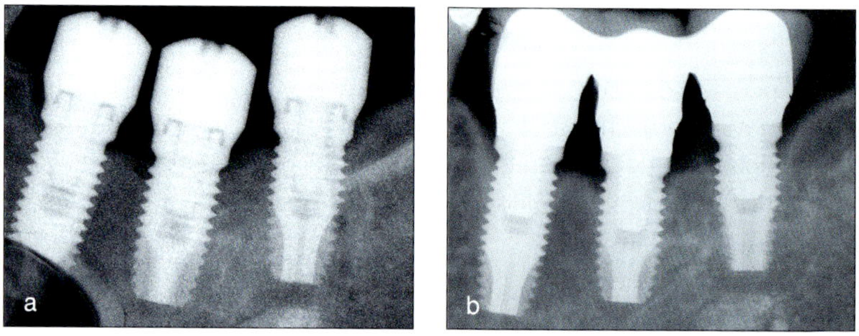

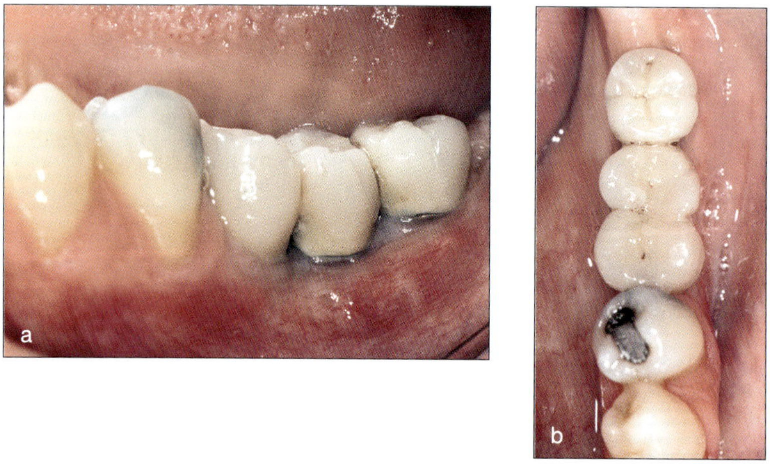

Figs 13-5a and 13-5b Buccal and occlusal views of three splinted crowns after 1 year of loading (restoration, Dr C. Raygot).

III. Principles for early loading

The reported success rates range from 80% to 97% for immediate loading and from 96% to 100% for conventional loading. The causes for immediate loading failure are:

—an insufficient primary implant anchorage
—transmission of micromovements to the implants
—occlusal overload

Early loading is a new treatment option using implants with a rough surface (acid etched, $HCl\text{-}H_2SO_4$). This concept answers time imperatives for clinicians, time and comfort imperatives for the patient, and optimizes the results obtained with immediate loading. Furthermore, the early fabrication of the prosthesis (8 weeks) allows loading of all types of implants (Figs 13-3 to 13-5). In the presence of insufficient bone quality (type IV), achieving inadequate primary stabilization often compromises osseointegration. A rough surface optimizes the primary anchorage of the implant. Dziedzic et al[20] show an improvement of bone anchorage with the acid-etched surface compared to smooth-surfaced implants. The force required to extract acid-etched implants (Osseotite, 3i) is 4 to 5 times higher than for smooth-surfaced implants.

A multicenter pilot study performed in humans compares the results of early loading (2 months) and conventional loading (4 to 6 months). All the used implants had an acid-etched surface (Osseotite). A success rate of 98.8% was obtained for the 716 implants loaded after 4 to 6 months of healing.

Mid- and long-term multicenter studies will have to confirm the efficacy of this treatment option.

References

1. Brånemark P-I, Zarb GA, Albrektsson T. Tissue-Integrated Prostheses. Chicago: Quintessence, 1985.
2. Adell R, Lekholm U, Rockler B, Brånemark P-I. A 15 year study of osseointegrated implants in the treatment of edentulous jaws. Int J Oral Surg 1981;10:387–416.
3. Schnitman PA, Wohrle PS, Rubenstein JE. Immediate fixed interim prostheses supported by two-stage threaded implants: Methodology and results. J Oral Implantol 1990;16:96–105.
4. Davarpanah M, Martínez H, Etienne D, Tecucianu JF, Porter SS, Lazzara RJ. Résultats préliminaires d'un nouvel implant à surface hybride. J Parodontol Implantol Orale 1999;1:51-60.
5. Brunski JB. Avoid pitfalls of overloading and micromotion of intraosseous implants. Dent Implantol Update 1993;4:77–81.
6. Donath K. Tissue reaction around loaded and unloaded titanium implants. J Hard Tissue Biol 1993;2:37–47.
7. Buser D, Weber HP, Lang NP. Tissue integration of nonsubmerged implants: 1-year results of a prospective study with 100 ITI hollow-cylinder and hollow-screw implants. Clin Oral Implants Res 1990;1:33–40.
8. Buser D. Mericske-Stern R, Bernard JP, et al. Long-term evaluation of non-submerged ITI implants. Clin Oral Implants Res 1997;8:161–172.
9. Becker W, Becker BE, Israelson H, et al. One-step surgical placement of Brånemark implants: A prospective multicenter clinical study. Int J Oral Maxillofac Implants 1997;12:454–462.
10. Bernard JP, Belser UC, Martinet JP, Borgis SA. Osseointegration of Brånemark fixtures using a single-step operating technique. A preliminary prospective one-year study in the edentulous mandible. Clin Oral Implants Res 1995;6:122–129.
11. Collaert B, De Bruyn H. Comparison of Brånemark fixture integration and short-term survival using one-stage or two-stage surgery in completely and partially edentulous mandibles. Clin Oral Implants Res 1998;9:131–135.
12. Ericsson I, Randow K, Glantz PO, Lindhe J, Nilner K. Clinical and radiographical features of submerged and non-submerged titanium implants. Clin Oral Implants Res 1994;5:185–189.
13. Ericsson I, Randow K, Nilner K, Petersson A. Some clinical and radiographical features of submerged and non-submerged titanium implants: A 5-year follow-up study. Clin Oral Implants Res 1997;8:422–426.
14. Piattelli A, Trisi P, Romasco N, Emanuelli M. Histologic analysis of screw implants retrieved from man: Influence of early loading and primary stability. J Oral Implantol 1993;19:303–306.
15. Salama H, Rose LF, Salama M, Bett NJ. Immediate loading of bilaterally splinted titanium root form implants in fixed prosthodontics—A technique reexamined: Two case reports. Int J Periodontics Restorative Dent 1995;15:345–361.
16. Schnitman PA, Wohrle PS, Rubenstein JE, DaSilva JD, Wang NH. Ten-year results for Brånemark implants immediately loaded with fixed prostheses at implant placement. Int J Oral Maxillofac Implants 1997;12:495–503.
17. Tarnow DP, Emtiaz S, Classi A. Immediate loading of threaded implants at stage I surgery in edentulous arches: Ten consecutive case reports with 1 to 5 year data. Int J Oral Maxillofac Implants 1997;12:319–324.
18. Wohrle PS, Schnitman PA, DaSilva JD, Wang NH, Koch GG. Brånemark implants placed into immediate function: 5-year results [abstract]. J Oral Implantol 1992;18:282.
19. Balshi TJ, Wolfinger GJ. Immediate loading of Brånemark implants in edentulous mandibles: A preliminary report. Implant Dent 1997;6:83–88.
20. Dziedzic DM, Beaty KD, Brown GR, Heylum T, Davies JE. Bone growth in metallic bone healing chambers. Faculty of Dentistry and Center for Biomaterials at the University of Toronto. Presented at the Fifth World Biomaterials Congress, Toronto, 1996.